One Hundred Orthopedic Cases

First Edition

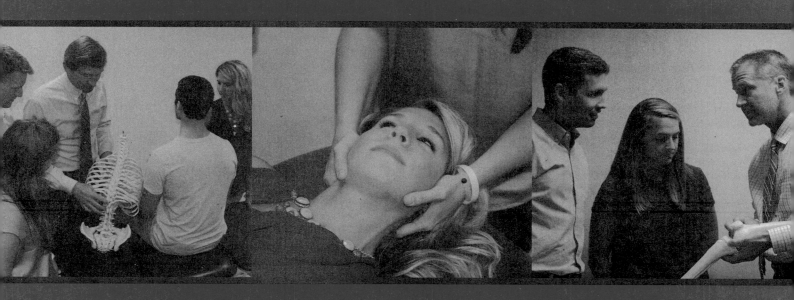

Ken Learman | Chad Cook
Youngstown State University | Duke University

PEARSON

Boston   Columbus   Indianapolis   New York   San Francisco   Upper Saddle River
Amsterdam   Cape Town   Dubai   London   Madrid   Milan   Munich   Paris   Montreal   Toronto
Delhi   Mexico City   Sao Paulo   Sydney   Hong Kong   Seoul   Singapore   Taipei   Tokyo

Publisher: Julie Levin Alexander
Publisher's Assistant: Regina Bruno
Executive Editor: John Goucher
Program manager: Nicole Ragonese
Editorial Assistant: Amanda Losonsky
Director of Marketing: David Gesell
Marketing Manager: Brittany Hammond
Marketing Specialist: Michael Sirinides
Project Management Lead: Cynthia Zonneveld
Project Manager: Patricia Gutierrez
Operations Specialist: Mary Ann Gloriande

Art Director: Mary Siener
Cover Designer: Cenveo Publisher Services
Cover Art: Anita Aiken/Jim Benedict
Media Director: Amy Peltier
Lead Media Project Manager: Lorena Cerisano
Full-Service Project Management: Rebecca Lazure, Laserwords
Private Ltd
Composition: Laserwords Private Ltd
Printer/Binder: Edwards Brothers Malloy Jackson Rd
Cover Printer: Phoenix Color/Hagerstown
Text Font: Times Ten LT Std 10/12

Credits and acknowledgments for content borrowed from other sources and reproduced, with permission, in this textbook appear on appropriate page within text.

Notice: The author and the publisher of this book have taken care to make certain that the information given is correct and compatible with the standards generally accepted at the time of publication. Nevertheless, as new information becomes available, changes in treatment and in the use of equipment and procedures become necessary. The reader is advised to carefully consult the instruction and information material included in each piece of equipment or device before administration. Students are warned that the use of any techniques must be authorized by their medical advisor, where appropriate, in accordance with local laws and regulations. The publisher disclaims any liability, loss, injury, or damage incurred as a consequence, directly or indirectly, of the use and application of any of the contents of this book.

Many of the designations by manufacturers and seller to distinguish their products are claimed as trademarks. Where those designations appear in this book, and the publisher was aware of a trademark claim, the designations have been printed in initial caps or all caps.

Library of Congress Cataloging-in-Publication Data
Learman, Ken, author.
100 orthopedic cases / Ken Learman, Chad Cook. — First edition.
    p. ; cm.
One hundred orthopedic cases
Includes bibliographical references.
ISBN 978-0-13-265306-0 — ISBN 0-13-265306-0
I. Cook, Chad, author. II. Title. III. Title: One hundred orthopedic cases.
[DNLM: 1. Musculoskeletal Diseases—diagnosis—Case Reports. 2. Diagnosis, Differential—Case Reports.
3. Physical Examination—methods—Case Reports. 4. Symptom Assessment—methods—Case Reports. WE 141]
RC925.7
616.7'075—dc23
                                                                                        2014031202

10 9 8 7 6 5 4 3 2 1

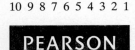

ISBN 10: 0-13-265306-0
ISBN 13: 978-0-13-265306-0

I would like to thank my wife Mary and sons Stephen and Shane for supporting me over the years. Without their patience, this project would not be possible. I would also like to thank the contributors who wrote cases from their extensive clinical experiences. They provided a wide variety of contextually rich orthopedic cases to serve as an educational platform for many students of the profession.

—*Ken Learman*

I would like to thank Amy, Zach, Jaeger and Simon for all the support they have provided me over the many years. I'd also like to dedicate this book to all of the new learners in the rehabilitation professions. Well done to you, you've picked noble and exciting fields of study.

—*Chad Cook*

Contents

Preface

As physical therapy educators, we've often struggled with creating new cases to use in lecture and laboratory classes as well as during practical examinations. We are sure we are not alone in this difficulty. It's not that creating cases is really that labor intensive, but remembering to provide enough information for the student to participate in the case correctly and taking the time to research the evidence behind the examination and treatment options can be daunting. The premise of *One Hundred Orthopedic Cases* is to provide physical therapy educators with a large assortment of orthopedic patient cases covering a wide variety of conditions for the purpose of challenging the clinical decision making of their students. It can also be effectively used by students or clinicians to stimulate their own clinical reasoning skills. Additionally, the text may serve as a basis for further clinical study in orthopedic study groups or in preparation for advanced credentialing certification examinations.

Creating a large repository of patient cases that covers a broad spectrum of diagnoses can take a fair amount of time and expertise, so we enlisted the help of many outstanding contributors to assist in searching the literature and creating the cases. Many of the patient cases were taken directly from case studies or modified from research studies in the literature; others were taken from patient case files and modified appropriately to fulfill the needs of the text.

Certainly, in any given case, the approach to care can take on many forms since evidenced-based practice incorporates any clinician's current level of experience and expertise as well considers each patient's beliefs and values. Therefore, the presented cases are based in current literature and represent a single method of clinical approach.

We are pleased to have set up the process that allows each case to be worked on without all the pertinent information immediately available. The online component, www.pearsonhighered.com/healthprofessionsresources, allows the entire case to be tied together but does so in an independent manner, preventing the student from reading ahead, thereby eliminating the need to give hints to the readers who are sorting through the cases. It is our hope that the cases improve learning opportunities for students of all genres. We are excited about the opportunity to provide *One Hundred Orthopedic Cases* to our learning colleagues and thank you for your service to our rehabilitation professions. Keep up the great work and we hope you enjoy solving each of the cases!

Ken Learman
Chad Cook

Contributors

EDITORS

Kenneth E. Learman, PT, PhD, OCS, COMT, FAAOMPT
Professor, Department of Physical Therapy
Youngstown State University
Youngstown, OH 44555

Chad Cook PT, PhD, FAAOMPT
Professor, Doctor of Physical Therapy
Duke University
Durham, NC 27708

CASE CONTRIBUTORS

Joseph Brence, PT, DPT, FAAOMPT, COMT, DAC
Vice President of Operations, Nxt Gen Institute of Physical
Therapy

Alyson R. Ellis, PT, DPT
Texas Physical Therapy Specialists
San Antonio, TX

Brittany Farber, PT, DPT
Alumnus, Walsh University
North Canton, OH

Lindsay Froman, PT, DPT
Alumnus, Walsh University
North Canton, OH

David Griswold, PT, DPT, COMT, CMP
Assistant Professor, Department of Physical Therapy
Youngstown State University
Youngstown, OH

Alicia Jadwisiak, PT, DPT
Alumnus, Walsh University
North Canton, OH

Emily Lonsway, PT, DPT
Alumnus, Walsh University
North Canton, OH

Kelly Mohn, PT, DPT
Alumnus, Walsh University
North Canton, OH

Jen Moore, PT, DPT
Alumnus, Walsh University
North Canton, OH

Ashley Neal, PT, DPT
Aegis Physical Therapy
Pittsburgh, PA

Jaime C. Paz, PT, DPT, MS
Program Director; Clinical Professor
Physical Therapy Program
Walsh University
North Canton, OH

Shannon M. Petersen, PT, DScPT, OCS, FAAOMPT, COMT
Associate Professor, Physical Therapy Program
Divine Providence
Des Moines University/Osteopathic Medical Center
Des Moines, IA

Kyle Rockwell, PT, DPT
Orthopedic and Neurological Rehabilitation
Divine Providence
Sleepy Eye, MN

Elyse Rolenz, PT, DPT
Alumnus, Walsh University
North Canton, OH

Lindsay Snyder, PT, DPT
Alumnus, Walsh University
North Canton, OH

McKenzi vanFossen, PT, DPT
Alumnus, Walsh University
North Canton, OH

Samantha Widder, PT, DPT
Alumnus, Walsh University
North Canton, OH

Jacob A. Wright, PT, DPT
Achieve Health and Wellness
Gray, TN

Reviewers

Josh Coram, PTA
Florida State College at Jacksonville
Jacksonville, FL

Janet Dolot, PT, DPT, OCS, COMPT
New York Medical College
Valhalla, NY

Robert Frampton, PT
University of Findlay
Findlay, OH

Kathleen Geist, PT, DPT, OCS, COMT
Emory University
Atlanta, GA

Jodi Gootkin, PT, MEd
Broward College
Davie, FL

Renae Gorman, PT, DPT, MTC, OCS
Springfield Technical Community College
Springfield, MA

Diana Hernandez, PT, MEd
South Texas College
McAllen, TX

John Jeziorowski, PT, PhD
Cleveland State University
Cleveland, OH

Karen Jones, PT, DPT
Herkimer County Community College
Herkimer, NY

Kristin Kjensrud, PT, MS
Mt. Hood Community College
Gresham, OR

Julianne Klepfer, BS Physical Therapy, MASS
Broome Community College
Binghamton, NY

Jacqueline Kopack, PT, DPT
Harcum Junior College
Bryn Mawr, PA

Heather MacKrell, PTA
Calhoun Community College
Tanner, AL

Julian Magee, PT, DPT, ATC
Alabama State University
Montgomery, AL

Nelson Marquez, PT, EdD
Polk Community College
Lakeland, FL

Ellen O'Keefe, PT, DPT
Athens Technical College
Elberton, GA

Jacob Thorp, PT, DHS, OCS, MTC
East Carolina University
Greenville, NC

Marcia Spoto, PT, DC, OCS
Nazareth College
Rochester, NY

Cameron Williams, PT, MS, DPT
Finlandia University
Hancock, MI

Nancy Wofford, DPT, OCS Cert MDT
Armstrong Atlantic State University
Savannah, GA

Peter Zawicki, PT, MS
Gateway Community College, Phoenix
Phoenix, AZ

How to Use This Handbook

Purpose of the Handbook

The handbook *One Hundred Orthopedic Patient Cases* is designed to assist learners in understanding the necessary ingredients in the clinical examination process for patients with orthopedic problems. Each case focuses on clinical situations that represent both mechanical and nonmechanical disorders that are commonly encountered by rehabilitative clinicians.

Clinical vignettes, or cases, are commonly used in the medical profession for decision making that requires judgment in situations of uncertainty.[1,2] The cases presented here will challenge the learner's decision making by requiring a synthesis of the material as well as an application of that synthesis. Although each case is built by using a sequential assessment method, all are designed to be used by learners of any orthopedic background.

The Learning Process

Although these 100 vignettes are likely to be used mostly by students in rehabilitation programs, the cases are germane for licensed rehabilitation clinicians who are interested in improving their overall knowledge. Because each case includes an explanation with evidence-based references, clinicians and learners can be confident that the "suggestions" for examination and treatment for each vignette are based on the best available evidence.

Example of the Material

General Information

Patient cases written within a context of an outpatient orthopedic, skilled nursing facility, acute care, and home health environment are provided. Each of the 100 cases provides standard "chart" criteria, including name, age, medical record number (MRN), home address, date of injury, determination of whether the injury is new, self-assessment of general health, self-report of exercise, occupation, household situation, and hand dominance. By including some situations in which patients have poor general health, clinicians and learners are more likely to address each case holistically.

Name:	*Mark Fontaine*	General Health:	*Good*
Age:	*49 years*	Amount of Exercise:	*0 hours/day, 0 days/week*
MRN:	*50507*	Occupation:	*Cable supplier*
Home Address:	*123 Becks Street, Durham, North Carolina*	Household:	*Lives with family*
		Hand Dominance:	*Right*
Date of Injury:	*2 months prior*	Race:	*White*
New Injury:	*Yes*		

Pain Drawings

A pain drawing and numeric pain scale provide the learner with a patient's self-assessment of the region and intensity of pain. Although pain drawings have been known to provide conflicting or inconsistent information for diagnosis,[3] it is generally accepted that the information gathered helps direct the patient care process of the clinician.

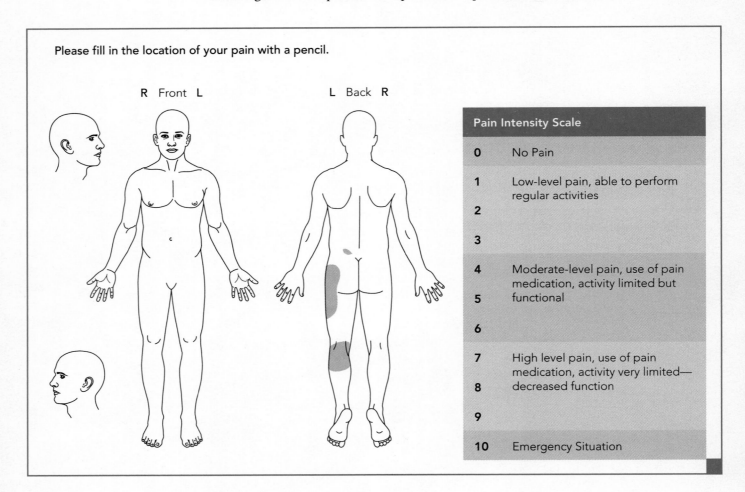

Please fill in the location of your pain with a pencil.

R Front L   L Back R

Pain Intensity Scale	
0	No Pain
1	Low-level pain, able to perform regular activities
2	
3	
4	Moderate-level pain, use of pain medication, activity limited but functional
5	
6	
7	High level pain, use of pain medication, activity very limited—decreased function
8	
9	
10	Emergency Situation

Further pain information is provided, including the number of days with pain in the last week and when the pain is at its worse.

In the last week, how many days have you had pain? *3*
Pain worst *Day (during exertion)*

Imaging

Within each case, imaging results (in the form of an impression only; no images) are provided when available. When imaging is absent, clinicians must decide whether "referring out" for appropriate imaging is warranted.

Medical History

Each case also includes a checklist representing a past medical history. A number of studies have shown that selected comorbidities can delay improvements or amplify the effect of certain conditions,[4] and these situations are worth investigating. By including these conditions, the clinician is required to consider the patient's health status as a whole.

Past Medical History (Please check any items that apply to you.)

Musculoskeletal:
- ○ Osteoarthritis
- ○ Rheumatoid Arthritis
- ○ Lupus/SLE
- ○ Fibromyalgia
- ○ Osteoporosis
- ○ Headaches
- ○ Bulging Disc
- ○ Leg Cramps
- ○ Restless Legs
- ○ Jaw Pain/TMJ
- ○ History of Falling
- ○ Use of Cane or Walker
- ○ Gout
- ○ Double Jointed

Other:_____

Neurological:
- ○ Stroke/TIA
- ○ Dementia

Neurological (continued)
- ○ Polio
- ○ Parkinson's Disease
- ○ Multiple Sclerosis
- ○ Epilepsy/Seizures
- ○ Concussion
- ○ Numbness
- ○ Tingling

Other:_____

Endocrine:
- ○ Diabetes
- ○ Kidney Dysfunction
- ○ Bladder Dysfunction
- ○ Liver Dysfunction
- ○ Thyroid Dysfunction

Other:_____

Cardiopulmonary:
- ○ Congestive Heart Failure
- ○ Heart Arrhythmia

Cardiopulmonary (continued)
- ○ Pacemaker
- ○ High Cholesterol
- ○ Blood Clots
- ○ Anemia
- ○ High Blood Pressure
- ○ Asthma
- ○ Shortness of Breath
- ○ COPD
- ○ HIV/AIDS

Other:_____

Other:
- ○ Anxiety
- ○ Depression
- ○ Cancer

Chief Complaint and Goals for Therapy

Also given in the cases are the patient's chief complaint and goals for therapy. This information is provided to further the understanding of the symptoms within the patient's framework.

General and Specific Outcomes Measures

A SANE[5] (Single Alpha Numeric Evaluation) functional rating allows the patient to self-report his or her current functional assessment during daily activities and during work and/or sports. The Patient-Specific Functional Scale allows each patient to document three activities he or she is currently struggling with and score each 0 to 10, which corresponds to the patient's ability to perform the activity.

SANE Functional Rating

Please rate your **ability** to use your injured area on a 0 to 100% scale with **0%** being unable to use the injured area and **100%** being normal use of injured area in your daily activity: _____

Also, if you exercise or have a sport activity or a job that requires special demands please rate your activity on the 0 to 100% scale: _____

The Patient Specific Function Scale[6] is a self-report instrument involving three activities (e.g., walking, sitting, shopping) identified by the patient during the initial visit that challenge her or his ability to fully function. The scale is scored from 0 ("unable to perform activity") to 10 ("able to perform activity at same level as before injury or problem"); a total score of 30 is possible. During each subsequent visit, the patient is queried again for her or his previously selected functional limitations to determine if there has been improvement.

Patient-Specific Functional Scale

Please list **3 activities** that you find are difficult because of this problem and circle the number that corresponds with your ability to perform the activity.

	Unable									No limitations
1.	1	2	3	4	5	6	7	8	9	10
2.	1	2	3	4	5	6	7	8	9	10
3.	1	2	3	4	5	6	7	8	9	10

Other unique outcomes measures are provided for each patient. For example, each case will often have a global score of well-being/quality of life, or a region-specific measure for function. In addition, each case may have a scale score associated with anxiety, depression, coping, or fear if these elements were identified in the patient history as a potential comorbidity.

Observation and patient history information are also provided for each patient. Within the patient history, the subdivisions of mechanism and description of injury, concordant movements or sign, the nature of the condition, and the behavior of the symptoms are identified. Under the patient's section, the responses of each testing sequence—(1) active physiological, (2) passive physiological, (3) passive accessory, and (4) special tests—are provided. For further explanation of these areas, please address Chapter 2 of this handbook.

Division of the Material

The *100 Orthopedic Patient Cases* handbook is designed for both sole use as well as use in an educational, laboratory setting. Consequently, each case has a *clinician's* section and a *patient's* section. The clinician section provides the details of the observation, patient history, and additional information (discussed previously) but does not include the results of the physical examination. The patient's section is separated from the clinician's section to allow students to role-play in a laboratory session and improve their examination capacities. If used by only one individual, the patient's section can be read by the single individual and combined with the clinician's section.

And finally, an explanation of each case is provided online. Once the handbook user has logged in and created an account on the companion website (*www.pearsonhighered .com/healthprofessionsresources*), the user can access an explanation of each of the 100 cases to further his or her understanding of the patients' conditions. The suggested process is referenced and detailed to improve the overall understanding of the proper clinical examination process. The material can be reviewed independently or by the learning team during a laboratory setting.

Endnotes

1. Bachmann LM, Mühleisen A, Bock A, ter Riet G, Held U, Kessels AG. Vignette studies of medical choice and judgement to study caregivers' medical decision behaviour: systematic review. BMC Med Res Methodol. 2008;8:50.

2. Donnon T, Paolucci EO. A generalizability study of the medical judgment vignettes interview to assess students' noncognitive attributes for medical school. BMC Med Educ. 2008;8:58.

3. Murphy DR, Hurwitz EL, Gerrard JK, Clary R. Pain patterns and descriptions in patients with radicular pain: Does the pain necessarily follow a specific dermatome? Chiropr Osteopat. 2009;17:9.

4. Baumeister H, Balke K, Härter M. Psychiatric and somatic comorbidities are negatively associated with quality of life in physically ill patients. J Clin Epidemiol. 2005;58:1090–100.

5. Hegedus EJ, Cook C, Fiander C, Wright A. Measures of arch height and their relationship to pain and dysfunction in people with lower limb impairments. Physiother Res Int. 2010 Feb 1. [Epub ahead of print]

6. Chatman AB, Hyams SP, Neel JM, Binkley JM, Stratford PW, Schomberg A, Stabler M. The Patient-Specific Functional Scale: measurement properties in patients with knee dysfunction. Phys Ther. 1997;77:820–9.

Elements of the Orthopedic Examination

Treatment Decision Making

The purpose of the orthopedic examination is to improve the ability of clinicians and learners to (1) recognize pertinent selection examination criteria, (2) identify the contributing causes to the patient's condition, (3) determine the ideal treatment for each individual patient, and (d) apply a pathoanatomical diagnosis to the patient's condition. To do so, clinicians use observational findings, patient history, and clinical tests and measures, as well as recognize potential contributing factors (such as comorbidities, psychological condition, chronicity of the disease, age, etc.) during their treatment decision-making process. Modern treatment decision-making models are built along a philosophy that patients, environments, pathologies, and clinicians are complex, and that the complexities suggest that there is no definitive right or wrong processes. Rather, there are mainly just variations in the correctness of the professionals' decision-making abilities.

All decision-making models are designed to provide clinicians with information that targets a threshold effect toward decision making. The *threshold approach* is a method of optimizing decision making by applying critical thinking during the solving of questions concerning directions toward treatment.[1] It is a given set of findings or a level of finding that triggers a reaction by the healthcare provider. A decision based on the threshold approach is sometimes referred to as *categorical reasoning.* A categorical decision is based on few findings, is unambiguous, and is easy to judge regarding importance.[2] This judgment may involve a decision to reduce the negative consequences associated with the suspected disorder (e.g., cauda equina or cancer) or may have an economical or potential benefit of morbidity reduction (e.g., breast cancer screening programs).

Effective treatment decision making requires judicious clinical reasoning and a tremendous amount of practice and experience. *Clinical reasoning* is a thinking process to direct a clinician to take "wise" action or to take the best judged action in a specific context.[3] It is a process in which the clinician, who interacts with the patient and other appropriate parties, helps the patient manage his or her own health strategies based on the clinician's unique findings and the patient's own response to his or her condition.[4]

Most clinicians use a mixed model for treatment decision making, which combines the elements of heurism and hypothetical-deductive thinking. *Heuristic decision making* is a process that assumes healthcare practitioners actively organize clinical perceptions into coherent wholes. This implies that clinicians have the ability to indirectly make clinical decisions in the absence of complete information by formulating patterns, and can create solutions that are characterized by generalizations that allow transfer from one problem to the next.[5] *Hypothetical-deductive decision making* involves the development of a hypothesis during the clinical examination, and the decision to refute or accept that hypothesis during the process of the examination. A decision is formulated after accumulation and processing clinical findings and confirming or refuting preexisting hypotheses. The process is considered a bottom-up approach, as it allows *any* pertinent finding to be a qualifier during the decision-making process. Both methods require careful data collection and a summation of the findings of the examination.

The Clinical Examination Process

The clinical examination is the most important component of treatment decision making. Although outside factors such as imaging and diagnosis do play a role in treatment decision making, the response to the examination and the contributing factors identified during the examination should be the most compelling elements when deciding appropriate treatment.

A sequential treatment decision-making process—involving three dedicated steps—is advocated in this handbook.[6]

Step 1: The first step involves the investigation of whether the patient's symptoms are reflective of a visceral disorder or a serious or potentially life-threatening illness. Examples include cancer, a fracture, a blood disorder, and an infection, among others, that are not routinely improved by an orthopedic-based treatment approach. By addressing this step, the clinician can identify disease processes that are outside the scope of the clinician's care and that require an intervention that is not within the skill set or practice pattern she or he holds. Primarily, however, recognition of a sinister problem can improve the likelihood of *appropriate* management of the patient.

Step 2: If the patient passes the first step of the treatment decision-making process, the clinician can move on to the second step, which is designed to determine from where the patient's pain arises. Test findings to isolate the lesion, for example, are used to further understand the cause of the condition and the likelihood of a dedicated diagnosis. Within this step, the clinician is also able to exclude or include selected diagnoses by using appropriate tests and measures.

Step 3: The final step of the treatment decision-making process involves determining what has gone wrong with this patient as a whole that would cause the pain experience (or whatever primary problem exists) to develop and persist. An understanding of the patient's full condition, classification of impairments, and likelihood of recovery are essential to her or his long-term care. This requires the use of information gathered within the medical history, outcomes measures assessment, and patient history. Use of this information allows the clinician to recognize conditions that will have a delayed recovery or that also require a dedicated approach to treat the comorbidity (e.g., depression, fear avoidance, etc.), which can indirectly influence the outcome of the primary problem.

Gregory Grieve[7] once wrote, "The meaning of each sign and symptom in itself has much greater importance for treatment indications than for diagnosis. It is not especially difficult to decide 'this is a degenerative joint condition.' We have to note how, and in what kind of patient . . . [do these examples of multiple variables associated with patient type have a] bearing on how we proceed, as does coexistent disease and past history." It is likely that outside step 1, step 3 is the most important step in the three-step process.

Clinical Examination Domains

The three different clinical examination domains—observation, patient history, and physical examination—impart essential information for treatment planning and endorse hypotheses of the type of physical impairment and related functional, physical, psychological, and social problems. Throughout the handbook, each region-specific case will provide information using this format:

1. Observation
2. Patient History
3. Physical Examination
    a. Active Physiological Findings
    b. Manual Muscle Testing
    c. Passive Physiological Findings
    d. Passive Accessory Findings
    e. Special Tests

Observation

The purpose of the observation is to examine visible static and movement-related defects for analysis during the patient history and physical examination. Commonly, the static general inspection consists of skin (integument) inspection, posture, and body symmetry. Skin inspection may yield valuable information on past injuries (scars), inflammatory processes (redness, swelling), and sympathetic contributions to pain. Although posture and body symmetry alone do not dictate the presence of impairment,[8,9] it is feasible to assume that these conditions may contribute to underlying pathologies. Dramatic postural faults are worth further investigation and can be the basis for future exploration in many anatomical regions, especially when examined in conjunction with other assessment concepts.[10,11]

Observation of functional movements such as walking and transfers are also useful when determining treatment planning. Observation can also pick up fearfulness of movement—a feature that can be linked to delayed recovery.

Patient History

Patient history is a useful guide in outlining the ease in which symptoms are aggravated, the activities that contribute to the chief complaint of the patient, and the relationship of the reported history to the physical measures assessed.[10] There are two primary goals in the early phase: The first is to characterize the problem and establish potential causes, and the second is to determine the affect of the problem on the patient's lifestyle.[11]

Although taking a patient history is often considered the most important aspect of a clinical evaluation, few studies have evaluated how subjective findings contribute to the problem solving for treatment application.[11] Nonetheless, those who have investigated history taking are also stratified into diagnostic and impairment-based methods. For clinicians who use a diagnostic-based examination method, history taking appears to play a favorable part in providing a significant value in the diagnostic process.[12,13]

Some evidence lends support to the idea that effective history taking is related to a desired outcome. Walker and colleagues[14] identified that subjective history—specifically, report of activity requirements—was associated with future outcome and performance. By means of systematically obtaining information, the clinician can obtain information regarding the origin, contribution, and potential prognosis of a condition.

There are four primary areas that should be covered during the patient history: (1) the mechanism and description of injury, (2) the concordant sign, (3) the nature of the condition, and (4) the behavior of the symptoms.

MECHANISM AND DESCRIPTION OF INJURY The mechanism of the injury is the detailed recital of what the patient was doing when he or she sustained the injury. In some circumstances, the mechanisms can provide useful information to the identification of the potential tissue. More importantly, the description of the injury provides a documentation of the essence of the problem. This involves two forms: (1) an explanation and description of the injury-related pain and (2) the timing of when the event occurred. The identification of the pain from the injury is further expounded during the discussion of the chief complaint and nature of the problem, whereas the timing of the event is closely associated with the stage of the disorder. Both components enable the patient to meet her or his expectations of discussing the condition at hand.

CONCORDANT SIGN The concordant pain response is an activity or movement that provokes the patient's "familiar sign" or chief complaint.[15] Laslett and colleagues[15] defined the concordant familiar sign as the pain or other symptoms identified on a pain drawing and verified by the patient as being the complaint that has prompted the person to seek diagnosis and treatment. Maitland[16] describes a similar focal point identified as the "comparable sign."

Laslett and colleagues[15] suggest that one should focus on the patient's concordant sign, and should distinguish this finding from other symptoms produced during the physical assessment. According to the researchers, a finding that may be painful or abnormal, but not related to the concordant sign, may be identified as a "discordant pain response." A discordant pain response is the provocation of a pain that is unlike the pain for which the patient is seeking treatment.

The concordant sign is queried during the patient history, but the phenomenon of discordant pain is also a physical response determined during the physical examination and requires further examination throughout the length of the intervention. The concordant sign is often used as a litmus test to determine both mechanical and pain-related changes over time.

THE NATURE OF THE CONDITION The nature of the condition is a reflection of the internalization of the patient's condition. It may alter how the examination and treatment are performed and may influence the aggressiveness of the clinician. Typically, there are three representative aspects explored by each: (1) severity, (2) irritability, and (3) stage.

Severity Discovering the *severity* of the disorder is the subjective identification of how significantly the problem has affected the patient. A severe problem will usually result in a reduction in activity of daily living functions, work-related problems, social disruption, and leisure activities. Severity may be associated with unwanted alterations or changes in lifestyle. The clinician should endeavor to determine where the patient's impairment lies on a continuum of nuisance or disability. Many functional outcomes scales are designed to measure the severity of the impairment and are effective in collecting aggregate data.

Irritability *Irritability*, or *reactivity*, is a term used to define the stability of a present condition. In essence, irritability denotes how quickly a stable condition degenerates in the presence of pain-causing inputs. Patients with irritability may often be leery of aggressive treatment because their conditions will typically worsen with selected activities.[16–18] Patients who exhibit irritable symptoms may respond poorly to an aggressive examination and treatment approaches. Irritability is operationally defined using three criteria: (1) What does the patient have to do to set off this condition? (2) Once the condition is triggered, how long do the symptoms last and how severe are the symptoms? and (3) What does the patient have to do to calm down the symptoms? The irritability of the patient will guide the comprehensiveness of the examination and will dictate the selection and aggressiveness of treatment procedures.

A common pitfall is the supposition that irritability is synonymous with a patient who is in a significant amount of pain. This thinking ignores that patients without pain, or without significant pain, can be irritable. Patients with serious pathology may not always present with significant pain. Likewise, patients with noteworthy neurological changes are often irritable and may demonstrate little or no pain.

Stage Most impairments change over time. A skilled clinician is able to understand the path or progression of the disorder, a concept identified as the *stage*.[16] The stage of an injury or impairment involves a snapshot of how the patient identifies his or her current level of dysfunction as compared to a given point in the past. This allows examination of whether the condition has stabilized, stagnated, or progressed. Consequently, there are only three potential reports for the stage of a disorder; worse, better, or the same, with variations in the level of "worse" or "better."

BEHAVIOR OF SYMPTOMS There are three aspects of the so-called behavior of pain: (1) time, (2) response to movements, and (3) area. First, it is critical to determine how the pain changes over a 24-hour period. Conditions associated with inflammation may worsen during rest or aggressive movements.[16] Noninflammatory conditions may worsen during very aggressive unguarded movements. Sinister problems (nonmechanical disorders that are potentially life threatening) often yield worsening symptoms at night. Second, the behavior of the symptoms is necessary to determine whether a specific movement pattern exists. Some conditions are worse in various postures or positions, whereas others demonstrate improvement or deterioration during repeated movements. Third, isolation of the area of the symptoms is necessary to determine potentially contributing structures. In some conditions, there may be more than one site of pain.[19] Regardless of the tissue diagnosis, the patient should be questioned regarding neighboring tissues. Failure to ascertain the total area of symptoms may lead to inappropriate or incomplete administration of treatment.

Physical Examination

The primary goal of the physical examination is to establish the influence of movement on the patient's concordant symptoms that were described during the patient history.[19] By assessing movement, the clinician is more likely to determine the contributory muscles, joint, or ligaments involved in the patient's condition. Most importantly, the use of movement to alter symptoms enables the clinician to determine the appropriate treatment method and how that method will positively or negatively contribute to the patient's condition. The following assessment elements are typically advocated during the physical examination:

1. *Active Movements* Includes active physiological techniques performed exclusively by the patient
2. *Passive Movements* Includes passive physiological, passive accessory, and occasionally combined passive movements performed exclusively by the clinician
3. *Special Tests* Includes palpation, muscle provocation testing, upper and lower motor screening, differentiation tests, neurological testing, and any specific clinical tests designed to implicate a lesion

ACTIVE MOVEMENTS Active movements are any form of physiological movement performed exclusively by the patient. In a clinical examination, the purpose of an active movement is to identify and examine the influence of selected active movements on the concordant sign. By determining the behavior of the concordant sign to selected movements, the clinician can identify potential active physiological treatment approaches.

There are several conjectures to examine when evaluating the influence of active movement on impairment. First, positive (or good) patient responses include an increase of range of motion, a reduction of pain, or both. The procedure (i.e., movement into flexion, abduction, internal rotation, etc.) that was responsible for the greatest abolition of pain or increase in range is considered the best potential selection for a treatment. Second, if symptoms were produced, how did the symptoms respond to single or repeated movements? Often, repeated movements will abolish symptoms especially during mechanical dysfunction.[20] Third, where within the range did the symptoms worsen? End-range pain is typically associated with a mechanical impairment, whereas mid- or through-range pain may be indicative of an inflammatory impairment or instability.[16] Fourth, it is imperative to investigate how the patient yields to a particular movement. Because the intent to treat may require repeated movements into a movement that is initially painful, it is important to consider how faithful the patient would commit to adoption of this potential strategy. And last, are there other factors that could potentially contribute to this problem? Is the movement sequential? Does there appear to be a range restriction or hypermobility? Is weakness a consideration?

PASSIVE MOVEMENTS Passive movements are any planar or physiological motions that are performed exclusively by the clinician. The purpose of a passive movement is to identify and examine the influence of selected passive movements (repeated or static) on the concordant sign. Passive movements include (1) passive physiological movements, (2) passive accessory movements, and (3) combined passive movements.

Passive physiological movements Passive physiological movements are "movements which are actively used in the many functions of the musculoskeletal system."[19] These movements are commonly defined in kinesiological literature as *osteokinematic motions* and generally are categorized using plane-based descriptors such as *flexion, extension, adduction, abduction,* and *medial* or *lateral rotation.* Passive physiological movements occur simultaneously with accessory motions; the degree of freedom and the availability of motion are a product of that accessory mobility.

Assessment of passive physiological movement is useful to differentiate total range of motion at a particular joint segment. Cyriax and Cyriax[21] claim that passive physiological movements are necessary to assess the contribution of ligaments, capsule, and other inert structures to the cause of the impairment. On occasions when patients are unable or fearful to move the joint to the end range, the apparent range may be mistakenly assessed as limited. To determine the true range of motion, a passive physiological movement is required.

Within-session changes in range or pain after use of passive physiological movements may be useful in the examination process. Within-session changes have been shown to correctly identify patients who are most likely to demonstrate between-session changes or carryover effects to the next treatment.[22]

Passive accessory movements Grieve[7] indicates that a passive accessory movement is "any movement mechanically or manually applied to a body with no voluntary muscular activity by the patient." Within the spine, the majority of mobilization procedures advocated within this textbook involve regional mobilizations. Posterior-anterior (PA) mobilizations involve three-point movements of the primary targeted and neighboring segments[23,24] and move the adjacent segments as well as the targeted segment.[25] When addressing peripheral dysfunction, passive accessory movements are effective for engaging selected components of the capsule and ligament. For optimum assessment, passive assessment should occur at multiple ranges throughout the physiological availability to determine range-pain behavior. Additionally, passive movements throughout the range of motion will provide range-pain behavior.

During the examination procedure for passive accessory movements, the articular movements are evaluated for reproduction of the concordant sign. Using either a translatory or rolling motion, the patient's segment is moved passively to the first point of pain identified by the patient; the intensity of the pain is then recorded by the clinician using some mechanism of scale. Repeated movements that describe pain or cause a within-session change may be useful as a treatment technique.

SPECIAL TESTS There are a number of purposes for a special clinical test, although two stand out for treatment decision making. First, special clinical tests are used to determine the level of functional impairment or disability of the patient (supportive information). For example, palpation and manual provocation tests lend support to the findings of certain impairments but yield little information in the absence of the movement examination.

The second, and potentially the most important, purpose for the use of special clinical tests is to provide a diagnostic value to a set of findings (using sensitivity and specificity values and the offshoots of these such as likelihood ratios, etc.). Tests and measures often are either sensitive or specific, indicating they are useful in eliminating or including a certain condition. Tests to rule out a condition are often used early in the examination and demonstrate strong sensitivity, whereas tests to include a condition have high specificity and are used later.

Outcome of Decision Making

At the end of each case the learner should consider whether to *treat* or *don't treat*. If the clinician decides to "don't treat," she or he should consider an effective alternative or referral source for the patient. If the clinician decides to "treat," she or he should consider which treatment classification would likely be most beneficial for the patient and what dosage of care is needed.

Because experience is a critical element of treatment decision making, and exposure to conditions is a considerable factor that differentiates expert clinicians from novel decision makers, this textbook provides a litany of different orthopedic cases. It is my hope you find this information useful.

Endnotes

1. Cahan A, Gilon D, Manor O, Paltiel O. Clinical experience did not reduce the variance in physicians' estimates of pretest probability in a cross-sectional survey. J Clin Epidemiol. 2005;58:1211–6.

2. Szolovits P, Patil RS, Schwartz WB. Artificial intelligence in medical diagnosis. Ann Intern Med. 1988;108:80–7.

3. Kabrhel C, Camargo CA, Goldhaber SZ. Clinical gestalt and the diagnosis of pulmonary embolism: Does experience matter? Chest. 2008;127:1627–30.

4. Norman G, Young M, Brooks L. Non-analytical models of clinical reasoning: the role of experience. Med Educ. 2007;41:1140–5.

5. Edwards I, Jones M, Carr J, Braunack-Mayer A, Jensen GM. Clinical reasoning strategies in physical therapy. Phys Ther. 2004;84:312–30; discussion 331–5.

6. Murphy D, Hurwitz E. A theoretical model for the development of a diagnosis-based clinical decision rule for the management of patients with spinal pain. BMC Musculoskeletal Disorders 2007;8:75.

7. Grieve G. Common Vertebral Joint Problems. 2nd ed. Edinburgh; Churchill Livingstone: 1988.

8. Fann A. The prevalence of postural asymmetry in people with and without chronic low back pain. Arch Phys Med Rehabil. 2002;83:1736–8.

9. Levangie PK. The association between static pelvic asymmetry and low back pain. Spine. 1999;15:1234–42.

10. Edwards B. Manual of Combined Movements. Oxford; Butterworth-Heinemann: 1999.

11. Woolf AD. How to assess musculoskeletal conditions. History and physical examination. Best Pract Res Clin Rheumatol. 2003;17:381–402.

12. McGregor AH, Dore CJ, McCarthy ID, Hughes SP. Are subjective clinical findings and objective clinical tests related to the motion characteristics of low back pain subjects? J Orthop Sports Phys Ther. 1998;28:370–7.

13. Luime J, Verhagen A, Miedema H, et al. Does this patient have an instability of the shoulder or a labrum lesion? JAMA. 2004;292:1989–99.

14. Walker W, Cifu D, Gardner M, Keyser-Marcus L. Functional assessment in patients with chronic pain: Can physicians predict performance? Spine. 2001;80:162–8.

15. Laslett M, Young S, Aprill C, McDonald B. Diagnosing painful sacroiliac joints: a validity study of a McKenzie evaluation and sacroiliac provocation tests. Aust J Physiother. 2003;49:89–97.

16. Maitland GD. Maitland's Vertebral Manipulation. 6th ed. London; Butterworth-Heinemann: 2001.

17. Zusman M. Irritability. Manual Ther. 1998;3:195–202.

18. Koury M, Scarpelli E. A manual therapy approach to evaluation and treatment of a patient with a chronic lumbar nerve root irritation. Phys Ther. 1994;74(6):548–59.

19. Maitland GD. Peripheral Manipulation. 3rd ed. London; Butterworth-Heinemann: 1986.

20. Niere KR, Torney SK. Clinicians' perceptions of minor cervical instability. Manual Ther. 2004;9:144–50.

21. Cyriax J, Cyriax P. Cyriax's illustrated manual of orthopaedic medicine. Oxford; Butterworth-Heinemann: 1993.

22. Tuttle N, Laasko L, Barrett R. Change in impairments in the first two treatments predicts outcome in impairments, but not in activity limitations, in subacute neck pain: an observational study. Aust J Physiother. 2006;52:281–5.

23. Lee R, Evans J. An in vivo study of the intervertebral movements produced by posteroanterior mobilization. Clin Biomech. 1997;12:400–8.

24. Lee R, Tsung BY, Tong P, Evans J. Bending stiffness of the lumbar spine subjected to posteroanterior manipulative force. J Rehabil Res Dev. 2005;42:167–74.

25. Kulig K, Powers CM, Landel RF, et al. Segmental lumbar mobility in individuals with low back pain: in vivo assessment during manual and self-imposed motion using dynamic MRI. BMC Musculoskel Disord. 2007;8:8.

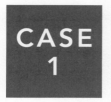

CASE 1

Setting: *Outpatient Orthopedics*

Date: *Present Day*

Medical Diagnosis: *Cervical Strain/Headaches*

Charted Data

Name:	*Libby Jacobson*	New Injury:	*Yes*
Age:	*22 years*	General Health:	*Good*
MRN:	*50501*	Amount of Exercise:	*30 minutes/day, 3 days/week*
Home Address:	*317 Eden Court, Trenton, New Jersey*	Occupation:	*Nursing student*
		Household:	*Single, lives alone*
Date of Injury:	*2 months ago*	Hand Dominance:	*Right*
		Race:	*Black*

Please fill in the location of your pain with a pencil.

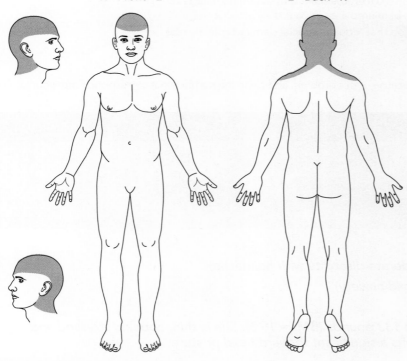

R Front L   L Back R

Pain Intensity Scale

0	No Pain
1	Low-level pain, able to perform regular activities
2	
3	
4	Moderate-level pain, use of pain medication, activity limited but functional
5	
6	
⑦	High-level pain, use of pain medication, activity very limited—decreased function
8	
9	
10	Emergency Situation

Imaging Results

A radiograph of the cervical spine yields no fractures and suggests only normal age-related degenerative changes (extremely minor in nature).

Medications

Zoloft, Ibuprofen (PRN)

Past Medical History (Please check any items that apply to you.)

Musculoskeletal:
- ○ Osteoarthritis
- ○ Rheumatoid Arthritis
- ○ Lupus/SLE
- ○ Fibromyalgia
- ○ Osteoporosis
- ⊗ Headaches

Musculoskeletal (continued)
- ○ Bulging Disc
- ○ Leg Cramps
- ○ Restless Legs
- ○ Jaw Pain/TMJ
- ○ History of Falling
- ○ Use of Cane or Walker

Musculoskeletal (continued)
- ○ Gout
- ○ Double Jointed
Other:_____

Neurological:
- ○ Stroke/TIA
- ○ Dementia

Neurological (continued)

- Polio
- Parkinson's Disease
- Multiple Sclerosis
- Epilepsy/Seizures
- Concussion
- Numbness
- Tingling

Other:_____

Endocrine:

- Diabetes
- Kidney Dysfunction

Endocrine (continued)

- Bladder Dysfunction
- Liver Dysfunction
- Thyroid Dysfunction

Other:_____

Cardiopulmonary:

- Congestive Heart Failure
- Heart Arrhythmia
- Pacemaker
- High Cholesterol
- Blood Clots
- Anemia

Cardiopulmonary (continued)

- High Blood Pressure
- Asthma
- Shortness of Breath
- COPD
- HIV/AIDS

Other:_____

Other:

- ⊗ Anxiety
- Depression
- Cancer

Chief Complaint: *Bilateral neck pain/headaches*

Goals for Therapy: *To reduce the headaches.*

In the last week, how many days have you had pain? *7*

Pain worst: *End of day (after studying)*

SANE Functional Rating

Please rate your **ability** to use your injured area on a 0 to 100% scale with **0%** being unable to use the injured area and **100%** being normal use of injured area in your daily activity: ___75%___

Also, if you exercise or have a sport activity or a job that requires special demands please rate your activity on the 0 to 100% scale: ___75%___

Patient-Specific Functional Scale

Please list 3 activities that you find are difficult because of this problem and circle the number that corresponds with your ability to perform the activity.

	Unable									No limitations
1. Reading	1	2	3	4	5	6	(7)	8	9	10
2. Using the computer	1	2	3	4	5	6	7	(8)	9	10
3. Using the smart phone	1	2	3	4	5	6	7	8	(9)	10

Unique Outcomes Measures

Neck Disability Index (NDI) = 23/50 (moderate disability with headache)

Hamilton Anxiety Scale Score = 18/56 (mild anxiety)

Observation

The patient is 5 feet 9 inches and weighs 133 pounds (BMI = 19.6). She is thin, appears stressed and concerned over her condition, and exhibits a significant forward head posture.

Patient History

The patient reports bilateral neck pain and the onset of headaches about 2 months ago, during the last semester of her nursing school requirements. She indicates that she does think the stress of her education and testing contributes to her neck pain and headaches, and that the two do seem to coincide.

Mechanism: *Although there was no specific incident, the patient did indicate that she has been stressed at school since she has been on academic probation and that this stress does seem to increase her neck and headache problems.*

Concordant Sign: *She indicates that her headache is initiated after long-term reading. Her neck pain is worse when using the computer.*

Nature of the Condition: *The 7/10 pain she reports occurs with the headaches and once the headaches start, the pain is too severe to continue reading or using the computer.*

Behavior of the Symptoms: *Symptoms worsen during sitting or using the computer and lessen once she lies down and sleeps.*

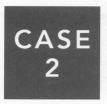

CASE 2

Setting: *Outpatient Orthopedics*

Date: *Present Day*

Medical Diagnosis: *Cervical Strain/Sprain*

Charted Data

Name:	*Mika Oh*	New Injury:	*No*
Age:	*67 years*	General Health:	*Fair*
MRN:	*50523*	Amount of Exercise:	*1 hour/day, 7 days/week*
Home Address:	*649 Strawberry Lane, Jackson, MO*	Occupation:	*Retired*
		Household:	*Married*
Date of Injury:	*Chronic*	Hand Dominance:	*Left*
		Race:	*Asian*

Please fill in the location of your pain with a pencil.

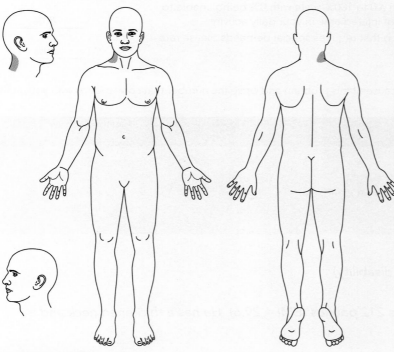

R Front L   L Back R

Pain Intensity Scale

0	No Pain
1	Low-level pain, able to perform regular activities
(2)	
3	
4	Moderate-level pain, use of pain medication, activity limited but functional
5	
6	
7	High-level pain, use of pain medication, activity very limited— decreased function
8	
9	
10	Emergency Situation

Imaging Results

A radiograph of the cervical spine yields significant degenerative changes at C5–C6, and C6–C7. An MRI was not ordered.

Medications:

Ibuprofen (PRN), Aspirin, Benzodiazepine

Past Medical History (Please check any items that apply to you.)

Musculoskeletal

- ⊗ Osteoarthritis
- ○ Rheumatoid Arthritis
- ○ Lupus/SLE
- ○ Fibromyalgia
- ○ Osteoporosis
- ○ Headaches

Musculoskeletal (continued)

- ○ Bulging Disc
- ⊗ Leg Cramps
- ○ Restless Legs
- ○ Jaw Pain/TMJ
- ○ History of Falling
- ○ Use of Cane or Walker

Musculoskeletal (continued)

- ○ Gout
- ○ Double Jointed
- Other:_____

Neurological:

- ○ Stroke/TIA
- ○ Dementia

Neurological (continued)

- ○ Polio
- ○ Parkinson's disease
- ○ Multiple Sclerosis
- ○ Epilepsy/Seizures
- ○ Concussion
- ○ Numbness
- ○ Tingling

Other:_____

Endocrine:

- ○ Diabetes
- ○ Kidney Dysfunction

Endocrine (continued)

- ○ Bladder Dysfunction
- ○ Liver Dysfunction
- ○ Thyroid Dysfunction

Other:_____

Cardiopulmonary:

- ○ Congestive Heart Failure
- ○ Heart Arrhythmia
- ○ Pacemaker
- ○ High Cholesterol
- ○ Blood Clots
- ○ Anemia

Cardiopulmonary (continued)

- ⊗ High Blood Pressure
- ○ Asthma
- ○ Shortness of Breath
- ○ COPD
- ○ HIV/AIDS

Other:_____

Other:

- ○ Anxiety
- ○ Depression
- ○ Cancer

Chief Complaint: *Right-sided neck pain*

Goals for Therapy: *To reduce the neck pain to allow him to perform hobbies such as woodworking and activities such as turning his head while driving.*

In the last week, how many days have you had pain? *7*

Pain worst: *During movements to the right side*

SANE Functional Rating

Please rate your **ability** to use your injured area on a 0 to 100% scale with **0%** being unable to use the injured area and **100%** being normal use of injured area in your daily activity: _____ 80% _____

Also, if you exercise or have a sport activity or a job that requires special demands please rate your activity on the 0 to 100% scale: _____ 70% _____

Patient-Specific Functional Scale

Please list 3 activities that you find are difficult because of this problem and circle the number that corresponds with your ability to perform the activity.

	Unable									No limitations
1. Woodwork	1	2	3	4	5	(6)	7	8	9	10
2. Driving	1	2	3	4	5	(6)	7	8	9	10
3. Yard work	1	2	3	4	5	6	(7)	8	9	10

Unique Outcomes Measures

Neck Disability Index = 18/50 (moderate disability)

Observation

The patient is 5 feet 11 inches and weighs 212 pounds (BMI = 29.6). He has a thickened neck and a flattened posterior neck posture.

Patient History

The patient reports right-sided neck pain that initiated about 4 weeks ago while helping his granddaughter build a doll house.

Mechanism: *The patient experienced long-term positioning into side flexion while building a doll house.*

Concordant Sign: *He indicates that his symptoms are triggered during right-side flexion (primarily) and right rotation (secondarily).*

Nature of the Condition: *He considers the problem more a nuisance than anything. He is very active and the "crick" in his neck has restricted his activity.*

Behavior of the Symptoms: *The symptoms are isolated to the right side of the neck and do not carry into the arms.*

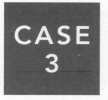

CASE 3

Setting: *Outpatient Orthopedics*

Date: *Present Day*

Medical Diagnosis: *Neck Strain*

Charted Data

Name:	*Larry McCallum*	New Injury:	*Yes*
Age:	*49 years*	General Health:	*Good*
MRN:	*50505*	Amount of Exercise:	*1 hour/day, 3 days/week*
Home Address:	*2900 Martinsville Corridor, St Lawrence, Nevada*	Occupation:	*Insurance salesman*
		Household:	*Married*
Date of Injury:	*4 weeks*	Hand Dominance:	*Left*
		Race:	*White*

Please fill in the location of your pain with a pencil.

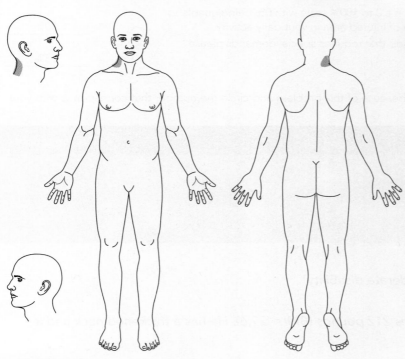

R Front L   L Back R

Pain Intensity Scale

0	No Pain
1	Low-level pain, able to perform regular activities
2	
3	
(4)	Moderate-level pain, use of pain medication, activity limited but functional
5	
6	
7	High-level pain, use of pain medication, activity very limited— decreased function
8	
9	
10	Emergency Situation

Imaging Results

A radiograph of the cervical spine yields mild degenerative changes at C5–C6 and C6–C7.

Medications

Ibuprofen (PRN), Aspirin

Past Medical History (Please check any items that apply to you.)

Musculoskeletal:
- ☒ Osteoarthritis
- ○ Rheumatoid Arthritis
- ○ Lupus/SLE
- ○ Fibromyalgia
- ○ Osteoporosis
- ○ Headaches

Musculoskeletal (continued)
- ○ Bulging Disc
- ☒ Leg Cramps*
- ☒ Restless Legs*
- ○ Jaw Pain/TMJ
- ○ History of Falling
- ○ Use of Cane or Walker

Musculoskeletal (continued)
- ○ Gout
- ○ Double Jointed
- Other:_____

Neurological:
- ○ Stroke/TIA
- ○ Dementia

Neurological (continued)

- ○ Polio
- ○ Parkinson's Disease
- ○ Multiple Sclerosis
- ○ Epilepsy/Seizures
- ○ Concussion
- ○ Numbness
- ○ Tingling

Other:_____

Endocrine:

- ○ Diabetes
- ○ Kidney Dysfunction

Endocrine (continued)

- ○ Bladder Dysfunction
- ○ Liver Dysfunction
- ○ Thyroid Dysfunction

Other:_____

Cardiopulmonary:

- ○ Congestive Heart Failure
- ○ Heart Arrhythmia
- ○ Pacemaker
- ○ High Cholesterol
- ○ Blood Clots
- ○ Anemia

Cardiopulmonary (continued)

- ⊗ High Blood Pressure
- ○ Asthma
- ○ Shortness of Breath
- ○ COPD
- ○ HIV/AIDS

Other:_____

Other:

- ○ Anxiety
- ○ Depression
- ○ Cancer

*At night only

Chief Complaint: *Right-sided neck pain*

Goals for Therapy: *To reduce the neck pain.*

In the last week, how many days have you had pain? 7

Pain worst: *During movements to the right side*

SANE Functional Rating

Please rate your **ability** to use your injured area on a 0 to 100% scale with **0%** being unable to use the injured area and **100%** being normal use of injured area in your daily activity: _80%_

Also, if you exercise or have a sport activity or a job that requires special demands please rate your activity on the 0 to 100% scale: _65%_

Patient-Specific Functional Scale

Please list **3 activities** that you find are difficult because of this problem and circle the number that corresponds with your ability to perform the activity.

	Unable								No limitations	
1. Golf	1	2	3	4	5	(6)	7	8	9	10
2. Reading (computer)	1	2	3	4	5	(6)	7	8	9	10
3. Yard work	1	2	3	4	5	6	(7)	8	9	10

Unique Outcomes Measures

Neck Disability Index (NDI) = 18/50 (moderate disability)

Observation

The patient is 5 feet 11 inches and weighs 212 pounds (BMI = 29.6). He has a thickened neck and a flattened posterior neck posture.

Patient History

The patient reports right-sided neck pain that initiated about 4 weeks ago after changing the garbage disposal unit at his daughter's apartment.

Mechanism: *The patient reports long-term positioning into side flexion while installing a garbage disposal unit.*

Concordant Sign: *He indicates that his symptoms are triggered during right-side flexion (primarily) and right rotation (secondarily).*

Nature of the Condition: *He considers the problem more a nuisance than anything. He is very active and the "crick" in his neck has restricted his activity.*

Behavior of the Symptoms: *The symptoms are isolated to the right side of the neck and do not carry into the arms.*

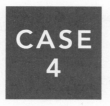

CASE 4

Setting: *Outpatient Orthopedics*

Date: *Present Day*

Medical Diagnosis: *Whiplash*

Charted Data

Name:	*Jen Logan*	New Injury:	*Yes*
Age:	*49 years*	General Health:	*Good*
MRN:	*50502*	Amount of Exercise:	*0 hours/day, 0 days/week*
Home Address:	*49 West Drive, Sommerville, New Jersey*	Occupation:	*Secretary*
		Household:	*Married with 3 children*
		Hand Dominance:	*Left*
Date of Injury:	*1 week*	Race:	*White*

Please fill in the location of your pain with a pencil.

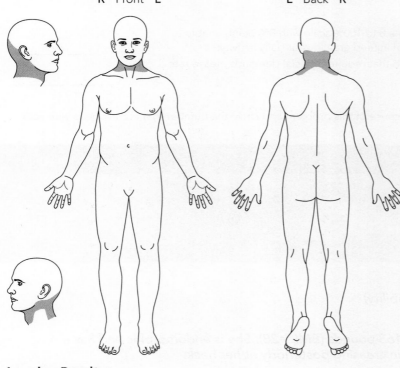

R Front L   L Back R

Pain Intensity Scale	
0	No Pain
1	Low-level pain, able to perform regular activities
2	
3	
(4)	Moderate-level pain, use of pain medication, activity limited but functional
5	
6	
7	High-level pain, use of pain medication, activity very limited—decreased function
8	
9	
10	Emergency Situation

Imaging Results

A radiograph of the cervical spine yields no fractures but does identify significant degenerative disc problems at C5–C6 and C6–C7.

Medications

Skelaxin, Ibuprofen (800 milligrams)

Past Medical History (Please check any items that apply to you.)

Musculoskeletal:
- ⊗ Osteoarthritis
- ○ Rheumatoid Arthritis
- ○ Lupus/SLE
- ○ Fibromyalgia
- ○ Osteoporosis
- ○ Headaches

Musculoskeletal (continued)
- ○ Bulging Disc
- ○ Leg Cramps
- ○ Restless Legs
- ○ Jaw Pain/TMJ
- ○ History of Falling
- ○ Use of Cane or Walker

Musculoskeletal (continued)
- ○ Gout
- ○ Double Jointed
- Other:_____

Neurological:
- ○ Stroke/TIA
- ○ Dementia

Neurological (continued)

- ○ Polio
- ○ Parkinson's Disease
- ○ Multiple Sclerosis
- ○ Epilepsy/Seizures
- ○ Concussion
- ○ Numbness
- ○ Tingling

Other:_____

Endocrine:

- ○ Diabetes
- ○ Kidney Dysfunction

Endocrine (continued)

- ○ Bladder Dysfunction
- ○ Liver Dysfunction
- ○ Thyroid Dysfunction

Other:_____

Cardiopulmonary:

- ○ Congestive Heart Failure
- ○ Heart Arrhythmia
- ○ Pacemaker
- ⊛ High Cholesterol
- ○ Blood Clots
- ○ Anemia

Cardiopulmonary (continued)

- ⊛ High Blood Pressure
- ○ Asthma
- ○ Shortness of Breath
- ○ COPD
- ○ HIV/AIDS

Other:_____

Other:

- ○ Anxiety
- ○ Depression
- ○ Cancer

Chief Complaint: *Bilateral neck and neck yoke pain*

Goals for Therapy: *To reduce the neck pain enough to allow the patient to work on her computer and drive her car. She would also like to be able to move her neck well enough to look over her shoulder and check for oncoming traffic without flaring up her neck pain.*

In the last week, how many days have you had pain? *7*

Pain worst: *End of day or when driving*

SANE Functional Rating

Please rate your **ability** to use your injured area on a 0 to 100% scale with **0%** being unable to use the injured area and **100%** being normal use of injured area in your daily activity: 70%

Also, if you exercise or have a sport activity or a job that requires special demands please rate your activity on the 0 to 100% scale: 0%

Patient-Specific Functional Scale

Please list 3 activities that you find are difficult because of this problem and circle the number that corresponds with your ability to perform the activity.

	Unable								No limitations	
1. Driving	1	2	3	(4)	5	6	7	8	9	10
2. Cooking (preparing food)	1	2	3	4	5	(6)	7	8	9	10
3. Using the computer	1	2	3	4	5	6	(7)	8	9	10

Unique Outcomes Measures

Neck Disability Index = 27/50 (severe disability)

Observation

The patient is 5 feet 4 inches and weighs 163 pounds (BMI = 28). She is endomorphic and has a forward head posture. Visually, she has skin creasing posteriorly at her neck.

Patient History

The patient reports bilateral neck pain after a motor vehicle accident two weeks ago. Prior to the accident, she had minor neck pain and had been diagnosed with osteoarthritis of the neck five years ago. This is her second motor vehicle accident in the last two years. She denies headaches.

Mechanism: *The patient was involved in a motor vehicle accident two weeks ago.*

Concordant Sign: *She indicates that side flexion and rotation (to both sides) elicit her concordant symptoms.*

Nature of the Condition: *The problem is restricting her work as a secretary. She has taken 6 days off in the last 10 workdays and is worried about her job.*

Behavior of the Symptoms: *The symptoms worsen with use of the computer but do not reach into the arms or thoracic region.*

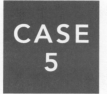

CASE 5

Setting: *Skilled Nursing Facility*
Date: *Present Day*
Medical Diagnosis: *Cervical Strain/Head Pain*

Charted Data

Name:	*Robert Missner*	New Injury:	*Yes*
Age:	*79 years*	General Health:	*Poor*
MRN:	*50503*	Amount of Exercise:	*0 hours/day, 0 days/week*
Home Address:	*506 Rose Lane, Ocala, Florida*	Occupation:	*Retired*
		Household:	*Institutionalized for 4 years*
Date of Injury:	*Insidious, 3 months*	Hand Dominance:	*Right*
		Race:	*White*

Please fill in the location of your pain with a pencil.

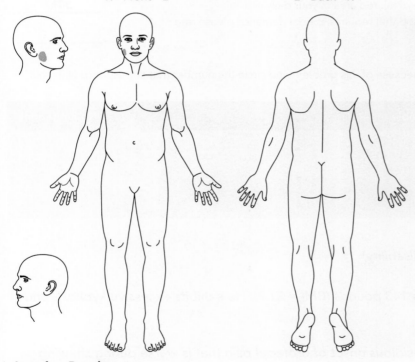

R Front L   L Back R

Pain Intensity Scale

0	No Pain
1	Low-level pain, able to perform regular activities
(2)	
3	
4	Moderate-level pain, use of pain medication, activity limited but functional
5	
6	
7	High-level pain, use of pain medication, activity very limited—decreased function
8	
9	
10	Emergency Situation

Imaging Results
No imaging has been performed.

Medications
Zocor, Azor, Betaxolol

Past Medical History (Please check any items that apply to you.)

Musculoskeletal:
- o **Osteoarthritis**
- o Rheumatoid Arthritis
- o Lupus/SLE
- o Fibromyalgia
- o Osteoporosis
- o Headaches

Musculoskeletal (continued)
- o Bulging Disc
- o Leg Cramps
- o Restless Legs
- o Jaw Pain/TMJ
- o History of Falling
- o Use of Cane or Walker

Musculoskeletal (continued)
- o Gout
- o Double Jointed
- Other:_____

Neurological:
- o Stroke/TIA
- ⊗ Dementia

Neurological (continued)

- o Polio
- o Parkinson's disease
- o Multiple Sclerosis
- o Epilepsy/Seizures
- o Concussion
- o Numbness
- o Tingling

Other:_____

Endocrine:

- o Diabetes
- o Kidney Dysfunction

Endocrine (continued)

- o Bladder Dysfunction
- o Liver Dysfunction
- o Thyroid Dysfunction

Other:_____

Cardiopulmonary:

- o Congestive Heart Failure
- o Heart Arrhythmia
- o Pacemaker
- ⊗ High Cholesterol
- o Blood Clots
- o Anemia

Cardiopulmonary (continued)

- o High Blood Pressure
- o Asthma
- ⊗ Shortness of Breath
- o COPD
- o HIV/AIDS

Other:_____

Other:

- o Anxiety
- o Depression
- o Cancer

Chief Complaint: *Orofacial pain with occasional headaches*

Goals for Therapy: *None*

In the last week, how many days have you had pain? *7*

Pain worst: *Symptoms are always present and do not change*

SANE Functional Rating

Please rate your **ability** to use your injured area on a 0 to 100% scale with **0%** being unable to use the injured area and **100%** being normal use of injured area in your daily activity: *30%*

Also, if you exercise or have a sport activity or a job that requires special demands please rate your activity on the 0 to 100% scale: *0%*

Patient-Specific Functional Scale

Please list 3 activities that you find are difficult because of this problem and circle the number that corresponds with your ability to perform the activity.

	Unable									No limitations
1. Eating	1	2	3	4	5	6	(7)	8	9	10
2. Watching TV	1	2	3	4	5	6	(7)	8	9	10
3. Concentrating while playing cards	1	2	3	4	5	6	(7)	8	9	10

Unique Outcomes Measures

Neck Disability Index = 14/50 (minimal disability)

Observation

The patient is 5 feet 8 inches and weighs 143 pounds (BMI = 21.7). He exhibits excessive kyphosis and asymmetry of the face.

Patient History

The patient and his caregivers note an insidious onset of orofacial pain that is worse during chewing and can cause unilateral headaches.

Mechanism: *Insidious.*

Concordant Sign: *Chewing, although pain is also present with no activity.*

Nature of the Condition: *The patient considers the condition an annoyance. His caregivers feel that early intervention may help eliminate the problem.*

Behavior of the Symptoms: *The symptoms have remained stationary over the last few months.*

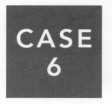

CASE 6

Setting: *Outpatient Orthopedics*

Date: *Present Day*

Medical Diagnosis: *Low Back Pain; Generalized Weakness*

Charted Data

Name:	*Linda Stewart*	New Injury:	*Yes*
Age:	*55 years*	General Health:	*Good*
MRN:	*67545*	Amount of Exercise:	*1 hour/day, 3 days/week*
Home Address:	*1923 Moonlight Drive, Gilbert, Arizona*	Occupation:	*Physical therapist*
		Household:	*Single, lives alone*
Date of Injury:	*3 months ago*	Hand Dominance:	*Right*
		Race:	*White*

Please fill in the location of your pain with a pencil.

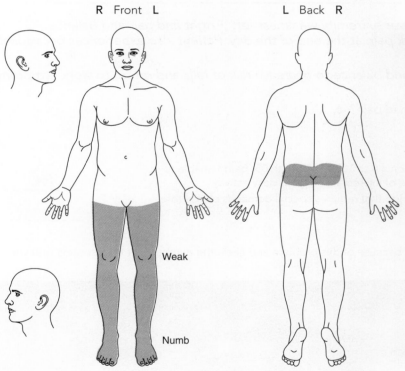

R Front L   L Back R

Weak

Numb

Pain Intensity Scale	
0	No Pain
1	Low-level pain, able to perform regular activities
2	
3	
4	Moderate-level pain, use of pain medication, activity limited but functional
5	
6	
⑦	High-level pain, use of pain medication, activity very limited— decreased function
8	
9	
10	Emergency Situation

Imaging Results

A radiograph of the lumbar spine yields no fractures and suggests only normal age-related degenerative changes (extremely minor in nature).

Medications

Prozac, Ibuprofen (PRN)

Past Medical History (Please check any items that apply to you.)

Musculoskeletal:
- ⊙ Osteoarthritis
- ⊙ Rheumatoid Arthritis
- ⊙ Lupus/SLE
- ⊙ Fibromyalgia
- ⊙ Osteoporosis
- ⊙ Headaches
- ⊗ Bulging Disc
- ⊙ Leg Cramps
- ⊙ Restless Legs
- ⊙ Jaw Pain/TMJ
- ⊗ History of Falling
- ⊙ Use of Cane or Walker
- ⊙ Gout
- ⊙ Double Jointed

Other:_____

Neurological:
- ⊙ Stroke/TIA
- ⊙ Dementia

- ⊙ Polio
- ⊙ Parkinson's Disease
- ⊙ Multiple Sclerosis
- ⊙ Epilepsy/Seizures
- ⊙ Concussion
- ⊗ Numbness
- ⊙ Tingling

Other:_____

Endocrine:
- ⊙ Diabetes
- ⊙ Kidney Dysfunction
- ⊙ Bladder Dysfunction
- ⊙ Liver Dysfunction
- ⊙ Thyroid Dysfunction

Other:_____

Cardiopulmonary:
- ⊙ Congestive Heart Failure
- ⊙ Heart Arrhythmia
- ⊙ Pacemaker

Cardiopulmonary (continued)
- ⊙ High Cholesterol
- ⊙ Blood Clots
- ⊙ Anemia
- ⊗ High Blood Pressure
- ⊙ Asthma
- ⊙ Shortness of Breath
- ⊙ COPD
- ⊙ HIV/AIDS

Other:_____

Other:
- ⊗ Anxiety
- ⊙ Depression
- ⊙ Cancer

Chief Complaint: *Patient has bilateral lower extremity weakness left > right and gait and balance impairments with complaints of low back pain at the end of the day. Patient also experiences occasional numbness in left foot.*

Goals for Therapy: *To improve strength and balance to decrease risk of falls and return to work symptom free.*

In the last week, how many days have you had pain? *6*

Pain worst: *End of day*

SANE Functional Rating

Please rate your **ability** to use your injured area on a 0 to 100% scale with **0%** being unable to use the injured area and **100%** being normal use of injured area in your daily activity: 75%

Also, if you exercise or have a sport activity or a job that requires special demands please rate your activity on the 0 to 100% scale: 60%

Patient-Specific Functional Scale

Please list **3 activities** that you find are difficult because of this problem and circle the number that corresponds with your ability to perform the activity.

	Unable									No limitations
1. Walking	1	2	3	4	⑤	6	7	8	9	10
2. Stairs	1	2	3	④	5	6	7	8	9	10
3. Dressing lower extremities	1	2	③	4	5	6	7	8	9	10

Unique Outcomes Measures

Functional Gait Assessment = 19/30

6-minute walk test = 1,075 feet with three episodes of loss of balance

Observation

The patient is 5 feet 7 inches and weighs 160 pounds (BMI = 25.1). In standing, she demonstrates forward head, rounded shoulders, and increased lumbar lordosis. During gait, patient intermittently hyperextends the left knee and demonstrates left ankle supination as she fatigues. Her left ankle exhibits decreased eccentric control as it slaps the ground at initial contact.

Patient History

Patient is a 55-year-old female who suffered a cervical injury following a motor vehicle accident 9.5 years ago, resulting in four cervical herniated discs. Nine years ago, she underwent a cervical discectomy and fusion of C6–C7 vertebrae. Two months ago the patient fell onto outstretched arms, bruising her left hip. Since that time she has experienced progressively worsening low back pain, lower extremity weakness, and gait and balance impairments.

Mechanism: *Patient states that she believes her symptoms initiated with her fall two months ago.*

Concordant Sign: *She indicates that her 7/10 low back pain is instigated at the end of the day. She notices that her lower extremity weakness and gait deviations—including left "foot slap"—initiate with short bouts of walking.*

Nature of the Condition: *The patient's lower extremity weakness and gait difficulties worsen with fatigue.*

Behavior of Symptoms: *Low back pain presents at the end of the day and improves with supine hook-lying position. Left foot numbness is occasional and is not triggered by any specific movement.*

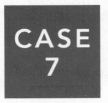

CASE 7

Setting: *Outpatient Orthopedics*

Date: *Present Day*

Medical Diagnosis: *Neck Pain*

Charted Data

Name:	*Joanne Marks*	General Health:	*Fair*
Age:	*53 years*	Amount of Exercise:	*30 minutes/week*
MRN:	*50501*	Occupation:	*Dental receptionist*
Home Address:	*910 Home Drive, New York City, New York*	Household:	*Married, lives with husband and two children*
Date of Injury:	*3 months ago*	Hand Dominance:	*Right*
New Injury:	*Yes*	Race:	*Black*

Please fill in the location of your pain with a pencil.

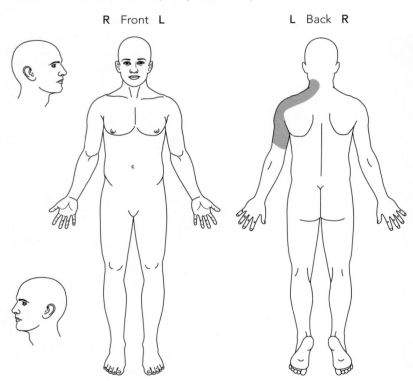

R   Front   L   L   Back   R

Pain Intensity Scale

0	No Pain
1	Low-level pain, able to perform regular activities
2	
③	
4	Moderate-level pain, use of pain medication, activity limited but functional
5	
6	
7	High-level pain, use of pain medication, activity very limited—decreased function
8	
9	
10	Emergency Situation

Imaging Results

A radiograph of left shoulder was unremarkable.

Medications:

Flexeril (PRN), Lopressor

Past Medical History (Please check any items that apply to you.)

Musculoskeletal

- ⊗ Osteoarthritis
- ○ Rheumatoid Arthritis
- ○ Lupus/SLE
- ○ Fibromyalgia
- ○ Osteoporosis
- ○ Headaches
- ○ Bulging Disc
- ○ Leg Cramps
- ○ Restless Legs
- ○ Jaw Pain/TMJ
- ○ History of Falling
- ○ Use of Cane or Walker
- ○ Gout
- ○ Double Jointed

Other:_____

Neurological:

- ○ Stroke/TIA
- ○ Dementia

Neurological (continued)

- ○ Polio
- ○ Parkinson's Disease
- ○ Multiple Sclerosis
- ○ Epilepsy/Seizures
- ○ Concussion
- ⊗ Numbness
- ⊗ Tingling

Other:_____

Endocrine:

- ○ Diabetes
- ○ Kidney Dysfunction
- ○ Bladder Dysfunction
- ○ Liver Dysfunction
- ○ Thyroid Dysfunction

Other:_____

Cardiopulmonary:

- ○ Congestive Heart Failure
- ○ Heart Arrhythmia

Cardiopulmonary (continued)

- ○ Pacemaker
- ○ High Cholesterol
- ○ Blood Clots
- ○ Anemia
- ⊗ High Blood Pressure
- ○ Asthma
- ○ Shortness of Breath
- ○ COPD
- ○ HIV/AIDS

Other:_____

Other:

- ○ Anxiety
- ○ Depression
- ○ Cancer

Chief Complaint: *Sharp pain, numbness and tingling into left arm*

Goals for Therapy: *To return to pain-free work.*

In the last week, how many days have you had pain? *7*

Pain worst: *Carrying items, sleeping on left side, and after completing workday*

SANE Functional Rating

Please rate your **ability** to use your injured area on a 0 to 100% scale with **0%** being unable to use the injured area and **100%** being normal use of injured area in your daily activity: *75%*

Also, if you exercise or have a sport activity or a job that requires special demands please rate your activity on the 0 to 100% scale: *75%*

Patient-Specific Functional Scale

Please list 3 activities that you find are difficult because of this problem and circle the number that corresponds with your ability to perform the activity.

	Unable									No limitations
1. Turning head when changing lanes	1	2	3	④	5	6	7	8	9	10
2. Using the computer	1	2	3	4	5	6	⑦	8	9	10
3. Carrying groceries	1	2	3	4	⑤	6	7	8	9	10

Unique Outcomes Measures

Neck Disability Index = 21/50 (moderate disability)

Fear Avoidance Beliefs Questionnaire (FABQ) = 6/42 in the work subscale and 15/24 in the physical activity (low level of fear)

Observation

The patient is 5 feet 2 inches and weighs 163 pounds (BMI = 29.8). She is overweight and exhibits forward head, rounded shoulder, and thoracic kyphosis. Patient demonstrates poor unsupported posture with increased thoracic kyphosis and forward posturing of head.

Patient History

The patient reports left arm pain that radiates into her forearm and occasionally into her left hand. She states that her pain started insidiously approximately 3 months ago. Her primary care physician diagnosed her with rotator cuff tendonitis and referred her for physical therapy evaluation and treatment.

Mechanism: *Although there was no specific incident that occurred to the patient, she did indicate that her pain increased after prolonged work at her computer station, or after talking on the telephone. Her symptoms began as a throbbing deep pain in her neck during rotation of the cervical spine and progressed into her arm.*

Concordant Sign: *The patient reports difficulty sleeping due to left shoulder pain. Her pain increases when carrying items, moving the left upper extremity, and making certain head movements, specifically flexion and rotation to the left.*

Nature of the Condition: *The patient reports her pain as a 2/10 on the numeric pain rating scale during the evaluation. The most intense pain that the patient has experienced in the last 24 hours is an 8/10. At best, her pain is a 2/10. Patient is unable to complete a full workday and has resorted to working half-days as a result of her pain. She reports increased pain after drinking coffee or when she sneezes.*

Behavior of the Symptoms: *Symptoms worsen during sitting or using the computer and lessen once she lies down on her back; the symptoms resume within approximately 15 minutes.*

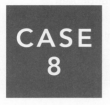

CASE 8

Setting: *Outpatient Orthopedic Clinic*

Date: *Present Day*

Medical Diagnosis: *Dizziness*

Charted Data

Name:	*Samantha DiGiovanni*	General Health:	*Excellent*
Age:	*22 years*	Amount of Exercise:	*2 hours/day, 6 days/week*
MRN:	*50578*	Occupation:	*University student/ Taekwondo instructor*
Home Address:	*134 East Street, Atlanta, Georgia*	Household:	*Resident in college dormitory*
Date of Injury:	*20-month history*	Hand Dominance:	*Right*
New Injury:	*Yes*	Race	*Caucasian*

Please fill in the location of your pain with a pencil.

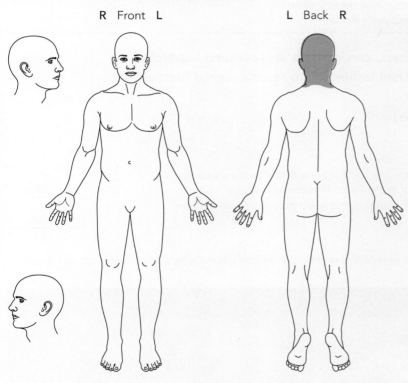

R   Front   L   L   Back   R

Pain Intensity Scale	
0	No Pain
1	Low-level pain, able to perform regular activities
2	
③	
4	Moderate-level pain, use of pain medication, activity limited but functional
5	
6	
7	High-level pain, use of pain medication, activity very limited— decreased function
8	
9	
10	Emergency Situation

Imaging Results

Radiological findings suggest two cervical disc herniations but level of herniations not known. No other imaging reported.

Medications

None documented

Past Medical History (Please check any items that apply to you.)

Unremarkable

Musculoskeletal:
- o Osteoarthritis
- o Rheumatoid Arthritis
- o Lupus/SLE
- o Fibromyalgia
- o Osteoporosis
- o Headaches
- o Bulging Disc
- o Leg Cramps
- o Restless Legs
- o Jaw Pain/TMJ
- o History of Falling
- o Use of Cane or Walker
- o Gout
- o Double Jointed

Other:_____

Neurological:
- o Stroke/TIA
- o Dementia

Neurological (continued)
- o Polio
- o Parkinson's Disease
- o Multiple Sclerosis
- o Epilepsy/Seizures
- o Concussion
- o Numbness
- o Tingling

Other:_____

Endocrine:
- o Diabetes
- o Kidney Dysfunction
- o Bladder Dysfunction
- o Liver Dysfunction
- o Thyroid Dysfunction

Other:_____

Cardiopulmonary:
- o Congestive Heart Failure
- o Heart Arrhythmia

Cardiopulmonary (continued)
- o Pacemaker
- o High Cholesterol
- o Blood Clots
- o Anemia
- o High Blood Pressure
- o Asthma
- o Shortness of Breath
- o COPD
- o HIV/AIDS

Other:_____

Other:
- o Anxiety
- o Depression
- o Cancer

Chief Complaint: *20-month history of dizziness, cervical pain, and occipital headache*

Goals for Therapy: *To reduce dizziness and headaches and to restore normal function.*

Outcomes Measures

In the last week, how many days have you had pain? *7*

Pain worst: *End of day or when driving*

SANE Functional Rating

Please rate your **ability** to use your injured area on a 0 to 100% scale with **0%** being unable to use the injured area and **100%** being normal use of injured area in your daily activity: *50%*

Also, if you exercise or have a sport activity or a job that requires special demands please rate your activity on the 0 to 100% scale: *30%*

Patient-Specific Functional Scale

Please list 3 activities that you find are difficult because of this problem and circle the number that corresponds with your ability to perform the activity.

	Unable								No limitations	
1. Reaching overhead	1	2	3	(4)	5	6	7	8	9	10
2. Sleeping	1	2	3	(4)	5	6	7	8	9	10
3. Taekwondo	1	2	(3)	4	5	6	7	8	9	10

Numerical Pain Rating Scale (NPRS)

Numeric pain rating scale (NPRS):[1] The patient is asked to rate their level of pain on an 11-point numerical scale 0–10 with 0 being "no pain" and 10 being the "worst possible pain."
The patient related this scale to her headaches, noting a constant 6/10 at rest and 8/10 at its worst.

Numeric scale for function: The patient is asked to rate the impact of their chief complaint on function on a 6-point scale with 0 being no impact and 5 being complete disability.
The patient reported a 3/5.

Unique Outcome Measures

Neck Disability Index[2] = 33/50 (moderate disability)

Dizziness Handicap Inventory[3] = 60/100

Observation

The patient is 5 feet 3 inches and weighs 130 pounds (BMI = 23.0). She presented with an asymmetrical cervical posture, positioning in right rotation. She was able to self-correct when cued to do so.

Patient History

The patient reports a 20-month history of dizziness, cervical pain, and occipital headache. She has received several different diagnoses from healthcare professionals, including ocular migraines, cervical disc herniations, and vertebral basilar insufficiency. The neurologist who had suggested her symptoms could be vascular in nature did not give clear or in-depth insight into this diagnosis. The patient describes her headache as a constant 6/10 at rest and 8/10 at its worst on a NPRS. The patient rated the overall impact of the dizziness on her functional abilities on a 6-point NPS as a 3/5. She also complains of bilateral tinnitus, a burning sensation of her right cervical spine and bilateral upper trap region, and numbness in her fourth and fifth digits of her right upper extremity. She reports a sense of "off balance" with quick rotational head movements, episodic blurry visual disturbances, and flashes of silver light in her visual field. Functional limitations caused by her chief complaint include reaching overhead, difficulty performing her work duties as a Taekwondo instructor, and the inability to sleep through the night secondary to neck pain. Previous treatment received by this patient was chiropractic management; however, it was unsuccessful at reducing her symptoms. The patient had also received three months of physical therapy consisting of myofascial release and craniosacral therapy with no change in status.

Mechanism: *No apparent reason.*

Concordant Sign: *Vestibular/Visual Testing: Vestibular-ocular reflex testing in the horizontal plane produced "floaters" in her visual field and "blurry vision" secondary to oscillopsia in the vertical plane. Saccadic movement testing produced blurry and double vision. Finally, smooth pursuit testing elicited blurry and double vision when the patient tracked in a superior direction. The manual orthopedic examination of the cervical spine elicited joint hypomobility for upper cervical flexion, left C0–C1, right C1–C2 rotation, and right C4–C5 side bending.*

Nature of the Condition: *Numerical rating for her headache was gauged by the patient as a constant 6/10 at rest and 8/10 at worst. Numerical rating for impact of dizziness on function was gauged to be a 3/5 on a 6-point scale.*

Behavior of the Symptoms: *Symptoms of dizziness appeared when the patient reached overhead and made quick head movements. Neck pain often awakens the patient at night while she is sleeping.*

Endnotes

1. Bolton JE. Accuracy of recall of usual pain intensity in back pain patients. Pain. 1999;83:533–9.

2. Vernon H, Mior S. The Neck Disability Index: a study of reliability and validity. J Manipulative Physiol Ther. 1991;14(7):409–15.

3. Jacobson, G.Newman, CW. The Development of the Dizziness Handicap Inventory. Arch Otolaryngol Head Neck Surg. 1990;116(4):424–7.

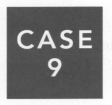

CASE 9

Setting: *Outpatient Orthopedics*

Date: *Present Day*

Medical Diagnosis: *Neck Strain*

Charted Data

Name:	*Nancy Stellar*	General Health:	*Good*
Age:	*32 years*	Amount of Exercise:	*3 hours of dancing/day, 6 days/week*
MRN:	*50505*		
Home Address:	*505 E. 43rd St., New York City, New York*	Occupation:	*Dancer, company director*
		Household:	*Married, 2 kids*
Date of Injury:	*8-year history*	Hand Dominance:	*Right*
New Injury:	*Yes*	Race:	*White*

Please fill in the location of you pain with a pencil.

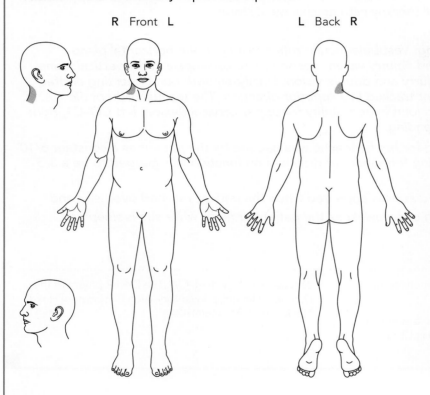

R Front L   L Back R

Pain Intensity Scale	
0	No Pain
1	Low-level pain, able to perform regular activities
2	
3	
(4)	Moderate-level pain, use of pain medication, activity limited but functional
5	
6	
7	High-level pain, use of pain medication, activity very limited— decreased function
8	
9	
10	Emergency Situation

Imaging Results
MRI 8 years ago post-traumatic fall that was determined to be unremarkable.

Medications
Advil (PRN)

Past Medical History (Please check any items that apply to you.)
Unremarkable

Musculoskeletal:
- o Osteoarthritis
- o Rheumatoid Arthritis
- o Lupus/SLE
- o Fibromyalgia
- o Osteoporosis
- o Headaches
- o Bulging Disc
- o Leg Cramps
- o Restless Legs
- o Jaw Pain/TMJ
- o History of Falling
- o Use of Cane or Walker
- o Gout
- o Double Jointed

Other:_____

Neurological:
- o Stroke/TIA
- o Dementia

Endocrine (continued)
- o Polio
- o Parkinson's Disease
- o Multiple Sclerosis
- o Epilepsy/Seizures
- o Concussion
- o Numbness
- o Tingling

Other:_____

Endocrine:
- o Diabetes
- o Kidney Dysfunction
- o Bladder Dysfunction
- o Liver Dysfunction
- o Thyroid Dysfunction

Other:_____

Cardiopulmonary:
- o Congestive Heart Failure
- o Heart Arrhythmia

Cardiopulmonary (continued)
- o Pacemaker
- o High Cholesterol
- o Blood Clots
- o Anemia
- o High Blood Pressure
- o Asthma
- o Shortness of Breath
- o COPD
- o HIV/AIDS

Other:_____

Other:
- o Anxiety
- o Depression
- o Cancer

Chief Complaint: *Right-sided neck and shoulder pain*

Goals for Therapy: *To improve neck mobility and pain and be able to return to normal function by improving the ability to carry items.*

In the last week, how many days have you had pain? *7*

Pain worst: *During movements of cervical right rotation and extension*

Numerical Pain Rating Scale (NPRS)

NPRS[1] for pain: The patient is asked to rate their level of pain on an 11-point numerical scale 0–10 with 0 being "no pain" and 10 being the "worst possible pain."

The patient noted a constant 6/10 neck pain.

Patient-Specific Functional Scale

Please list 3 activities that you find are difficult because of this problem and circle the number that corresponds with your ability to perform the activity

	Unable									No limitations
1. Turning head when driving	1	2	3	4	(5)	6	7	8	9	10
2. Reaching up overhead	1	2	3	(4)	5	6	7	8	9	10
3. Carrying groceries	1	(2)	3	4	5	6	7	8	9	10

Unique Outcomes Measures

Neck Disability Index (NDI) = 12%

Neck and upper limb index = 27%

Fear Avoidance Belief Questionnaire Physical Activity = 9/24

Observation

The patient is a slender 110 pounds and is 5 feet 3 inches. Her postural assessment showed a forward head position and a flexed lower cervical spine. Thoracic kyphosis also was noted.

Patient History

The patient reports a traumatic incident while dancing eight years ago when she was dropped onto her shoulder during a dance routine. She reports constant neck pain and limitations since. Upon the initial evaluation, the patient complained of a constant 6/10 neck pain that worsened with specific movements. The only activity that relieved her symptoms involved placing heat on her neck at home.

Mechanism: *Traumatic fall onto the right shoulder during a dance routine.*

Concordant Sign: *Limited neck mobility with right rotation while driving and neck pain with neck extension when looking up and reaching into a cabinet.*

Nature of the Condition: *The patient considers her condition somewhat disabling since she has been unable to do activities such as carry bags, groceries, children, etc. and must use a cart. This was not reflective on her NDI score of 12% indicating a mild disability.[2]*

Behavior of the Symptoms: *The symptoms are a constant 6/10 pain that do not worsen much throughout the day since she has modified her activities.*

Endnotes

1. Bolton JE. Accuracy of recall of usual pain intensity in back pain patients. Pain. 1999;83:533–9.

2. Vernon, H. The Neck Disability Index: State-of-the-Art, 1991–2008. J Manipulative Physiol Ther. 2008;31(7):491–502.

CASE 10

Setting: *Outpatient Orthopedic Office*

Date: *Present Day*

Medical Diagnosis: *Double Crush Syndrome (Bilateral Carpal Tunnel Symptoms and Cervical Stiffness)*

Charted Data

Name:	*Brenda Tillotson*	New Injury:	*Yes*
Age:	*39 years*	General Health:	*Good*
MRN:	*93284*	Amount of Exercise:	*1 hour/day, 3 days/week*
Home Address:	*1717 Wheatland Drive, Segunda Hills, California*	Occupation:	*Occupational therapist*
		Household:	*Married, 1 young child*
		Hand Dominance:	*Right*
Date of Injury:	*3 weeks ago*	Race:	*Asian*

Please fill in the location of your pain with a pencil.

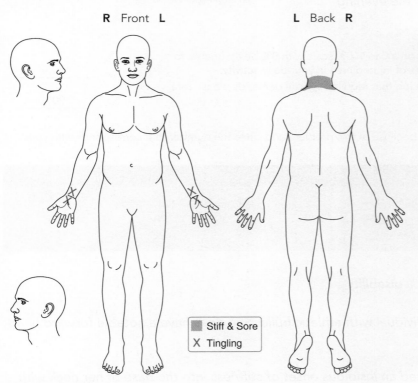

R Front L   L Back R

Stiff & Sore
X Tingling

Pain Intensity Scale

0	No Pain
1	Low-level pain, able to perform regular activities
2	
(3)	
4	Moderate-level pain, use of pain medication, activity limited but functional
5	
6	
7	High-level pain, use of pain medication, activity very limited— decreased function
8	
9	
10	Emergency Situation

Imaging Results
No imaging was performed.

Medications:
Celexa (anti-depressant)

Past Medical History (Please check any items that apply to you.)

Musculoskeletal:
- o Osteoarthritis
- o Rheumatoid Arthritis
- o Lupus/SLE
- o Fibromyalgia
- o Osteoporosis
- o Headaches

Musculoskeletal (continued)
- o Bulging Disc
- o Leg Cramps
- o Restless Legs
- o Jaw Pain/TMJ
- o History of Falling
- o Use of Cane or Walker

Musculoskeletal (continued)
- o Gout
- o Double Jointed
- Other:_____

Neurological:
- o Stroke/TIA
- o Dementia

Neurological (continued)

- ○ Polio
- ○ Parkinson's disease
- ○ Multiple Sclerosis
- ○ Epilepsy/Seizures
- ○ Concussion
- ○ Numbness
- ○ Tingling

Other: _Migraines_

Endocrine:

- ○ Diabetes
- ○ Kidney Dysfunction

Endocrine (continued)

- ○ Bladder Dysfunction
- ○ Liver Dysfunction
- ○ Thyroid Dysfunction

Other:_____

Cardiopulmonary:

- ○ Congestive Heart Failure
- ○ Heart Arrhythmia
- ○ Pacemaker
- ○ High Cholesterol
- ○ Blood Clots
- ○ Anemia

Cardiopulmonary (continued)

- ○ High Blood Pressure
- ○ Asthma
- ○ Shortness of Breath
- ○ COPD
- ○ HIV/AIDS

Other:_____

Other:

- ○ Anxiety
- ⊗ Depression
- ○ Cancer
- ○ Bipolar Disorder

Chief Complaint: _Stiffness into the base of the neck, bilateral palmar wrist sensation changes (described as numbness/tingling)_

Goals for Therapy: _To reduce neck stiffness and wrist symptoms._

In the last week, how many days have you had pain? _Patient does not have significant complaints of "pain" but does report daily occurrences of her chief complaint._

Pain worst: _In the morning and later into the evening_

Pain best: _During the day_

SANE Functional Rating

Please rate your **ability** to use your injured area on a 0 to 100% scale with **0%** being unable to use the injured area and **100%** being normal use of injured area in your daily activity: **90%**

Also, if you exercise or have a sport activity or a job that requires special demands please rate your activity on the 0 to 100% scale: **90%**

Patient-Specific Functional Scale

Please list 3 activities that you find are difficult because of this problem and circle the number that corresponds with your ability to perform the activity

	Unable									No limitations
1. Sleeping	1	2	(3)	4	5	6	7	8	9	10
2. Reading	1	2	3	4	5	6	(7)	8	9	10
3. Housework	1	2	3	4	5	6	(7)	8	9	10

Unique Outcomes Measures

Neck Disability Index (NDI) = 10/50; 20% disability

Observation

The patient appears to be a healthy individual with athletic build. She does have a notable forward head and rounded shoulders posture at rest.

Patient History

The patient reported that she had noticed an insidious onset of stiffness into the base of her neck with bilateral palmar wrist sensation changes, approximately 3 weeks prior to seeking physical therapy care. She described these symptoms as occurring in the morning, decreasing into the afternoon, and returning in the evening. She is currently working as an occupational therapist and reports that she was performing a significant number of chart reviews and computer work at this time of onset. She states this was the first time she had experienced these symptoms, but reports she has a long-standing history of migraines, which is medically controlled. She hasn't experienced a migraine in over a year.

Mechanism: _At the time of onset, the patient was performing work that forced her to assume sustained postures over a computer terminal._

Concordant Sign: _The patient's chief complaint of cervical stiffness was reproduced when she assumed end-range flexion and extension. She also had a positive upper limb neurodynamic test for the median nerve that reproduced her palmar symptoms bilaterally._

Nature of the Condition: _This condition is a nuisance for the patient. She continues to work and perform physical activities but is avoiding activities such as reading for pleasure._

Behavior of the Symptoms: _The patient's symptoms are reproducible but are not irritable._

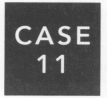

CASE 11

Setting: *Outpatient Orthopedics*

Date: *Present Day*

Medical Diagnosis: *Shoulder Impingement*

Charted Data

Name:	*Robert Swanson*	New Injury:	*Yes*
Age:	*59 years*	General Health:	*Fair*
MRN:	*50517*	Amount of Exercise:	*0 hours/day, 0 days/week*
Home Address:	*45 West Court, Apartment 12, Asheboro, North Carolina*	Occupation:	*Salesman*
		Household:	*Divorced, lives alone*
		Hand Dominance:	*Right*
Date of Injury:	*3 days*	Race:	*White*

Please fill in the location of your pain with a pencil.

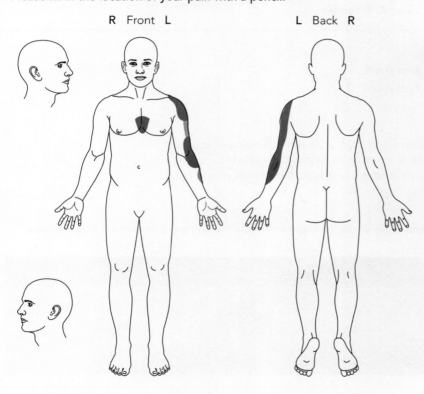

R Front L   L Back R

Pain Intensity Scale

0	No Pain
1	Low-level pain, able to perform regular activities
2	
3	
4	Moderate-level pain, use of pain medication, activity limited but functional
5	
6	
(7)	High-level pain, use of pain medication, activity very limited— decreased function
8	
9	
10	Emergency Situation

Imaging Results

A radiograph of his shoulder indicates degeneration of the glenohumeral joint and possible sub-acromial bursitis.

Past Medical History (Please check any items that apply to you)

Musculoskeletal:
- ⊗ Osteoarthritis
- ○ Rheumatoid Arthritis
- ○ Lupus/SLE
- ○ Fibromyalgia
- ○ Osteoporosis
- ○ Headaches
- ⊗ Bulging Disc
- ○ Leg Cramps
- ○ Restless Legs
- ○ Jaw Pain/TMJ
- ○ History of Falling
- ○ Use of Cane or Walker
- ○ Gout
- ○ Double Jointed

Other:_____

Neurological:
- ○ Stroke/TIA
- ○ Dementia

Neurological (continued)
- ○ Polio
- ○ Parkinson's Disease
- ○ Multiple Sclerosis
- ○ Epilepsy/Seizures
- ○ Concussion
- ○ Numbness
- ○ Tingling

Other:_____

Endocrine:
- ○ Diabetes
- ○ Kidney Dysfunction
- ○ Bladder Dysfunction
- ○ Liver Dysfunction
- ○ Thyroid Dysfunction

Other:_____

Cardiopulmonary:
- ○ Congestive Heart Failure
- ⊗ Heart Arrhythmia

Cardiopulmonary (continued)
- ○ Pacemaker
- ⊗ High Cholesterol
- ○ Blood Clots
- ○ Anemia
- ⊗ High Blood Pressure
- ○ Asthma
- ⊗ Shortness of Breath
- ○ COPD
- ○ HIV/AIDS

Other:_____

Other:
- ○ Anxiety
- ⊗ Depression
- ○ Cancer

Chief Complaint: *Left arm pain*

Goals for Therapy: *To get rid of the left arm pain.*

In the last week, how many days have you had pain? *3*

Pain worst: *Day (during exertion)*

SANE Functional Rating

Please rate your **ability** to use your injured area on a 0 to 100% scale with **0%** being unable to use the injured area and **100%** being normal use of injured area in your daily activity: *85%*

Also, if you exercise or have a sport activity or a job that requires special demands please rate your activity on the 0 to 100% scale: *50%*

Patient-Specific Functional Scale

Please list 3 activities that you find are difficult because of this problem and circle the number that corresponds with your ability to perform the activity.

	Unable								No limitations	
1. Walking	1	2	3	4	(5)	6	7	8	9	10
2. Climbing stairs	1	2	3	(4)	5	6	7	8	9	10
3. Carrying suitcase	1	2	3	4	(5)	6	7	8	9	10

Unique Outcomes Measures

DASH (disability of the arm, shoulder, and hand) score = 64/100

Positive on both depression questions (both answered with a yes or a no)

1. *During the past month, have you often been bothered by feeling down, depressed, or hopeless?*
2. *During the past month, have you often been bothered by little interest or pleasure in doing things?*

Observation

The patient is 5 feet 9 inches and weighs 232 pounds (BMI = 34.3). He is overweight and looks unhealthy. The patient breathes heavily during the interview and sweats during the examination without exertion.

Patient History

The patient notes that his arm pain began just 3 days ago after lifting and carrying several display cases from his van to the hotel symposium. He reports that his shoulder pain now hurts with any form of exertion and decreases when he sits or lies down. He has never had a history of shoulder problems before and is discouraged because his sales job requires a lot of lifting and carrying.

Mechanism: *The specific incident was associated with carrying display cases from the patient's van to the hotel. The pain began immediately after the lifting.*

Concordant Sign: *The patient is unable to fully reproduce his arm pain and he describes it as a deep throb that is worse during lifting or any form of activity.*

Nature of the Condition: *The patient indicates that the pain is very significant. He notes that it is slightly less than it was 3 days ago and there are periods where the pain is absent. He indicates that he cannot lift items and therefore cannot do his job.*

Behavior of the Symptoms: *This aspect of his history is vague but it appears that when the patient lifts something or performs any form of aggressive activity (including walking or stair climbing), his shoulder and arm pain worsen.*

CASE 12

Setting: *Outpatient Orthopedics*

Date: *Present Day*

Medical Diagnosis: *Multidirectional Shoulder Instability*

Charted Data

Name:	*Maria Garcia*	Amount of Exercise:	*1 hour/day, 5 days/week*
Age:	*18 years*	Occupation:	*High school student, member of high school swim team, works at Walmart stocking shelves*
MRN:	*68452*		
Home Address:	*2018 Adams Road, Montpelier, Vermont*		
		Household:	*Single, lives at home with mom, dad, and 2 sisters*
Date of Injury:	*2 months ago*		
New Injury:	*Yes*	Hand Dominance:	*Right*
General Health:	*Good*	Race:	*Hispanic*

Please fill in the location of your pain with a pencil.

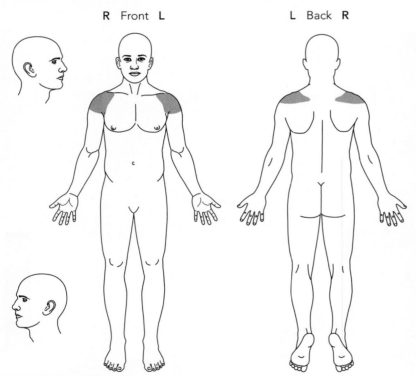

R   Front   L   L   Back   R

Pain Intensity Scale

0	No Pain
1	Low-level pain, able to perform regular activities
2	
3	
4	Moderate-level pain, use of pain medication, activity limited but functional
5	
6	
⑦	High-level pain, use of pain medication, activity very limited—decreased function
8	
9	
10	Emergency Situation

Imaging Results

The patient has not had any imaging completed for right shoulder pathology at this time.

Medications

Zoloft, Ibuprofen (PRN), Dexasone injection (received 1 year ago)

Past Medical History *(Please check any items that apply to you.)*

Musculoskeletal:
- o Osteoarthritis
- o Rheumatoid Arthritis
- o Lupus/SLE
- o Fibromyalgia
- o Osteoporosis
- o Headaches
- o Bulging Disc
- o Leg Cramps
- o Restless Legs
- o Jaw Pain/TMJ
- o History of Falling
- o Use of Cane or Walker
- o Gout
- o Double Jointed

Other: *Hx of Bilateral Shoulder Tendinitis*

Neurological:
- o Stroke/TIA
- o Dementia

Neurological (continued)
- o Polio
- o Parkinson's Disease
- o Multiple Sclerosis
- o Epilepsy/Seizures
- o Concussion
- o Numbness
- o Tingling

Other:_____

Endocrine:
- o Diabetes
- o Kidney Dysfunction
- o Bladder Dysfunction
- o Liver Dysfunction
- o Thyroid Dysfunction

Other:_____

Cardiopulmonary:
- o Congestive Heart Failure
- o Heart Arrhythmia

Cardiopulmonary (continued)
- o Pacemaker
- o High Cholesterol
- o Blood Clots
- o Anemia
- o High Blood Pressure
- o Asthma
- o Shortness of Breath
- o COPD
- o HIV/AIDS

Other:_____

Other:
- ⊗ Anxiety
- o Depression
- o Cancer

Chief Complaint: *Pain in bilateral shoulders*

Goals for Therapy: *To reduce the pain and be able to participate in swimming.*

In the last week, how many days have you had pain? *5*

Pain worst: *7–8/10*

SANE Functional Rating

Please rate your **ability** to use your injured area on a 0 to 100% scale with **0%** being unable to use the injured area and **100%** being normal use of injured area in your daily activity: ___75%___

Also, if you exercise or have a sport activity or a job that requires special demands please rate your activity on the 0 to 100% scale: ___50%___

Patient-Specific Functional Scale

Please list **3 activities** that you find are difficult because of this problem and circle the number that corresponds with your ability to perform the activity.

	Unable									No limitations
1. Swimming	1	2	3	(4)	5	6	7	8	9	10
2. Washing hair	1	2	3	4	(5)	6	7	8	9	10
3. Reaching high shelves at work	1	2	3	(4)	5	6	7	8	9	10

Unique Outcomes Measures

DASH = 30.0

Sports/Performing arts module = 50.0 (higher number indicates greater disability)

Observation

The patient is 5 feet 9 inches and weighs 133 pounds (BMI = 19.6). She exhibits a slight forward head and rounded shoulders posture in sitting and a slight winging of her scapula bilaterally.

Patient History

The patient reports pain in her right shoulder beginning approximately 2 months ago when she was swimming. She has been swimming for the past 6 years on various swim teams. She reports a history of recurring bilateral shoulder tendinitis and received conservative management, including Dexasone injections use with symptom resolution approximately 1 year ago. The patient also notes that both her shoulders feel "loose" and that both shoulders occasionally "pop out" when she is swimming or lifting her arms in front of her and above her head, and both sides are painful. Currently she reports needing frequent rest breaks throughout swim practice due to the pain.

Mechanism: *Although there was no specific incident, the patient did indicate that she has recently increased the amount of time spent in the pool with swim practice, and shortly after is when she noticed the pain in both of her shoulders.*

Concordant Sign: *The patient indicates that her shoulder pain is initiated during swim practice and worsens by the end of practice as well as when she is stocking high shelves at work.*

Nature of the Condition: *The 6/10 pain the patient reports occurs with overhead movements with swimming and work.*

Behavior of the Symptoms: *Symptoms worsen with repetitive overhead activities in all directions and lessen with rest.*

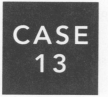

CASE 13

Setting: *Outpatient Orthopedics*

Date: *Present Day*

Medical Diagnosis: *Shoulder Pain*

Charted Data

Name:	*Mike McGee*	New Injury:	*Yes*
Age:	*52 years*	General Health:	*Fair*
MRN:	*34532*	Amount of Exercise:	*1 hour/day, 3 days/week*
Home Address:	*3136 Eshelman Road, Austin, Texas*	Occupation:	*Farmer*
		Household:	*Married*
Date of Injury:	*2 months ago*	Hand Dominance:	*Right*
		Race:	*White*

Please fill in the location of your pain with a pencil.

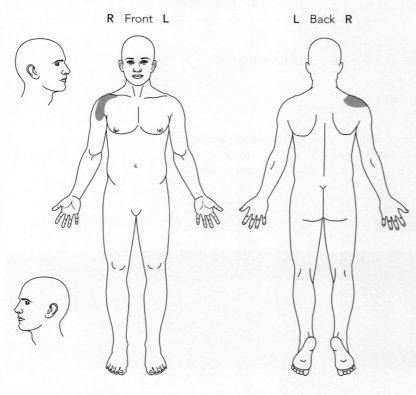

R   Front   L   L   Back   R

Pain Intensity Scale	
0	No Pain
1	Low-level pain, able to perform regular activities
2	
3	
4	Moderate-level pain, use of pain medication, activity limited but functional
(5)	
6	
7	High-level pain, use of pain medication, activity very limited—decreased function
8	
9	
10	Emergency Situation

Imaging Results
A radiograph of the cervical spine yields no fractures and suggests degenerative changes.

Medications
Ibuprofen, Lopressor, Lipitor

Past Medical History (Please check any items that apply to you.)

Musculoskeletal:
- ⊗ Osteoarthritis
- ○ Rheumatoid Arthritis
- ○ Lupus/SLE
- ○ Fibromyalgia
- ○ Osteoporosis
- ○ Headaches
- ○ Bulging Disc
- ○ Leg Cramps
- ○ Restless Legs
- ○ Jaw Pain/TMJ
- ○ History of Falling
- ○ Use of Cane or Walker
- ○ Gout
- ○ Double Jointed

Other:_____

Neurological:
- ○ Stroke/TIA
- ○ Dementia

Neurological (continued)
- ○ Polio
- ○ Parkinson's Disease
- ○ Multiple Sclerosis
- ○ Epilepsy/Seizures
- ○ Concussion
- ○ Numbness
- ○ Tingling

Other:_____

Endocrine:
- ⊗ Diabetes
- ○ Kidney Dysfunction
- ○ Bladder Dysfunction
- ○ Liver Dysfunction
- ○ Thyroid Dysfunction

Other:_____

Cardiopulmonary:
- ○ Congestive Heart Failure
- ○ Heart Arrhythmia

Cardiopulmonary (continued)
- ○ Pacemaker
- ⊗ High Cholesterol
- ⊗ Blood Clots
- ○ Anemia
- ⊗ High Blood Pressure
- ○ Asthma
- ○ Shortness of Breath
- ○ COPD
- ○ HIV/AIDS

Other:_____

Other:
- ⊗ Anxiety
- ○ Depression
- ○ Cancer

Chief Complaint: *Right shoulder pain*

Goals for Therapy: *To reduce shoulder pain and improve function in arm.*

In the last week, how many days have you had pain? *7*

Pain worst: *During overhead reaching activities*

SANE Functional Rating

Please rate your **ability** to use your injured area on a 0 to 100% scale with **0%** being unable to use the injured area and **100%** being normal use of injured area in your daily activity: _____ *75%*

Also, if you exercise or have a sport activity or a job that requires special demands please rate your activity on the 0 to 100% scale: _____ *75%*

Patient-Specific Functional Scale

Please list 3 activities that you find are difficult because of this problem and circle the number that corresponds with your ability to perform the activity.

	Unable									No limitations
1. Combing hair	1	2	3	(4)	5	6	7	8	9	10
2. Putting on coat	1	2	(3)	4	5	6	7	8	9	10
3. Tucking in shirt	1	2	(3)	4	5	6	7	8	9	10

Unique Outcomes Measures

DASH = 52/100

Shoulder Pain and Disability Index (SPADI) = 52/100

Observation

The patient is 5 feet 7 inches and weighs 236 pounds (BMI = 37). He is morbidly obese with a forward head and kyphotic posture observed with sitting. Atrophy of the infraspinatus and supraspinatus is observed with upright sitting.

Patient History

The patient reports right shoulder pain that has increased over the past several months. He does not recall any specific injury that contributed to his pain but states pain is increased with overhead activities.

Mechanism: *The patient cannot remember a specific incident that contributed to the pain in his right shoulder. He states pain is increased with overhead activities and he has limited ability to perform his job duties at the farm.*

Concordant Sign: *The patient complains of a dull ache that radiates into his upper and lower arm. He reports the ache is worse with activity, at night when he lies on his affected shoulder, and when putting his right arm into his coat.*

Nature of the Condition: *The 6/10 pain the patient reports occurs with overhead activities. He also reports difficulty over the past several days with tucking in his shirt and thus requires his wife's help.*

Behavior of the Symptoms: *Symptoms worsen as the day progresses and the patient notices pain is worse at night. Pain is also increased with lying on the affected shoulder, thus he is unable to sleep on his right side due to pain.*

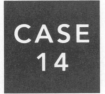

CASE 14

Setting: *Outpatient Orthopedics*

Date: *Present Day*

Medical Diagnosis: *Shoulder Pain*

Charted Data

Name:	*Maria Wallen*	General Health:	*Fair*
Age:	*52*	Amount of Exercise:	*Sedentary*
MRN:	*430193*	Occupation:	*School transportation*
Home Address:	*490 Kaster Road, Houston, Texas*	Household:	*Married, lives with husband and two children*
Date of Injury:	*10 months ago*	Hand Dominance:	*Right*
New Injury:	*Yes*	Race:	*White*

Please fill in the location of your pain with a pencil.

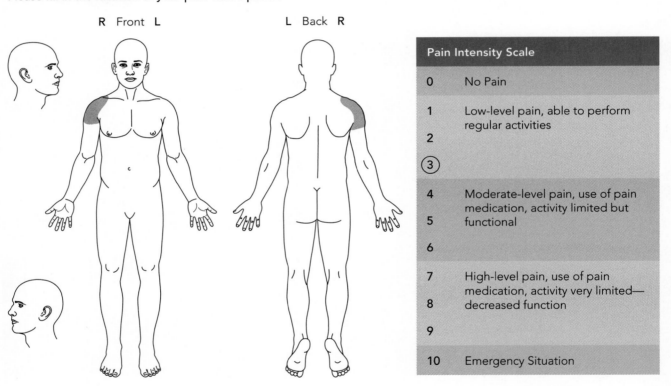

Imaging Results

A radiograph of the spine presents with normal age-related changes. Radiograph of right shoulder displays no signs of acute fracture.

Medications

Atenolol, Lovastatin, Insulin, Albuterol, Lyrica

Past Medical History: (Please check any items that apply to you.)

Musculoskeletal:
- ○ Osteoarthritis
- ○ Rheumatoid Arthritis
- ○ Lupus/SLE
- ⊗ Fibromyalgia
- ○ Osteoporosis
- ○ Headaches
- ○ Bulging Disc
- ○ Leg Cramps
- ○ Restless Legs
- ○ Jaw Pain/TMJ
- ○ History of Falling
- ○ Use of Cane or Walker
- ○ Gout
- ○ Double Jointed

Other:_____

Neurological:
- ○ Stroke/TIA
- ○ Dementia

Neurological (continued)
- ○ Polio
- ○ Parkinson's disease
- ○ Multiple Sclerosis
- ○ Epilepsy/Seizures
- ○ Concussion
- ○ Numbness
- ○ Tingling

Other:_____

Endocrine:
- ⊗ Diabetes
- ○ Kidney Dysfunction
- ○ Bladder Dysfunction
- ○ Liver Dysfunction
- ○ Thyroid Dysfunction

Other:_____

Cardiopulmonary:
- ○ Congestive Heart Failure
- ○ Heart Arrhythmia

Cardiopulmonary (continued)
- ○ Pacemaker
- ⊗ High Cholesterol
- ○ Blood Clots
- ○ Anemia
- ⊗ High Blood Pressure
- ⊗ Asthma
- ○ Shortness of Breath
- ○ COPD
- ○ HIV/AIDS

Other:_____

Other:
- ○ Anxiety
- ○ Depression
- ○ Cancer

Chief Complaint: *Right shoulder pain with decreased use of shoulder*

Goals for Therapy: *To be able to use the shoulder without pain again so that patient will have less difficulty working the school bus door, applying her seatbelt, and performing and self-care activities.*

In the last week, how many days have you had pain? *7*

Pain worst: *With right shoulder activity*

SANE Functional Rating

Please rate your **ability** to use your injured area on a 0 to 100% scale with **0%** being unable to use the injured area and **100%** being normal use of injured area in your daily activity: _____ **75%**

Also, if you exercise or have a sport activity or a job that requires special demands please rate your activity on the 0 to 100% scale: _____ **75%**

Patient-Specific Functional Scale

Please list **3 activities** that you find are difficult because of this problem and circle the number that corresponds with your ability to perform the activity.

	Unable								No limitations	
1. Using right arm to dress (hook bra)	1	②3	4	5	6	7	8	9	10
2. Brushing hair	1	②3	4	5	6	7	8	9	10
3. Reaching seatbelt	1	②3	4	5	6	7	8	9	10

Unique Outcomes Measures

Quick disability of arm, hand, and shoulder = 40 (moderate disability).

Observation

The patient is 5 feet 3 inches and weighs 164 pounds (BMI = 29). She presents with mild forward head posture. There is decreased thoracic kyphosis. She also presents with asymmetrical shoulder girdles, with the left being more superior than the right.

Patient History

The patient reports that her symptoms have been progressively getting worse. Initially, the pain was felt only at night or when she reached too far behind her back. Throughout the last few weeks, she has been noticing significant decreases in the amount of motion she has available with her right shoulder. The pain has also increased and is present during the majority of the day.

Mechanism: *The patient does not recall any specific incident or trauma that initiated her symptoms. She states that initially the pain was greatest during sleep and with repetitive motions such as vacuuming. She states she is severely limited in her ability to move her right shoulder.*

Concordant Sign: *The patient does not state any specific motion or position that decreases her pain. She reports she has the most limitations with brushing and washing her hair, hooking her bra, and tucking in her shirt. All of these activities are significantly painful and she is no longer able to complete them without help.*

Nature of the Condition: *The patient reports that her pain is a 3/10 at rest. When attempting to complete a challenging motion, like hooking her bra or vacuuming, her pain escalates to a 6–7/10. She is unable to lie on her right side due to the pain. Operating the school bus door to let students in and out of the bus also increases her pain.*

Behavior of the Symptoms: *Symptoms worsen during repetitive shoulder movements, lying on her affected side, and reaching behind her back or above her head. The symptoms are decreased with rest; however, the patient reports there is always some pain that lingers.*

CASE 15

Setting: *Outpatient Orthopedics*

Date: *Present Day*

Medical Diagnosis: *Right Shoulder Dislocation*

Charted Data

Name:	*Anthony Jones*	Amount of Exercise:	*2 hours/day, 5 days/week*
Age:	*18 years*	Occupation:	*High school senior baseball player*
MRN:	*43657*		
Home Address:	*2600 Brown Street, Columbus, Ohio*	Household:	*Lives in a single-story home with parents and younger brother*
Date of Injury:	*2 days ago*		
New Injury:	*Yes*	Hand Dominance:	*Right*
General Health:	*Good*	Race:	*White*

Please fill in the location of your pain with a pencil.

R   Front   L   L   Back   R

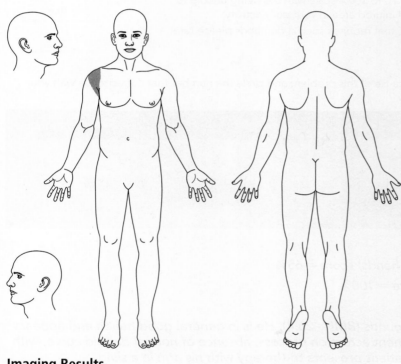

Pain Intensity Scale

0	No Pain
1	Low-level pain, able to perform regular activities
2	
3	
4	Moderate-level pain, use of pain medication, activity limited but functional
5	
6	
(7)	High-level pain, use of pain medication, activity very limited—decreased function
8	
9	
10	Emergency Situation

Imaging Results

Radiographs of the right shoulder were unremarkable.

Medications

Ibuprofen (PRN)

Past Medical History (Please check any items that apply to you.)

Unremarkable

Musculoskeletal:	Musculoskeletal (continued)	Musculoskeletal (continued)
○ Osteoarthritis	○ Headaches	○ History of Falling
○ Rheumatoid Arthritis	○ Bulging Disc	○ Use of Cane or Walker
○ Lupus/SLE	○ Leg Cramps	○ Gout
○ Fibromyalgia	○ Restless Legs	○ Double Jointed
○ Osteoporosis	○ Jaw Pain/TMJ	Other:_____

Neurological:

- o Stroke/TIA
- o Dementia
- o Polio
- o Parkinson's Disease
- o Multiple Sclerosis
- o Epilepsy/Seizures
- o Concussion
- o Numbness
- o Tingling

Other:_____

Endocrine:

- o Diabetes
- o Kidney Dysfunction

Endocrine (continued)

- o Bladder Dysfunction
- o Liver Dysfunction
- o Thyroid Dysfunction

Other:_____

Cardiopulmonary:

- o Congestive Heart Failure
- o Heart Arrhythmia
- o Pacemaker
- o High Cholesterol
- o Blood Clots
- o Anemia
- o High Blood Pressure
- o Asthma

Cardiopulmonary (continued)

- o Shortness of Breath
- o COPD
- o HIV/AIDS

Other:

Other:

- o Anxiety
- o Depression
- o Cancer

Chief Complaint: *Anterior right shoulder pain with movement and a feeling of instability*

Goals for Therapy: *To decrease pain in right shoulder and improve function in order to return to baseball and to work out without pain.*

In the last week, how many days have you had pain? *2 (incident occurred 2 days ago)*

Pain worst: *With movement*

SANE Functional Rating

Please rate your **ability** to use your injured area on a 0 to 100% scale with **0%** being unable to use the injured area and **100%** being normal use of injured area in your daily activity: _____75%_____

Also, if you exercise or have a sport activity or a job that requires special demands please rate your activity on the 0 to 100% scale: _____30%_____

Patient-Specific Functional Scale

Please list 3 activities that you find are difficult because of this problem and circle the number that corresponds with your ability to perform the activity.

	Unable								No limitations	
1. Lift weights	(1)	2	3	4	5	6	7	8	9	10
2. Play baseball	(1)	2	3	4	5	6	7	8	9	10
3. Donning shirt	1	2	3	4	(5)	6	7	8	9	10

Unique Outcomes Measures

DASH (disability of the arm, shoulder, and hands) score = 65%

DASH sports/performing arts module score = 100%

Observation

The patient is 6 feet tall and weighs 195 pounds (BMI = 26.4). He is in general good health and appears fit. His right shoulder demonstrates prominent acromion process, absence of normal deltoid curve, with anterior bulge of the humeral head. The patient presents to therapy with his arm in a sling.

Patient History

The patient is an 18-year-old male with an unremarkable medical history and no previous history of shoulder pathology. He reports onset of right shoulder pain following a fall on an outstretched arm playing baseball.

Mechanism: *The patient states that two days ago while playing baseball he dove for a ball; he describes landing on an abducted and externally rotated right arm. The patient indicated going to the emergency room to relocate the articulation and radiographs were taken.*

Concordant Sign: *The patient indicates that pain is initiated with shoulder abduction, internal rotation, and horizontal adduction.*

Nature of the Condition: *The 7/10 pain the patient reports occurs with movement.*

Behavior of the Symptoms: *Symptoms worsen with shoulder movement and lessen with ice and rest.*

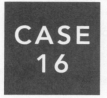

CASE 16

Setting: *Outpatient Orthopedic Clinic*

Date: *Present Day*

Medical Diagnosis: *Shoulder Impingement*

Charted Data

Name:	*Jonathan Smith*	General Health:	*Good*
Age:	*40 years*	Amount of Exercise:	*1 hour/day, 5 days/week*
MRN:	*50556*	Occupation:	*Laboratory research technician*
Home Address:	*34 N. Main Street, Jacksonville, Florida*	Household:	*Home with wife and one child (age 10)*
Date of Injury:	*8 months*	Hand Dominance:	*Right*
New Injury:	*Yes*	Race	*African American*

Please fill in the location of your pain with a pencil.

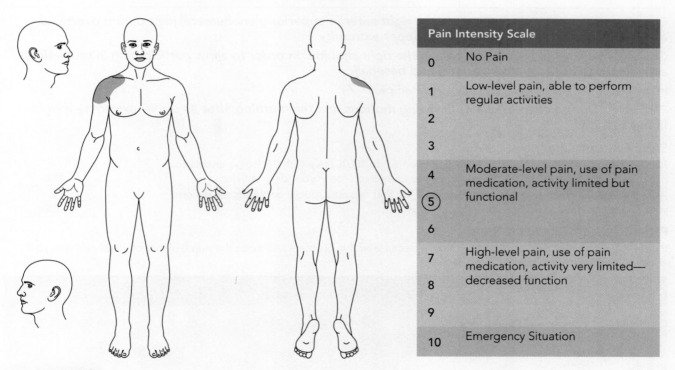

R   Front   L   L   Back   R

Pain Intensity Scale	
0	No Pain
1	Low-level pain, able to perform regular activities
2	
3	
4	Moderate-level pain, use of pain medication, activity limited but functional
(5)	
6	
7	High-level pain, use of pain medication, activity very limited—decreased function
8	
9	
10	Emergency Situation

Imaging Results

Radiographs of shoulder complex were negative for evidence of a fracture or moderate to severe ligamentous disruption.

Medications

Naprosyn (prescribed NSAID) 2 times/day

Past Medical History (Please check any items that apply to you.)

Unremarkable

Musculoskeletal:

- o Osteoarthritis
- o Rheumatoid Arthritis
- o Lupus/SLE
- o Fibromyalgia
- o Osteoporosis
- o Headaches
- o Bulging Disc
- o Leg Cramps
- o Restless Legs
- o Jaw Pain/TMJ
- o History of Falling
- o Use of Cane or Walker
- o Gout
- o Double Jointed

Other:_____

Neurological:

- o Stroke/TIA
- o Dementia

Neurological (continued)

- o Polio
- o Parkinson's Disease
- o Multiple Sclerosis
- o Epilepsy/Seizures
- o Concussion
- o Numbness
- o Tingling

Other:_____

Endocrine:

- o Diabetes
- o Kidney Dysfunction
- o Bladder Dysfunction
- o Liver Dysfunction
- o Thyroid Dysfunction

Other:_____

Cardiopulmonary:

- o Congestive Heart Failure
- o Heart Arrhythmia

Cardiopulmonary (continued)

- o Pacemaker
- o High Cholesterol
- o Blood Clots
- o Anemia
- o High Blood Pressure
- o Asthma
- o Shortness of Breath
- o COPD
- o HIV/AIDS

Other:_____

Other:

- o Anxiety
- o Depression
- o Cancer

Chief Complaint: *Intermittent pain in the right anterior-superior glenohumeral joint during overhead activities requiring the use of the right upper extremity*

Goals for Therapy: *To reduce the pain in the right shoulder in order to allow participation in recreational activities such as racquetball, tennis, and baseball.*

In the last week, how many days have you had pain? *7*

Pain worst: *During over-head and throwing motions and the morning after an upper extremity weight-lifting session*

SANE Functional Rating

Please rate your **ability** to use your injured area on a 0 to 100% scale with **0%** being unable to use the injured area and **100%** being normal use of injured area in your daily activity: _____ **45%** _____

Also, if you exercise or have a sport activity or a job that requires special demands please rate your activity on the 0 to 100% scale: _____ **20%** _____

Patient-Specific Functional Scale

Please list **3 activities** that you find are difficult because of this problem and circle the number that corresponds with your ability to perform the activity.

	Unable								No limitations	
1. Tennis	1	2	③	4	5	6	7	8	9	10
2. Weight training	1	2	3	4	⑤	6	7	8	9	10
3. Baseball	1	2	3	④	5	6	7	8	9	10

Unique Outcomes Measures

Disabilities of the arm, shoulder, and hand (DASH)[1] = 35

Shoulder Pain and Disability Index (SPADI)[2] = 30%

Observation

The patient is 5 feet 10 inches and weighs 175 pounds (BMI = 25.1). He exhibits bilateral anteriorly directed shoulders, with the right shoulder more anterior than the left shoulder. The right scapula appears more abducted than the left scapula. Bilateral scapular winging is evident with right winging greater than left. He favors his right upper extremity by holding the glenohumeral joint in adduction, and internal rotation and the elbow in flexion during independent ambulation.[3]

Patient History

The patient indicates an 8-month history of progressively worsening symptoms. He reports no direct trauma. He trains with weights regularly, with pain in the right shoulder minimal during training but maximal the morning following training.

Mechanism: *Over 8 months progressively worsening. No direct trauma.*

Concordant Sign: *The patient's pain is reproduced during 150° to 180° of right glenohumeral flexion and 140° to 170° of right glenohumeral abduction.*

Nature of the Condition: *The condition moderately limits the patient's ability to perform recreational sports, such as tennis and baseball, but only minimally limits his ability to perform daily activities, such as showering and doing dishes.*

Behavior of the Symptoms: *Pain worsens during high-velocity over-head activities and lifting heavy objects. The pain persists and worsens on the mornings following activity involving the right upper extremity.*

Endnotes

1. Hudak PL, Amadio PC, Bombardier C, Beaton D, Cole D, Davis A, Hawker G, et al. Development of an upper extremity outcome measure: The DASH (Disabilities of the Arm, Shoulder, and Head). Am J Ind Med. 1996;29(6):602–8.

2. Roach K, Budiman-Mak E, Songsiridej N, Lertratanakul Y. Development of a shoulder pain and disability index. Arthritis Care Res. 1991 Dec;4(4):143–9.

3. Host H. Scapular taping in the treatment of anterior shoulder impingement. Phys Ther. 1995;75:803–12.

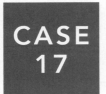

CASE 17

Setting: *Outpatient*

Date: *Present Day*

Medical Diagnosis: *Type II Posterior SLAP Lesion*

Charted Data

Name:	*Mike Jones*	New Injury:	*Yes*
Age:	*18 years*	General Health:	*Excellent*
MRN:	*50911*	Amount of Exercise:	*2–3 hours/day, 5 days/week*
Home Address:	*136 Circle Drive, Bismarck, North Dakota*	Occupation:	*College student*
		Household:	*2-bedroom apartment on third floor*
Date of Injury:	*7 days ago*	Hand Dominance:	*Right*

Please fill in the location of your pain with a pencil.

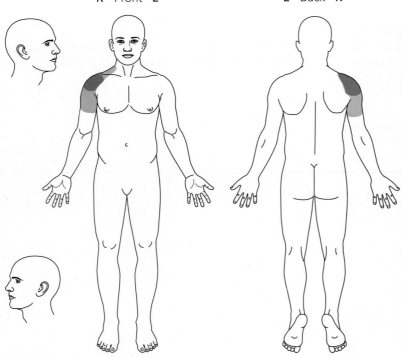

R Front L   L Back R

Pain Intensity Scale	
0	No Pain
1	Low-level pain, able to perform regular activities
2	
3	
4	Moderate-level pain, use of pain medication, activity limited but functional
5	
6	
(7)	High-level pain, use of pain medication, activity very limited—decreased function
8	
9	
10	Emergency Situation

Imaging Results

The patient has received no imaging.

Medications

Humalog with meals using sliding scale, Lantus 1 time/day, and Ibuprofen

Past Medical History (Please check any items that apply to you.)

Musculoskeletal:

- o Osteoarthritis
- o Rheumatoid Arthritis
- o Lupus/SLE
- o Fibromyalgia
- o Osteoporosis
- o Headaches

Musculoskeletal (continued)

- o Bulging Disc
- o Leg Cramps
- o Restless Legs
- o Jaw Pain/TMJ
- o History of Falling
- o Use of Cane or Walker

Musculoskeletal (continued)

- o Gout
- o Double Jointed

Other:_____

Neurological:

- o Stroke/TIA
- o Dementia
- o Polio
- o Parkinson's Disease
- o Multiple Sclerosis
- o Epilepsy/Seizures
- o Concussion
- o Numbness
- o Tingling

Other:_____

Endocrine:

- ⊗ Diabetes
- o Kidney Dysfunction

Endocrine (continued)

- o Bladder Dysfunction
- o Liver Dysfunction
- o Thyroid Dysfunction

Other:_____

Cardiopulmonary:

- o Congestive Heart Failure
- o Heart Arrhythmia
- o Pacemaker
- o High Cholesterol
- o Blood Clots
- o Anemia
- o High Blood Pressure
- o Asthma

Cardiopulmonary (continued)

- o Shortness of Breath
- o COPD
- o HIV/AIDS

Other:_____

Other:

- o Anxiety
- o Depression
- o Cancer

Chief Complaint: *Right shoulder pain that is diffuse in nature and located anteriorly and posteriorly in the GH joint. Pain located deep in the joint with sudden sharp pain and weakness with arm movements, such as reaching out to the side.*

Goals for Therapy: *To reduce pain and return to playing tennis full time as soon as possible.*

In the last week, how many days have you had pain? *7*

Pain worst: *9/10 on visual analog scale (VAS) with over-head serves and forehand strokes*

SANE Functional Rating

Please rate your **ability** to use your injured area on a 0 to 100% scale with **0%** being unable to use the injured area and **100%** being normal use of injured area in your daily activity: ___85%___

Also, if you exercise or have a sport activity or a job that requires special demands please rate your activity on the 0 to 100% scale: ___20%___

Patient-Specific Functional Scale

Please list 3 activities that you find are difficult because of this problem and circle the number that corresponds with your ability to perform the activity.

	Unable									No limitations
1. Tennis	1	(2)	3	4	5	6	7	8	9	10
2. Weight training	1	2	(3)	4	5	6	7	8	9	10
3. Over-head reaching	1	2	3	4	(5)	6	7	8	9	10

Unique Outcomes Measures

Disability of arm, shoulder, and hand (DASH)

- *Disability/pain section score = 20.8*
- *Sport section = 87.5*

UCLA shoulder scale = 17/35

Observation

The patient is 5 feet 11 inches and weighs 175 pounds (BMI = 24.4). He appears to be in good overall health with slight lumbar lordosis.

Patient History

An 18-year-old right-handed scholarship tennis player in the local elite training system referred himself to physical therapy for evaluation and treatment, complaining of recurrent right shoulder pain. He recalled having had no major trauma to his right shoulder. Pain is minimal at rest, but increases with reaching and over-head activities.

Mechanism: *Repeated over-head serves and forehand strokes with tennis.*

Concordant Sign: *Sharp with abduction and forward flexion.*

Nature of the Condition: *Patient is able to do light activity and activities of daily living (ADLs), but has had to discontinue court activities secondary to right shoulder pain.*

Behavior of the Symptoms: *Pain worsens with over-head activities and forehand strokes.*

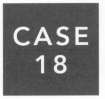

CASE 18

Setting: *Outpatient Orthopedic Clinic*

Date: *Present Day*

Medical Diagnosis: *Total Shoulder Arthroplasty (TSA)*

Charted Data

Name:	*Mary Jo Jenkins*	General Health:	*Fair*
Age:	*66 years*	Amount of Exercise:	*30 minutes/day, 3 days/week*
MRN:	*50533*		
Home Address:	*21 N. Main Street, Tampa, Florida*	Occupation:	*Librarian*
		Household:	*Lives with husband in one-level home*
Date of Injury:	*15 months ago*		
New Injury:	*15 months chronic*	Hand Dominance:	*Right*

Please fill in the location of your pain with a pencil.

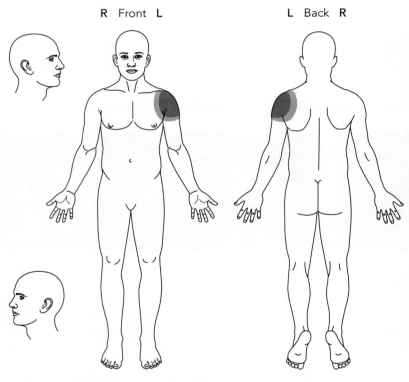

R Front L   L Back R

Pain Intensity Scale	
0	No Pain
1	Low-level pain, able to perform regular activities
2	
3	
4	Moderate-level pain, use of pain medication, activity limited but functional
(5)	
6	
7	High-level pain, use of pain medication, activity very limited—decreased function
8	
9	
10	Emergency Situation

Imaging Results

Initial radiographs of shoulder complex show total joint degeneration and severe osteoarthritis. Postoperative radiographs.

Medications

Celebrex and Vasotec daily

Past Medical History (Please check any items that apply to you.)

Musculoskeletal:

- ⊗ Osteoarthritis
- ⊗ Rheumatoid Arthritis
- ○ Lupus/SLE
- ○ Fibromyalgia
- ⊗ Osteoporosis
- ○ Headaches
- ○ Bulging Disc
- ○ Leg Cramps
- ○ Restless Legs
- ○ Jaw Pain/TMJ
- ⊗ History of Falling
- ○ Use of Cane or Walker
- ○ Gout
- ○ Double Jointed

Other:_____

Neurological:

- ○ Stroke/TIA
- ○ Dementia

Neurological (continued)

- ○ Polio
- ○ Parkinson's Disease
- ○ Multiple Sclerosis
- ○ Epilepsy/Seizures
- ○ Concussion
- ○ Numbness
- ○ Tingling

Other:_____

Endocrine:

- ○ Diabetes
- ○ Kidney Dysfunction
- ○ Bladder Dysfunction
- ○ Liver Dysfunction
- ○ Thyroid Dysfunction

Other:_____

Cardiopulmonary:

- ○ Congestive Heart Failure
- ○ Heart Arrhythmia

Cardiopulmonary (continued)

- ○ Pacemaker
- ○ High Cholesterol
- ○ Blood Clots
- ○ Anemia
- ⊗ High Blood Pressure
- ○ Asthma
- ○ Shortness of Breath
- ○ COPD
- ○ HIV/AIDS

Other:_____

Other:

- ○ Anxiety
- ○ Depression
- ○ Cancer

Chief Complaint: *Constant dull, aching pain in left shoulder*

Goals for Therapy: *To reduce the pain in the left shoulder in order to allow reaching over-head activities for return to work as a librarian.*

In the last week, how many days have you had pain? *7*

Pain worst: *8/10 pain with any left shoulder movement; 4/10 pain when at rest*

SANE Functional Rating

Please rate your **ability** to use your injured area on a 0 to 100% scale with **0%** being unable to use the injured area and **100%** being normal use of injured area in your daily activity: *85%*

Also, if you exercise or have a sport activity or a job that requires special demands please rate your activity on the 0 to 100% scale: *80%*

Patient-Specific Functional Scale

Please list 3 activities that you find are difficult because of this problem and circle the number that corresponds with your ability to perform the activity.

	Unable								No limitations	
1. Overhead activities	1	②	3	4	5	6	7	8	9	10
2. Reaching	1	2	③	4	5	6	7	8	9	10
3. Dressing	1	2	3	④	5	6	7	8	9	10

Unique Outcomes Measures

Disabilities of the arm, shoulder, and hand (DASH)[1] = 87%

Shoulder pain and disability index (SPADI)[2] = 76%

Observation

The patient is 5 feet 4 inches and weighs 156 pounds (BMI = 26.8). She currently has her left shoulder in sling and swath for immobilization postoperative TSA. The surgical incision is intact and bandaged, showing no signs of infection. She has kyphotic posture with forward head and rounded shoulders.

Patient History

The patient indicates a 15-month history of progressively worsening symptoms. No direct trauma reported by the patient, but she does have a history of osteo- or rheumatoid arthritis (OA/RA). The patient is s/p TSA yesterday. She also has a history of hypertension and falls. She does not have a regular exercise routine and has a BMI of 26.8.

Mechanism: *Progressively worsening after 15 months. No direct trauma or mechanism of injury.*

Concordant Sign: *Patient's pain is produced with any active or passive physiologic movement.*

Nature of the Condition: *The condition currently severely limits the patient's ability to perform ADLs and work-related activities, such as reaching overhead, showering, and doing dishes.*

Behavior of the Symptoms: *Pain worsens during active and passive range of motion.*

Endnotes

1. Hudak PL, Amadio PC, Bombardier C, Pamela L, Peter C, Beaton D, et al. Development of an upper extremity outcome measure: the DASH (disabilities of the arm, shoulder, and head). Am J Ind Med. 1996;29(6):602–8.

2. Roach KE, Budiman-Mak E, Songsiridej N, Lertratanakul Y. Development of a shoulder pain and disability index. Arthritis Care Res. 1991;4(4):143–9.

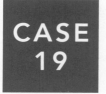

CASE 19

Setting: *Outpatient Orthopedic Clinic*

Date: *Present Day*

Medical Diagnosis: *Supraspinatus Tendinopathy* ⫶ Impingement

Charted Data

Name:	*Susan Alexis*	New Injury:	*Yes*
Age:	*20 years*	General Health:	*Excellent*
MRN:	*50533*	Amount of Exercise:	*3 hours/day, 6 days/week*
Home Address:	*5156 17th Street, Chicago, Illinois*	Occupation:	*Swimmer*
		Household:	*Lives with parents in one-level home*
Date of Injury:	*3 days ago*	Hand Dominance:	*Left*

Please fill in the location of your pain with a pencil.

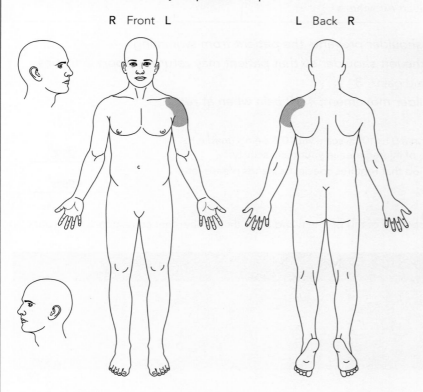

R   Front   L   L   Back   R

Pain Intensity Scale	
0	No Pain
1	Low-level pain, able to perform regular activities
2	
3	
4	Moderate-level pain, use of pain medication, activity limited but functional
⑤	
6	
7	High-level pain, use of pain medication, activity very limited—decreased function
8	
9	
10	Emergency Situation

Imaging Results

Radiographs of the left shoulder are normal. MRI shows a Bigliani Type I acromion and Type 2 hypersignal in the supraspinatus tendon.[1]

Medications

Tylenol

Past Medical History (Please check any items that apply to you.)

Musculoskeletal:
- ○ Osteoarthritis
- ○ Rheumatoid Arthritis
- ○ Lupus/SLE
- ○ Fibromyalgia
- ○ Osteoporosis
- ○ Headaches
- ○ Bulging Disc
- ○ Leg Cramps
- ○ Restless Legs
- ○ Jaw Pain/TMJ
- ○ History of Falling
- ○ Use of Cane or Walker
- ○ Gout
- ○ Double Jointed

Other:_____

Neurological:
- ○ Stroke/TIA
- ○ Dementia

Neurological (continued)
- ○ Polio
- ○ Parkinson's Disease
- ○ Multiple Sclerosis
- ○ Epilepsy/Seizures
- ○ Concussion
- ○ Numbness
- ○ Tingling

Other:_____

Endocrine:
- ○ Diabetes
- ○ Kidney Dysfunction
- ○ Bladder Dysfunction
- ○ Liver Dysfunction
- ○ Thyroid Dysfunction

Other:_____

Cardiopulmonary:
- ○ Congestive Heart Failure
- ○ Heart Arrhythmia

Cardiopulmonary (continued)
- ○ Pacemaker
- ○ High Cholesterol
- ○ Blood Clots
- ○ Anemia
- ○ High Blood Pressure
- ○ Asthma
- ○ Shortness of Breath
- ○ COPD
- ○ HIV/AIDS

Other:_____

Other:
- ⊗ Anxiety
- ○ Depression
- ○ Cancer

Chief Complaint: *Debilitating pain in left shoulder prevents the patient from swimming.*

Goals for Therapy: *To reduce the pain in the left shoulder so that patient may return to sport activities.*

In the last week, how many days have you had pain? *3*

Pain worst: *9.5/10 pain with any left shoulder movement; 4/10 pain when at rest.*

SANE Functional Rating

Please rate your **ability** to use your injured area on a 0 to 100% scale with **0%** being unable to use the injured area and **100%** being normal use of injured area in your daily activity: _____*25%*_____

Also, if you exercise or have a sport activity or a job that requires special demands please rate your activity on the 0 to 100% scale: _____*90%*_____

Patient-Specific Functional Scale

Please list 3 activities that you find are difficult because of this problem and circle the number that corresponds with your ability to perform the activity.

	Unable									No limitations
1. Over-head activities	1	②	3	4	5	6	7	8	9	10
2. Reaching	1	2	③	4	5	6	7	8	9	10
3. Dressing	1	2	3	4	⑤	6	7	8	9	10

Unique Outcomes Measures
Disabilities of the arm, shoulder, and hand (DASH)[2]
- *Disability/Pain section = 26.6*
- *Sports = 68.75*

Observation

The patient is 5 feet 4 inches and weighs 121 pounds (BMI = 20.8). She has forward head position and protracted shoulders with a Kibler type III scapula, in which excessive migration of the upper angle of the scapula occurs during movement with greater than 90° of flexion.[3] *Bone palpation revealed pain in the AC (acromioclavicular) joint, coracoid process, greater tuberosity of the humerus, upper and lower angle of the scapula, and cervical spine at C5, C6, and C7. Palpation of the musculature revealed pain in the upper- and mid-trapezius, levator scapulae, sternocleidomastoid, scalene, and rhomboid muscles.*[4]

Patient History

The patient is a female competitive swimmer with a training frequency of 6 times a week, 3 hours per day. She reports feeling strong pain in the anterior region of the left dominant shoulder during a practice session. She was able to finish the session, but was unable to practice the following day due to pain in the shoulder.

Mechanism: *No direct trauma or mechanism of injury.*

Concordant Sign: *The patient's pain is produced with any active physiologic movement.*

Nature of the Condition: *The condition currently severely limits the patient's ability to perform sport-related activities.*

Behavior of the Symptoms: *Pain worsens during repetitive active range of motion.*

Endnotes

1. Collipal E, Silva H, Ortega L, Espinoza E, Martínez C. The acromion and its different forms. Int J Morphol. 2010;28(4):1189–92.

2. Hudak PL, Amadio PC, Bombardier C, Pamela L, Peter C, Beaton D, et al. Development of an upper extremity outcome measure: The DASH (disabilities of the arm, shoulder, and head). Am J Ind Med. 1996;29(6):602–8.

3. Kibler WB. The role of the scapula in athletic shoulder function. Am J Sports Med. 1998;26(2):325–37.

4. Leão Almeida GP, De Souza VL, Barbosa G, Santos MB, Saccol MF, Cohen M. Swimmer's shoulder in young athlete: rehabilitation with emphasis on manual therapy and stabilization of shoulder complex. Man Ther. 2011;16:510–5.

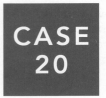

CASE 20

Setting: *Outpatient Orthopedics*

Date: *Present Day*

Medical Diagnosis: *Shoulder Pain*

Charted Data

Name: *Taylor Banks*

Age: *16 years*

MRN: *08442*

Home Address: *1482 Cloud Street, Bloomington, Minnesota*

Date of Injury: *Gradual onset over the past 2 weeks*

New Injury: *Yes*

General Health: *Good*

Amount of Exercise: *Participates in volleyball practice 3 times per week and volleyball games 1–2 times per week. No other sports or athletic hobbies. Plays trombone in jazz band. Outside of school spends most time on her laptop computer.*

Occupation: *High school student*

Household: *Lives with parents*

Please fill in the location of your pain with a pencil.

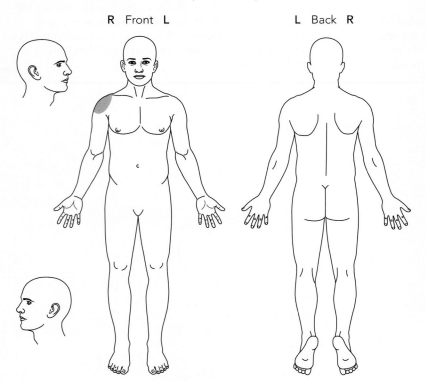

R Front L   L Back R

Pain Intensity Scale	
0	No Pain
1	Low-level pain, able to perform regular activities
2	
3	
(4)	Moderate-level pain, use of pain medication, activity limited but functional
5	
6	
7	High-level pain, use of pain medication, activity very limited— decreased function
8	
9	
10	Emergency Situation

Imaging Results

No imaging tests have been performed.

Medications

Ibuprofen (PRN)

Past Medical History (Please check any items that apply to you.)

Musculoskeletal:

- ○ Osteoarthritis
- ○ Rheumatoid Arthritis
- ○ Lupus/SLE
- ○ Fibromyalgia
- ○ Osteoporosis
- ○ Headaches
- ○ Bulging Disc
- ○ Leg Cramps
- ○ Restless Legs
- ○ Jaw Pain/TMJ
- ○ History of Falling
- ○ Use of Cane or Walker
- ○ Gout
- ○ Double Jointed

Other:_____

Neurological:

- ○ Stroke/TIA
- ○ Dementia

Neurological (continued)

- ○ Polio
- ○ Parkinson's Disease
- ○ Multiple Sclerosis
- ○ Epilepsy/Seizures
- ○ Concussion
- ○ Numbness
- ○ Tingling

Other:_____

Endocrine:

- ○ Diabetes
- ○ Kidney Dysfunction
- ○ Bladder Dysfunction
- ○ Liver Dysfunction
- ○ Thyroid Dysfunction

Other:_____

Cardiopulmonary:

- ○ Congestive Heart Failure
- ○ Heart Arrhythmia

Cardiopulmonary (continued)

- ○ Pacemaker
- ○ High Cholesterol
- ○ Blood Clots
- ○ Anemia
- ○ High Blood Pressure
- ○ Asthma
- ○ Shortness of Breath
- ○ COPD
- ○ HIV/AIDS

Other:_____

Other:

- ⊗ Anxiety
- ○ Depression
- ○ Cancer

Chief Complaint: *Shoulder pain*

Goals for Therapy: *Serve the volleyball without shoulder pain during or after practice.*

In the last week, how many days have you had pain? *4*

Pain worst: *5/10*

Pain best: *0/10*

SANE Functional Rating

Please rate your **ability** to use your injured area on a 0 to 100% scale with **0%** being unable to use the injured area and **100%** being normal use of injured area in your daily activity: _____ *70%*

Also, if you exercise or have a sport activity or a job that requires special demands please rate your activity on the 0 to 100% scale: _____ *40%*

Patient-Specific Functional Scale

Please list 3 activities that you find are difficult because of this problem and circle the number that corresponds with your ability to perform the activity.

	Unable									No limitations
1. Serving in volleyball	1	2	③	4	5	6	7	8	9	10
2. Fixing hair	1	2	3	4	⑤	6	7	8	9	10
3. Reaching into cabinet	1	2	3	4	5	6	7	⑧	9	10

Unique Outcomes Measures

Quick Disabilities of the arm, shoulder, and hand (QuickDASH) = 25

Sports module = 68.75.[1]

Observation

The patient is 5 feet 4 inches and weighs 106 pounds (BMI = 18.2). No observable redness or swelling is present in the shoulder region.

Patient History

The patient reports gradual onset of intermittent shoulder aching following volleyball practice over the past week. The season began 2 weeks ago. Symptoms have worsened over the past 2 days and have become more limiting with over-head activities.

Mechanism: *Two days ago, the patient attended a 1-hour individual volleyball lesson focusing on serving the ball; during this time she noticed pain in the superior aspect of the shoulder each time she raised her arm to serve the ball over-head and an increase in pain when she would strike the ball. She reports concluding the lesson early due to pain with attempts at further serves.*

Concordant Sign: *The most intense pain is present in the superior and anterior region of the shoulder with over-head use of the right upper extremity and volleyball.*

Nature of the Condition: *The shoulder continues to ache following practice. More intense and localized pain is present with over-head use.*

Behavior of the Symptoms: *No symptoms are present at rest. The patient experiences anterior and superior shoulder pain each day at volleyball practice when she serves the ball over-head; pain increases in intensity as the practice goes on. Pain level while serving the ball over-head is 6/10 and decreases to 3/10 in intensity and lasts 2–3 hours following practice. Pain with over-head activity such as fixing her hair is 3/10 and subsides upon bringing the upper extremity down to resting position.*

Endnotes

1. Gummesson C, Ward M, Atroshi I. The shortened disabilities of the arm, shoulder and hand questionnaire (QuickDASH): validity and reliability based on responses within the full-length DASH. BMC Musculoskeletal Disorders. 2006; 7(44):1–7. www .biomedcentral.com.

CASE 21

Setting: *Outpatient Orthopedics*

Date: *Present Day*

Medical Diagnosis: *Right Wrist Pain*

Charted Data

Name:	*Tommy Moyer*	General Health:	*Good*
Age:	*22 years*	Amount of Exercise:	*1 hour/day, 6 days/week*
MRN:	*444333*	Occupation:	*College student, collegiate-level baseball player*
Home Address:	*868 Redcrest Lane, Portland, Maine*	Household:	*Lives in dorm room with 3 colleagues*
Date of Injury:	*2 days ago*	Hand Dominance:	*Right*
New Injury:	*Yes*	Race	*White*

Please fill in the location of your pain with a pencil.

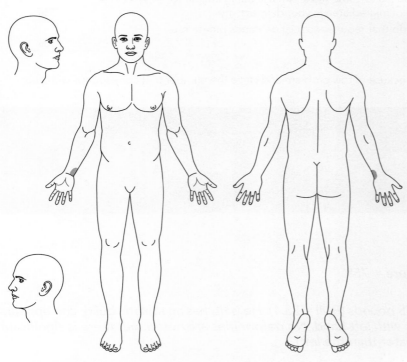

R Front L   L Back R

Pain Intensity Scale	
0	No Pain
1	Low-level pain, able to perform regular activities
2	
3	
4	Moderate-level pain, use of pain medication, activity limited but functional
5	
6	
7	High-level pain, use of pain medication, activity very limited—decreased function
(8)	
9	
10	Emergency Situation

Imaging Results

No imaging is available at this time.

Medications

Ibuprofen (PRN)

Past Medical History (Please check any items that apply to you.)

Musculoskeletal:
- o Osteoarthritis
- o Rheumatoid Arthritis
- o Lupus/SLE
- o Fibromyalgia
- o Osteoporosis

Musculoskeletal (continued)
- o Headaches
- o Bulging Disc
- o Leg Cramps
- o Restless Legs
- o Jaw Pain/TMJ

Musculoskeletal (continued)
- o History of Falling
- o Use of Cane or Walker
- o Gout
- o Double Jointed
- Other:_____

Neurological:

- ○ Stroke/TIA
- ○ Dementia
- ○ Polio
- ○ Parkinson's Disease
- ○ Multiple Sclerosis
- ○ Epilepsy/Seizures
- ⊗ Concussion
- ○ Numbness
- ○ Tingling

Other:_____

Endocrine:

- ○ Diabetes
- ○ Kidney Dysfunction

Endocrine (continued)

- ○ Bladder Dysfunction
- ○ Liver Dysfunction
- ○ Thyroid Dysfunction

Other:_____

Cardiopulmonary:

- ○ Congestive Heart Failure
- ○ Heart Arrhythmia
- ○ Pacemaker
- ○ High Cholesterol
- ○ Blood Clots
- ○ Anemia
- ○ High Blood Pressure
- ○ Asthma

Cardiopulmonary (continued)

- ○ Shortness of Breath
- ○ COPD
- ○ HIV/AIDS

Other:_____

Other:

- ○ Anxiety
- ○ Depression
- ○ Cancer

Chief Complaint: *Right medial wrist pain*

Goals for Therapy: *To reduce wrist pain and return to baseball.*

In the last week, how many days have you had pain? *2*

Pain worst: *When waking up this morning*

SANE Functional Rating

Please rate your **ability** to use your injured area on a 0 to 100% scale with **0%** being unable to use the injured area and **100%** being normal use of injured area in your daily activity: _75%_

Also, if you exercise or have a sport activity or a job that requires special demands please rate your activity on the 0 to 100% scale: _25%_

Patient-Specific Functional Scale

Please list 3 activities that you find are difficult because of this problem and circle the number that corresponds with your ability to perform the activity.

	Unable								No limitations	
1. Baseball	(1)	2	3	4	5	6	7	8	9	10
2. Using the computer	1	2	3	4	(5)	6	7	8	9	10
3. Using iPhone	1	2	3	(4)	5	6	7	8	9	10

Unique Outcomes Measures

DASH score = 38.1%

DASH Sports/Performing arts module score = 75%

Observation

The patient is 6 feet 1 inch and weighs 175 pounds (BMI = 23.1). He is fit, has an athletic build, and appears to be in pain. He is holding his right wrist with left hand. No deformities are noted, but there is significant swelling on right medial wrist (2.5cm greater than the left).

Patient History

The patient reports right medial wrist pain that began during baseball practice two days prior. He reports that he swung the bat to hit a ball and felt instant pain in his right wrist. He did not report any snapping sensation during this time. He has grown up playing sports and has never had an upper extremity injury. The patient experienced 1 minor concussion when playing high school football; no issues followed.

Mechanism: *He was swinging the bat with a twisting motion of the wrist when this pain began.*

Concordant Sign: *The patient complained of concordant pain with ulnar deviation and supination/pronation. He is experiencing his concordant sign when using his computer, taking notes in class, and using his cell phone.*

Nature of the Condition: *The patient experiences 8/10 pain when waking up in morning, when typing, and when using his phone. It remains at 6/10 consistently during other times.*

Behavior of the Symptoms: *Symptoms worsen when he uses the computer or phone; symptoms decrease when he sits with right arm relaxed.*

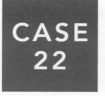

CASE 22

Setting: *Outpatient Orthopedics*

Date: *Present Day*

Medical Diagnosis: *Colles' Fracture*

Charted Data

Name:	*Brenda Bullough*	Amount of Exercise:	*Walks on lunch breaks ~ 20 minutes/day, 2–3 days/ week*
Age:	*48*		
MRN:	*986028347*		
Home Address:	*7384 Agave Avenue, Albuquerque, New Mexico*	Occupation:	*Receptionist and office manager*
Date of Injury:	*6 weeks prior*	Household:	*Married, lives with spouse*
New Injury:	*No*	Hand Dominance:	*Right*
General Health:	*Fair*	Race:	*Asian*

Please fill in the location of your pain with a pencil.

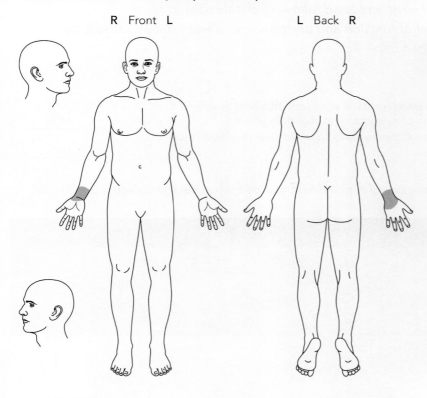

R Front L   L Back R

Pain Intensity Scale	
0	No Pain
1	Low-level pain, able to perform regular activities
2	
3	
(4)	Moderate-level pain, use of pain medication, activity limited but functional
5	
6	
7	High-level pain, use of pain medication, activity very limited— decreased function
8	
9	
10	Emergency Situation

Imaging Results

A radiograph of the right wrist shows that the fracture is now healed with good alignment of bony structures.

Medications

None

Past Medical History (Please check any items that apply to you.)

Musculoskeletal:
- ○ Osteoarthritis
- ○ Rheumatoid Arthritis
- ○ Lupus/SLE
- ⊗ Fibromyalgia
- ○ Osteoporosis
- ○ Headaches
- ○ Bulging Disc
- ○ Leg Cramps
- ○ Restless Legs
- ○ Jaw Pain/TMJ
- ○ History of Falling
- ○ Use of Cane or Walker
- ○ Gout
- ○ Double Jointed

Other:_____

Neurological:
- ○ Stroke/TIA
- ○ Dementia

Neurological (continued)
- ○ Polio
- ○ Parkinson's Disease
- ○ Multiple Sclerosis
- ○ Epilepsy/Seizures
- ○ Concussion
- ○ Numbness
- ○ Tingling

Other:_____

Endocrine:
- ○ Diabetes
- ○ Kidney Dysfunction
- ○ Bladder Dysfunction
- ○ Liver Dysfunction
- ○ Thyroid Dysfunction

Other:_____

Cardiopulmonary:
- ○ Congestive Heart Failure
- ○ Heart Arrhythmia

Cardiopulmonary (continued)
- ○ Pacemaker
- ○ High Cholesterol
- ○ Blood Clots
- ○ Anemia
- ○ High Blood Pressure
- ○ Asthma
- ○ Shortness of Breath
- ○ COPD
- ○ HIV/AIDS

Other:_____

Other:
- ⊗ Anxiety
- ⊗ Depression
- ○ Cancer

Chief Complaint: *Multi-range stiffness of wrist and hand following distal radial fracture*

Goals for Therapy: *To return to prior level of function and performance of work duties without pain.*

In the last week, how many days have you had pain? *7*

Pain worst: *When lifting objects*

SANE Functional Rating

Please rate your **ability** to use your injured area on a 0 to 100% scale with **0%** being unable to use the injured area and **100%** being normal use of injured area in your daily activity: _____ **60%**

Also, if you exercise or have a sport activity or a job that requires special demands please rate your activity on the 0 to 100% scale: _____ **60%**

Patient-Specific Functional Scale

Please list 3 activities that you find are difficult because of this problem and circle the number that corresponds with your ability to perform the activity.

	Unable									No limitations
1. Typing on keyboard	1	2	3	4	5	(6)	7	8	9	10
2. Writing	1	2	3	(4)	5	6	7	8	9	10
3. Carrying objects	1	2	3	(4)	5	6	7	8	9	10

Unique Outcomes Measures
Quick DASH = 68%

Observation

The patient is a female of 5 feet 1 inch weighing 100 pounds (BMI = 18.9) who presents to therapy with guarded right upper extremity. Initially, the patient was wearing an over-the-counter wrist cock-up splint. Her right forearm and thenar eminence show general atrophy compared to left. The patient appears anxious and smells heavily of cigarette smoke.

Patient History

The patient presents to therapy after having wrist cast removed two days prior. She reports that she slipped on an icy sidewalk at a grocery store eight weeks prior, sustaining a Colles' fracture. She was treated in a local emergency department where the fracture was reduced and immobilized with a cast. She is eager to describe the lawsuit that she has filed against the store for neglecting to clear ice from sidewalks on the store's property. The patient reports that she purchased the splint after getting the cast removed because she feels the fracture is "not healed." She complains she can no longer perform work duties due to her wrist stiffness and pain, and she has minor limitations with home activities and self-care—"but not as much as work duties."

Mechanism: The patient fell on an icy sidewalk with reaction of reaching posteriorly to brace herself, resulting in right distal radial fracture.

Concordant Sign: The patient has pain with all wrist movements and lifting objects with right hand.

Nature of the Condition: The patient experiences a dull, aching pain while performing ADLs, and compensates primarily with the use of her left hand.

Behavior of the Symptoms Pain is induced easily upon active range of motion (AROM) with high irritability of symptoms.

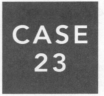

CASE 23

Setting: *Outpatient Orthopedics*

Date: *Present Day*

Medical Diagnosis: *Elbow Strain*

Charted Data

Name:	*Noah Jackson*	New Injury:	*Yes*
Age:	*21 years*	General Health:	*Good*
MRN:	*43423*	Amount of Exercise:	*2 hours/day; 6 days/week*
Home Address:	*323 Opal Drive, Sacramento, California*	Occupation:	*Student, baseball player*
		Household:	*Single*
Date of Injury:	*4 weeks ago*	Hand Dominance:	*Right*
		Race:	*Black*

Please fill in the location of your pain with a pencil.

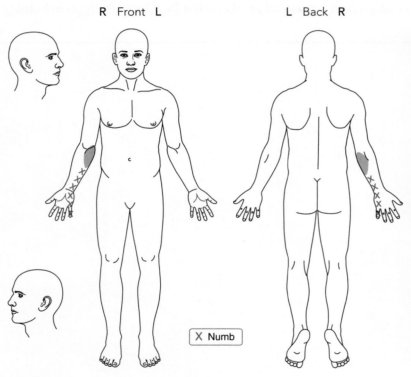

R   Front   L   L   Back   R

X   Numb

Pain Intensity Scale	
0	No Pain
(1)	Low-level pain, able to perform regular activities
2	
3	
4	Moderate-level pain, use of pain medication, activity limited but functional
5	
6	
7	High-level pain, use of pain medication, activity very limited—decreased function
8	
9	
10	Emergency Situation

Imaging Results

No radiographs have been taken. Patient is seen via direct access.

Medications

Ibuprofen (PRN)

Past Medical History (Please check any items that apply to you.)

Musculoskeletal:
- ○ Osteoarthritis
- ○ Rheumatoid Arthritis
- ○ Lupus/SLE
- ○ Fibromyalgia
- ○ Osteoporosis
- ○ Headaches
- ○ Bulging Disc
- ○ Leg Cramps
- ○ Restless Legs
- ○ Jaw Pain/TMJ
- ○ History of Falling
- ○ Use of Cane or Walker
- ○ Gout
- ○ Double Jointed

Other:_____

Neurological:
- ○ Stroke/TIA
- ○ Dementia

Neurological (continued)
- ○ Polio
- ○ Parkinson's Disease
- ○ Multiple Sclerosis
- ○ Epilepsy/Seizures
- ○ Concussion
- ⊗ Numbness
- ⊗ Tingling

Other:_____

Endocrine:
- ○ Diabetes
- ○ Kidney Dysfunction
- ○ Bladder Dysfunction
- ○ Liver Dysfunction
- ○ Thyroid Dysfunction

Other:_____

Cardiopulmonary:
- ○ Congestive Heart Failure
- ○ Heart Arrhythmia

Cardiopulmonary (continued)
- ○ Pacemaker
- ○ High Cholesterol
- ○ Blood Clots
- ○ Anemia
- ○ High Blood Pressure
- ○ Asthma
- ○ Shortness of Breath
- ○ COPD
- ○ HIV/AIDS

Other:_____

Other:
- ○ Anxiety
- ○ Depression
- ○ Cancer

Chief Complaint: *Decreased sensation along the medial forearm and decreased motor function in hand and wrist*

Goals for Therapy: *To return to playing baseball.*

In the last week, how many days have you had pain? *1*

Pain worst: *He reports vague pain in right arm and is unable to report an exact location of pain. Patient's main complaint is numbness and tingling into forearm and fourth and fifth digits. When symptoms are present, he has difficulty buttoning his shirt.*

SANE Functional Rating

Please rate your **ability** to use your injured area on a 0 to 100% scale with **0%** being unable to use the injured area and **100%** being normal use of injured area in your daily activity: 75%

Also, if you exercise or have a sport activity or a job that requires special demands please rate your activity on the 0 to 100% scale: 75%

Patient-Specific Functional Scale

Please list **3 activities** that you find are difficult because of this problem and circle the number that corresponds with your ability to perform the activity.

	Unable								No limitations	
1. Overhead throwing	(1)	2	3	4	5	6	7	8	9	10
2. Gripping a cup	1	2	3	4	(5)	6	7	8	9	10
3. Buttoning shirt	1	2	3	(4)	5	6	7	8	9	10

Unique Outcome Measures

Quick-DASH (disability of arm, shoulder and hand) = 40 (moderate disability)

Observation

The patient is 5 feet 9 inches and weighs 200 pounds (BMI = 29.5). He is in good shape with a forward head and kyphotic posture observed in sitting. No swelling, discoloration, or deformity are noted in the right elbow and shoulder.

Patient History

The patient complains of decreased sensation along the medial forearm and decreased motor function in the right hand and wrist. He reported symptoms have been occurring for approximately four weeks, progressively increasing. He states "a lack of control of his arm" and is unable to throw over-head when the symptoms are present.

Mechanism: *Although he cannot remember a specific incident that caused his current symptoms, the patient does report a baseball blow to his right elbow, approximately four weeks ago. His symptoms have progressed since then.*

Concordant Sign: *Point tenderness is found along the medial mid-shaft of the humerus, the medial epicondyle, and the olecranon process. Palpation of the ulnar nerve elicited radiating pain.*

Nature of the Condition: *Numbness and tingling have limited the patient's ability to participate in baseball. He reports when symptoms are present he has limited function of his wrist and hand and is unable to grip objects in his right hand.*

Behavior of the Symptoms *Symptoms have limited the patient's ability to throw over-head in baseball. The patient is upset with the fact that he is unable to pitch at this time. He reports symptoms also increase when talking on his cell phone with his elbow flexed.*

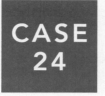

CASE 24

Setting: *Outpatient Orthopedic Clinic*

Date: *Present Day*

Medical Diagnosis: *Lunotriquetral Ligament Tear*

Charted Data

Name:	*Bob Jimvonovich*	New Injury:	*Yes*
Age:	*33 years*	General Health:	*Excellent*
MRN:	*66221*	Amount of Exercise:	*1 hour/day, 5 days/week*
Home Address:	*12345 Pine Lake Road, Dexter, Michigan*	Occupation:	*Tree trimmer*
		Household:	*Lives with his wife in 2-story home*
Date of Injury:	*3 days*	Hand Dominance:	*Left*

Please fill in the location of your pain with a pencil.

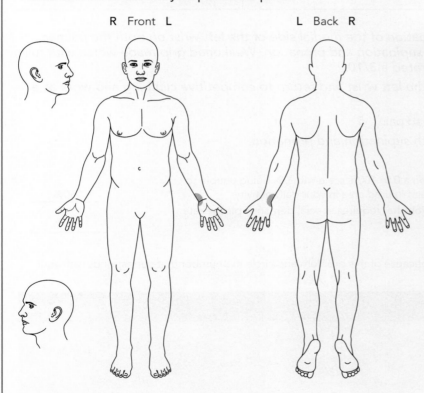

R Front L   L Back R

Pain Intensity Scale	
0	No Pain
1	Low-level pain, able to perform regular activities
2	
3	
4	Moderate-level pain, use of pain medication, activity limited but
(5)	functional
6	
7	High-level pain, use of pain medication, activity very limited—
8	decreased function
9	
10	Emergency Situation

Imaging Results

The MRI showed no convincing injury to the TFCC and no other injuries were noted, so a MRA was scheduled. The MRA revealed a tear to the lunotriquetral ligament.

Medications

Advil 200 mg when needed

Past Medical History (Please check any items that apply to you.)

Musculoskeletal:
- ○ Osteoarthritis
- ○ Rheumatoid Arthritis
- ○ Lupus/SLE
- ○ Fibromyalgia
- ○ Osteoporosis
- ⊗ Headaches
- ○ Bulging Disc
- ○ Leg Cramps
- ○ Restless Legs
- ○ Jaw Pain/TMJ
- ○ History of Falling
- ○ Use of Cane or Walker
- ○ Gout
- ○ Double Jointed

Other:_____

Neurological:
- ○ Stroke/TIA
- ○ Dementia

Neurological (continued)
- ○ Polio
- ○ Parkinson's Disease
- ○ Multiple Sclerosis
- ○ Epilepsy/Seizures
- ○ Concussion
- ○ Numbness
- ○ Tingling

Other:_____

Endocrine:
- ○ Diabetes
- ○ Kidney Dysfunction
- ○ Bladder Dysfunction
- ○ Liver Dysfunction
- ○ Thyroid Dysfunction

Other:_____

Cardiopulmonary:
- ○ Congestive Heart Failure
- ○ Heart Arrhythmia

Cardiopulmonary (continued)
- ○ Pacemaker
- ○ High Cholesterol
- ○ Blood Clots
- ○ Anemia
- ○ High Blood Pressure
- ○ Asthma
- ○ Shortness of Breath
- ○ COPD
- ○ HIV/AIDS

Other:_____

Other:
- ○ Anxiety
- ○ Depression
- ○ Cancer

Chief Complaint: *Mild tenderness on palpation of the medial side of the left wrist on both the palmar and dorsal apects. Pain upon end-range supination and pronation. Weakened grip made worse with full pronation. Pain sharp and discrete, and rated a 3/10.*

Goals for Therapy: *To reduce the pain in the left wrist and return to competitive climbing and work as a tree trimmer.*

In the last week, how many days have you had pain? *5*

Pain worst: *3/10 pain at rest and 7/10 with supination and pronation*

SANE Functional Rating

Please rate your **ability** to use your injured area on a 0 to 100% scale with **0%** being unable to use the injured area and **100%** being normal use of injured area in your daily activity: *60%*

Also, if you exercise or have a sport activity or a job that requires special demands please rate your activity on the 0 to 100% scale: *30%*

Patient-Specific Functional Scale

Please list **3 activities** that you find are difficult because of this problem and circle the number that corresponds with your ability to perform the activity.

	Unable									No limitations
1. Climbing	1	(2)	3	4	5	6	7	8	9	10
2. Writing	1	2	3	4	(5)	6	7	8	9	10
3. Eating	1	2	3	4	5	6	(7)	8	9	10

Unique Outcomes Measures
Disability of arm, shoulder, and hand (DASH)

- *Disability/pain section score = 32.8%*
- *Sport section = 82%*

Observation

The patient is 6 feet 1 inch and weighs 162 pounds (BMI: 21.4). His left wrist demonstrates mild edema when compared to the right wrist (1.5 cm). There is slight lumbar lordosis, but no other postural abnormalities were noted.

Patient History

The patient indicates the injury occurred while bouldering (a type of competitive climbing) on an overhanging ledge. His feet swung out, causing him to have forceful ulnar deviation of the left wrist. The patient reports feeling a crunch and immediate pain that lasted several minutes. He also states that after the injury something felt out of place on the medial aspect of the wrist. He was unable to continue to climb secondary to pain.

Mechanism: *Forceful ulnar deviation from fall.*

Concordant Sign: *Patient's pain is reproduced with end-range supination and pronation. Gripping in forearm pronation also causes pain.*

Nature of the Condition: *The current condition has severely limited the patient in his competitive climbing. ADLs such as squeezing dish soap, rolling over in bed, and pulling back a shower curtain are moderately limited.*

Behavior of the Symptoms: *Pain worsens during active and passive ROM.*

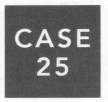

CASE 25

Setting: *Skilled Nursing Facility*

Date: *Present Day*

Medical Diagnosis: *Elbow Dislocation*

Charted Data

Name:	*Susan O'Donald*	New Injury:	*Yes*
Age:	*82 years*	General Health:	*Poor*
MRN:	*45654*	Amount of Exercise:	*0 hours/day, 0 days/week*
Home Address:	*314 4th Street, Orlando, Florida*	Occupation:	*Retired*
		Household:	*Resident in skilled nursing facility*
Date of Injury:	*10 days ago*	Hand Dominance:	*Left*

Please fill in the location of you pain with a pencil

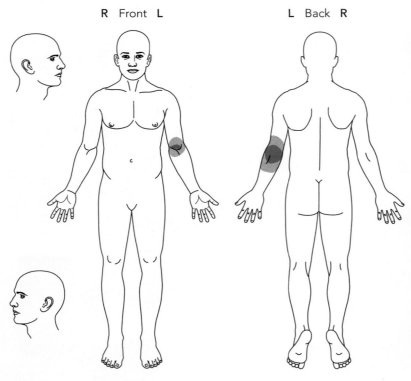

R   Front   L   L   Back   R

Pain Intensity Scale	
0	No Pain
1	Lowlevel pain, able to perform regular activities
2	
3	
4	Moderate-level pain, use of pain medication, activity limited but functional
5	
6	
⑦	High-level pain, use of pain medication, activity very limited— decreased function
8	
9	
10	Emergency Situation

Imaging Results

A radiograph revealed a simple elbow dislocation on the patient's left side. MRI confirmed there was no tear in the UCL or LCL of the elbow.

Medications

500 mg Percocet every 6 hours; Sectral and Ibuprofen

Past Medical History (Please check any items that apply to you.)

Musculoskeletal:

- ⊗ Osteoarthritis
- ○ Rheumatoid Arthritis
- ○ Lupus/SLE
- ○ Fibromyalgia
- ○ Osteoporosis
- ○ Headaches
- ○ Bulging Disc
- ○ Leg Cramps
- ○ Restless Legs
- ○ Jaw Pain/TMJ
- ⊗ History of Falling
- ○ Use of Cane or Walker
- ○ Gout
- ○ Double Jointed

Other:_____

Neurological:

- ○ Stroke/TIA
- ○ Dementia

Neurological (continued)

- ○ Polio
- ○ Parkinson's Disease
- ○ Multiple Sclerosis
- ○ Epilepsy/Seizures
- ○ Concussion
- ○ Numbness
- ○ Tingling

Other:_____

Endocrine:

- ○ Diabetes
- ○ Kidney Dysfunction
- ○ Bladder Dysfunction
- ○ Liver Dysfunction
- ○ Thyroid Dysfunction

Other:_____

Cardiopulmonary:

- ○ Congestive Heart Failure
- ○ Heart Arrhythmia

Cardiopulmonary (continued)

- ○ Pacemaker
- ○ High Cholesterol
- ○ Blood Clots
- ○ Anemia
- ⊗ High Blood Pressure
- ○ Asthma
- ○ Shortness of Breath
- ○ COPD
- ○ HIV/AIDS

Other:_____

Other:

- ○ Anxiety
- ○ Depression
- ○ Cancer

Chief Complaint: *Pain in the left posterior medial elbow*

Goals for Therapy: *To reduce pain and get out of the sling as soon as possible.*

In the last week, how many days have you had pain? *7*

Pain worst: *With movement and at night*

SANE Functional Rating

Please rate your **ability** to use your injured area on a 0 to 100% scale with **0%** being unable to use the injured area and **100%** being normal use of injured area in your daily activity: _____86%_____

Also, if you exercise or have a sport activity or a job that requires special demands please rate your activity on the 0 to 100% scale: _____N/A_____

Patient-Specific Functional Scale

Please list 3 activities that you find are difficult because of this problem and circle the number that corresponds with your ability to perform the activity.

	Unable								No limitations	
1. Reaching*	(1)	2	3	4	5	6	7	8	9	10
2. Eating*	(1)	2	3	4	5	6	7	8	9	10
3. Writing	1	2	3	4	5	6	(7)	8	9	10

*Mostly due to sling/immobilizer.

Unique Outcomes Measures

Short Form 36 (SF-36) = 42[1]

The Mini Mental State Examination = 26[2]

DASH = 82.2% (DASH)[3]

Observation

The patient is 5 feet 1 inch and weighs 146 pounds (BMI) = 27.6). She demonstrates kyphosis with rounded shoulders and appears to be overweight. No use of any assistive device for ambulation. The patient's left shoulder is in a sling for immobilization.

Patient History

The patient states that the injury happened 10 days ago when she got up to use the bathroom and lost her balance. She tried to catch herself with her left arm, but the arm gave way as she landed. She was rushed to the emergency room, where imaging was taken and the ER doctor reduced the dislocation. She has been in a sling for 10 days. She also reports the pain is 2/10 at rest, but awakes at night when the pain is 7/10.

Mechanism: *The pain initiated immediately after her fall.*

Concordant Sign: *When the patient is lying on the affected side.*

Nature of the Condition: *The condition is debilitating and she has had difficulty sleeping due to pain at night. The Percocet helps with pain management.*

Behavior of the Symptoms: *Pain worsens with any elbow movement, but she states the pain has lessened over the past few days. Pain also awakens her at night.*

Endnotes

1. Ware JE, Sherbourne CD. The MOS 36-Item Short-Form Health Survey (SF-36): I. Conceptual framework and item selection. Med Care 1992;30:473–83.

2. Kukull WA, Larson EB, Teri L, Bowen J, McCormick W, Pfanschmidt ML. The Mini-Mental State Examination Score and the clinical diagnosis of dementia. J Clin Epidemiol 1994;47(9):1061–7.

3. Hudak PL, Amadio PC, Bombardier C, Pamela L, Peter C, Beaton D, et al. Development of an upper extremity outcome measure: The DASH (disabilities of the arm, shoulder, and head). Am J Indust Med 1996;29(6):602–8.

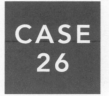

CASE 26

Setting: *Outpatient Orthopedic Clinic*

Date: *Present Day*

Medical Diagnosis: *UCL Tear of the Elbow*

Charted Data

Name:	*Billy Bob Mancovich*	New Injury:	*1 week status post*
Age:	*19 years*	General Health:	*Excellent*
MRN:	*50533*	Amount of Exercise:	*1–2 hours/day, 5 days/week*
Home Address:	*27 N. State Street, Buffalo, New York*	Occupation:	*Student*
		Household:	*Lives with another student in dorm room*
Date of Injury:	*1 week ago*	Hand Dominance:	*Left*

Please fill in the location of your pain with a pencil.

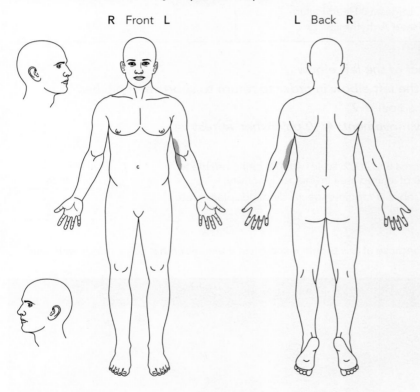

R Front L   L Back R

Pain Intensity Scale	
0	No Pain
1	Low-level pain, able to perform regular activities
2	
3	
4	Moderate-level pain, use of pain medication, activity limited but functional
(5)	
6	
7	High-level pain, use of pain medication, activity very limited— decreased function
8	
9	
10	Emergency Situation

Imaging Results

All radiographs of the elbow were unremarkable with the exception of mild cartilage irregularities seen along the posteromedial aspect of the trochlea and the medial aspect of the olecranon. An MRI was read as negative for any ligamentous disruption or other tissue damage.

Medications

Tylenol

Past Medical History (Please check any items that apply to you.)

Unremarkable

Musculoskeletal:

- o Osteoarthritis
- o Rheumatoid Arthritis
- o Lupus/SLE
- o Fibromyalgia
- o Osteoporosis
- o Headaches
- o Bulging Disc
- o Leg Cramps
- o Restless Legs
- o Jaw Pain/TMJ
- o History of Falling
- o Use of Cane or Walker
- o Gout
- o Double Jointed

Other:_____

Neurological:

- o Stroke/TIA
- o Dementia

Neurological (continued)

- o Polio
- o Parkinson's Disease
- o Multiple Sclerosis
- o Epilepsy/Seizures
- o Concussion
- o Numbness
- o Tingling

Other:_____

Endocrine:

- o Diabetes
- o Kidney Dysfunction
- o Bladder Dysfunction
- o Liver Dysfunction
- o Thyroid Dysfunction

Other:_____

Cardiopulmonary:

- o Congestive Heart Failure
- o Heart Arrhythmia

Cardiopulmonary (continued)

- o Pacemaker
- o High Cholesterol
- o Blood Clots
- o Anemia
- o High Blood Pressure
- o Asthma
- o Shortness of Breath
- o COPD
- o HIV/AIDS

Other:_____

Other:

- o Anxiety
- o Depression
- o Cancer

Chief Complaint: *Pain in the medial aspect of the left elbow*

Goals for Therapy: *To reduce the pain in the left elbow in order to return to sports as a pitcher.*

In the last week, how many days have you had pain? *7*

Pain worst: *6/10 pain with any left elbow movement; 4/10 pain when at rest*

SANE Functional Rating

Please rate your **ability** to use your injured area on a 0 to 100% scale with **0%** being unable to use the injured area and **100%** being normal use of injured area in your daily activity: *85%*

Also, if you exercise or have a sport activity or a job that requires special demands please rate your activity on the 0 to 100% scale: *80%*

Patient-Specific Functional Scale

Please list **3 activities** that you find are difficult because of this problem and circle the number that corresponds with your ability to perform the activity.

	Unable									No limitations
1. Overhead throwing	1	(2)	3	4	5	6	7	8	9	10
2. Weight Lifting	1	2	3	4	(5)	6	7	8	9	10
3. Carrying gear bag	1	2	3	4	(5)	6	7	8	9	10

Unique Outcomes Measures

Disabilities of the arm, shoulder, and hand (DASH)[1] = 84%

Mayo elbow performance score[2] = 60 (fair)

Observation

The patient is 5 feet 9 inches and weighs 170 pounds (BMI = 25). He presents with a mild palpable swelling over the medial aspect of his left elbow with tenderness to touch at the insertion of the UCL on the ulna as well as the mid-substance region of the ligament.

Patient History

The patient has an unremarkable past medical history, and is a collegiate athlete who exercises regularly.

Mechanism *During over-head throwing in a bullpen session, the patient reported a popping sensation in his throwing arm followed by medial elbow pain.*

Concordant Sign *The patient's pain is produced with any over-head activity or valgus stress at the elbow.*

Nature of the Condition *The patient's condition currently severely limits his ability to perform any throwing activities or over-head weight lifting using the left arm.*

Behavior of the Symptoms *His pain worsens with forceful over-head throwing activities and any active or passive physiologic movements causing a valgus stress at the elbow.*

Endnotes

1. Hudak PL, Amadio PC, Bombardier C, Pamela L, Peter C, Beaton D, et al. Development of an upper extremity outcome measure: The DASH (disabilities of the arm, shoulder, and head). Am J Industrial Med 1996;29(6):602–8.

2. Turchin DC, Beaton DE, Richards RR. Validity of observer-based aggregate scoring systems as descriptors of elbow pain, function, and disability. J Bone Joint Surg 1998;80(2):154–62.

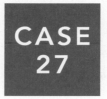

CASE 27

Setting: *Outpatient Orthopedic Clinic*

Date: *Present Day*

Medical Diagnosis: *Common Extensor Tendinopathy* · *lateral epicondalgia*

Charted Data

Name:	*Casey Halton*	General Health:	*Good*
Age:	*39 years*	Amount of Exercise:	*30–60 minutes/day, 6 days/week*
MRN:	*507321*	Occupation:	*Teacher*
Home Address:	*1333 Lost Creek Road, Smithtown, Massachusetts*	Household:	*Single-story house on large rural property*
Date of Injury:	*3 months ago*	Hand Dominance:	*Right*
New Injury:	*No*	Race	*Caucasian*

Please fill in the location of your pain with a pencil.

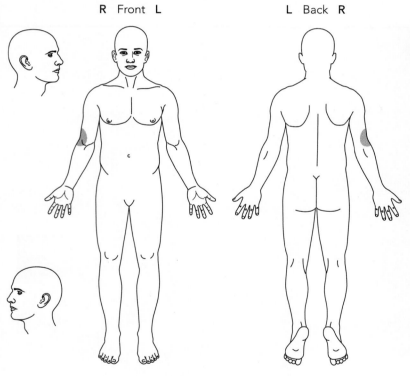

R   Front   L   L   Back   R

Pain Intensity Scale

0	No Pain
1	Low-level pain, able to perform regular activities
2	
3	
4	Moderate-level pain, use of pain medication, activity limited but functional
5	
(6)	
7	High-level pain, use of pain medication, activity very limited— decreased function
8	
9	
10	Emergency Situation

Imaging Results

Radiograph and MRI results revealed normal findings. Imaging was negative for evidence of a fracture or moderate to severe ligamentous disruption.

Medications

Aleve PRN

Past Medical History (Please check any items that apply to you.)

Unremarkable

Musculoskeletal:

- o Osteoarthritis
- o Rheumatoid Arthritis
- o Lupus/SLE
- o Fibromyalgia
- o Osteoporosis
- o Headaches
- o Bulging Disc
- o Leg Cramps
- o Restless Legs
- o Jaw Pain/TMJ
- o History of Falling
- o Use of Cane or Walker
- o Gout
- o Double Jointed

Other:_____

Neurological:

- o Stroke/TIA
- o Dementia

Neurological (continued)

- o Polio
- o Parkinson's Disease
- o Multiple Sclerosis
- o Epilepsy/Seizures
- o Concussion
- o Numbness
- o Tingling

Other:_____

Endocrine:

- o Diabetes
- o Kidney Dysfunction
- o Bladder Dysfunction
- o Liver Dysfunction
- o Thyroid Dysfunction

Other:_____

Cardiopulmonary:

- o Congestive Heart Failure
- o Heart Arrhythmia

Cardiopulmonary (continued)

- o Pacemaker
- o High Cholesterol
- o Blood Clots
- o Anemia
- o High Blood Pressure
- o Asthma
- o Shortness of Breath
- o COPD
- o HIV/AIDS

Other:_____

Other:

- o Anxiety
- o Depression
- o Cancer

Chief Complaint: *Intermittent sharp pain with occasional aching over the lateral right elbow.*

Goals for Therapy: *To reduce/eliminate lateral elbow pain in order to continue working on rural property.*

In the last week, how many days have you had pain? *7*

Pain worst: *When lifting heavy objects (stone)*

SANE Functional Rating

Please rate your **ability** to use your injured area on a 0 to 100% scale with **0%** being unable to use the injured area and **100%** being normal use of injured area in your daily activity: *50%*

Also, if you exercise or have a sport activity or a job that requires special demands please rate your activity on the 0 to 100% scale: *10%*

Patient-Specific Functional Scale

Please list **3 activities** that you find are difficult because of this problem and circle the number that corresponds with your ability to perform the activity.

	Unable									No limitations
1. Lifting bricks	(1)	2	3	4	5	6	7	8	9	10
2. Gardening	1	2	(3)	4	5	6	7	8	9	10
3. Carrying books	1	2	3	4	(5)	6	7	8	9	10

Unique Outcomes Measures

Patient-rated tennis elbow evaluation (PRTEE)[1] = 56/150

Disability of the arm, shoulder, and hand (DASH)[2] = 28

Observation

The patient is 5 feet 7 inches and weighs 150 pounds (BMI = 23.5). She presents with slight forward shoulders bilaterally and minimal cervical kyphosis. The patient also presents with hyperalgesia to palpation of the area just distal to the right lateral epicondyle. Resisted wrist extension, gripping, and third digit extension revealed marked pain. There was no visible edema or redness.

Patient History[3]

The patient indicates onset of initial pain 3 months ago after several days of engaging in extremely heavy lifting while building a stone wall at her rural property. The pain was so intense that it forced her to stop working on the wall. Pain is worse during heavy lifting and gardening. The pain can often be described as intermittent sharp pain with aching over the lateral right elbow. The patient indicated feeling a burning sensation over the posterior lateral elbow and intermittent stiffness over the wrist. She is usually very active doing housework and maintaining her rural property. Currently, she is working as a teacher but has not been able to do work around the house as usual due to the pain. She has no history of elbow injury or surgery of any kind.

Mechanism: *Intermittent symptoms have lasted for 3 months. No direct trauma was experienced; activity aggravates symptoms.*

Concordant Sign: *Reproduction of pain with heavy lifting (>10 lbs.). Pain is also reproduced by active, end-range right elbow extension/abduction.*

Nature of the Condition *The condition mildly limits daily activities such as cooking, cleaning, and teaching, but severely limits gardening, household upkeep, and lifting of any kind.*

Behavior of the Symptoms: *Pain worsens during activity, especially when lifting heavy objects or the elbow is placed in an end-range extension position. The pain is alleviated by rest.*

Endnotes

1. Rompe J, Overend T, MacDermid J. Validation of the patient-rated tennis elbow evaluation questionnaire. J Hand Ther. 2007;20(1):3–10.

2. Hudak P, Amadio P, Bombardier C, Beaton D, Cole D, Davis A, Hawker G, et al. Development of an upper extremity outcome measure: The DASH (disabilities of the arm, shoulder, and head). Am J Ind Med. 1996;29(6):602–8.

3. Vicenzino B, Wright A. Effects of a novel manipulative physiotherapy technique on tennis elbow: a single case study. Man Ther. 1995;1:30–5.

CASE 28

Setting: *Outpatient*

Date: *Present Day*

Medical Diagnosis: *Medial Elbow Pain*

Charted Data

Name:	*James Finnigan*	New Injury:	*Yes*
Age:	*22*	General Health:	*Excellent*
MRN:	*50699*	Amount of Exercise:	*1–2 hours/day, 5 days/week*
Home Address:	*224 Market Street, Youngstown, Ohio*	Occupation:	*College student*
		Household:	*3-bedroom apartment on the 6th floor*
Date of Injury:	*4 weeks ago*	Hand Dominance:	*Right*

Please fill in the location of your pain with a pencil.

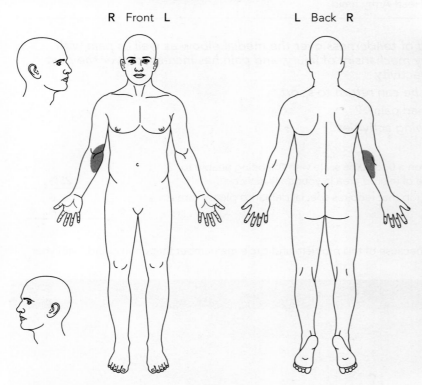

R Front L   L Back R

Pain Intensity Scale	
0	No Pain
1	Low-level pain, able to perform regular activities
2	
3	
4	Moderate-level pain, use of pain medication, activity limited but functional
5	
6	
(7)	High-level pain, use of pain medication, activity very limited—decreased function
8	
9	
10	Emergency Situation

Imaging Results

No imaging has been done at this time.

Medications

1000 mg of Tylenol and Albuterol

Past Medical History (Please check any items that apply to you.)

Musculoskeletal:
- o Osteoarthritis
- o Rheumatoid Arthritis
- o Lupus/SLE
- o Fibromyalgia
- o Osteoporosis
- o Headaches
- o Bulging Disc
- o Leg Cramps
- o Restless Legs
- o Jaw Pain/TMJ
- o History of Falling
- o Use of Cane or Walker
- o Gout
- o Double Jointed

Other:_____

Neurological:
- o Stroke/TIA
- o Dementia

Neurological (continued)
- o Polio
- o Parkinson's Disease
- o Multiple Sclerosis
- o Epilepsy/Seizures
- o Concussion
- o Numbness
- o Tingling

Other:_____

Endocrine:
- o Diabetes
- o Kidney Dysfunction
- o Bladder Dysfunction
- o Liver Dysfunction
- o Thyroid Dysfunction

Other:_____

Cardiopulmonary:
- o Congestive Heart Failure
- o Heart Arrhythmia

Cardiopulmonary (continued)
- o Pacemaker
- o High Cholesterol
- o Blood Clots
- o Anemia
- o High Blood Pressure
- ⊗ Asthma
- o Shortness of Breath
- o COPD
- o HIV/AIDS

Other:_____

Other:
- o Anxiety
- o Depression
- o Cancer

Chief Complaint: *The patient complained of tenderness over the medial elbow as well as pain with foream pronation. He does not recall any mechansim of injury, and pain has increased over the past week. Pain is 4/10 at rest and 9/10 with activity.*

Goals for Therapy: *To reduce the pain so he can return to sport.*

In the last week, how many days have you had pain? *7*

Pain worst: *When doing over-head throwing activities*

SANE Functional Rating

Please rate your **ability** to use your injured area on a 0 to 100% scale with **0%** being unable to use the injured area and **100%** being normal use of injured area in your daily activity: _____ 25%_____

Also, if you exercise or have a sport activity or a job that requires special demands please rate your activity on the 0 to 100% scale: _____ N/A_____

Patient-Specific Functional Scale

Please list **3 activities** that you find are difficult because of this problem and circle the number that corresponds with your ability to perform the activity.

	Unable								No limitations	
1. Overhead throwing	1	(2)	3	4	5	6	7	8	9	10
2. Gripping	1	2	3	(4)	5	6	7	8	9	10
3. Writing	1	2	3	4	5	6	7	8	(9)	10

Unique Outcomes Measures
Disability of arm, shoulder, and hand (DASH)[1]

- *Disability/pain section score = 40.2%*
- *Sport section = 95%*
- *Mayo elbow performance score[2] = 65—Fair*

Observation

The patient is 6 feet tall and weighs 175 pounds (BMI = 23.7), and demonstrates rounded shoulders and a forward head, as well as slight winging of the right scapula. No discoloration or deformity are noted at the site of the pain.

Patient History

The patient is a division 1 college pitcher who is experiencing extreme pain in his medial elbow with over-head activity; his pain has now become constant. He indicates that the pain started about 4 weeks ago and has gotten dramatically worse over the past 7 days. He does not recall a mechanism of injury. His pain is so bad that he discontinued all pitching activities.

Mechanism: *No mechanism of injury (MOI); pain has been chronic for 4 weeks.*

Concordant Sign: *Sharp pain with pitching and pronation and flexion cause a dull aching pain.*

Nature of the Condition: *The condition made the patient discontinue all throwing activities and now the pain is constant. He is taking 1000 mg of Tylenol for better sleep at night.*

Behavior of the Symptoms: *The pain worsens with flexion and pronation and increases with repetitive motions.*

Endnotes

1. Hudak PL, Amadio PC, Bombardier C, Beaton D, Cole D, Davis A, Hawker G, et al. Development of an upper extremity outcome measure: The DASH (disabilities of the arm, shoulder, and head). Am J Ind Med. 1996;29(6):602–8.

2. Turchin DC Validity of observer-based aggregate scoring systems as descriptors of elbow pain, function, and disability. J Bone Joint Surg. 1998;80-A(2):154–62.

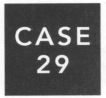

CASE 29

Setting: *Outpatient Orthopedics*

Date: *Present Day*

Medical Diagnosis: *Bilateral Wrist Pain*

Charted Data

Name:	*Jeannette Mathews*	New Injury:	*No*
Age:	*52*	General Health:	*Good*
MRN:	*59369*	Amount of Exercise:	*30 minutes/day, 2 days/week*
Home Address:	*1921 E. Delavan, Bellevue, Washington*	Occupation:	*Administrative assistant*
		Household:	*3-bedroom house*
Date of Injury:	*Symptoms for 4 years, worsening over past 6 weeks*	Hand Dominance:	*Right*
		Race	*Caucasian*

Please fill in the location of your pain with a pencil.

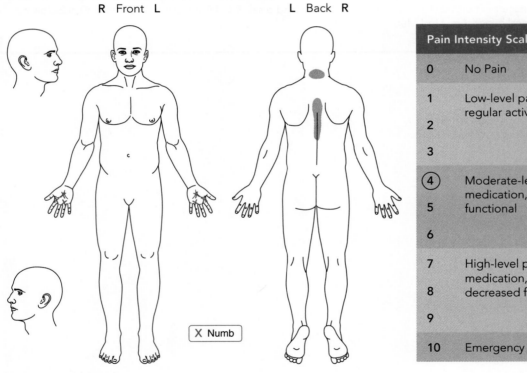

R   Front   L   L   Back   R

Pain Intensity Scale	
0	No Pain
1	Low-level pain, able to perform regular activities
2	
3	
(4)	Moderate-level pain, use of pain medication, activity limited but functional
5	
6	
7	High-level pain, use of pain medication, activity very limited— decreased function
8	
9	
10	Emergency Situation

X Numb

Imaging Results

Radiographs of the cervical spine reveal moderate degeneration at multiple levels. Nerve conduction velocity (NCV) of the upper extremities showed conduction velocity slowing across both wrists.

Medications

1000 mg of Tylenol and Albuterol

Past Medical History (Please check any items that apply to you.)

Musculoskeletal:
- ○ Osteoarthritis
- ○ Rheumatoid Arthritis
- ○ Lupus/SLE
- ○ Fibromyalgia
- ○ Osteoporosis
- ⊗ Headaches
- ⊗ Bulging Disc
- ○ Leg Cramps
- ○ Restless Legs
- ○ Jaw Pain/TMJ
- ○ History of Falling
- ○ Use of Cane or Walker
- ○ Gout
- ○ Double Jointed

Other:_____

Neurological:
- ○ Stroke/TIA
- ○ Dementia

Neurological (continued)
- ○ Polio
- ○ Parkinson's Disease
- ○ Multiple Sclerosis
- ○ Epilepsy/Seizures
- ○ Concussion
- ⊗ Numbness
- ⊗ Tingling

Other:_____

Endocrine:
- ○ Diabetes
- ○ Kidney Dysfunction
- ○ Bladder Dysfunction
- ○ Liver Dysfunction
- ○ Thyroid Dysfunction

Other:_____

Cardiopulmonary:
- ○ Congestive Heart Failure
- ○ Heart Arrhythmia

Cardiopulmonary (continued)
- ○ Pacemaker
- ○ High Cholesterol
- ○ Blood Clots
- ○ Anemia
- ⊗ High Blood Pressure
- ⊗ Asthma
- ○ Shortness of Breath
- ○ COPD
- ○ HIV/AIDS

Other:_____

Other:
- ○ Anxiety
- ○ Depression
- ○ Cancer

Chief Complaint: *The patient reports pain in both wrists and hands with intermittent numbness and tingling in the middle 2 fingers of the right hand and the 3 fingers of the left. The pain is aggravated by prolonged sitting at work and when she is on Facebook.*

Goals for Therapy: *To reduce the pain and numbness so that the patient can surf the Internet, perform job tasks, and return to the gym for exercising without so much discomfort.*

In the last week, how many days have you had pain? *7*

Pain worst: *When in prolonged sitting postures*

SANE Functional Rating

Please rate your **ability** to use your injured area on a 0 to 100% scale with **0%** being unable to use the injured area and **100%** being normal use of injured area in your daily activity: *75%*

Also, if you exercise or have a sport activity or a job that requires special demands please rate your activity on the 0 to 100% scale: *60%*

Patient-Specific Functional Scale

Please list 3 activities that you find are difficult because of this problem and circle the number that corresponds with your ability to perform the activity.

	Unable									No limitations
1. Surfing the Internet	1	2	3	4	5	⑥	7	8	9	10
2. Gripping during weight lifting	1	2	3	④	5	6	7	8	9	10
3. Writing	1	2	3	4	5	⑥	7	8	9	10

Unique Outcomes Measures

The symptom severity scale (SSS) = 2.6, and the functional status scale (FSS)[1] = 2.8.

Observation

The patient is 5 feet 6 inches tall and weighs 175 pounds (BMI = 28.2). She has rounded shoulders and a forward head with a mild Dowager's hump. She does not appear to be in any distress but does rub her hands together and shake them frequently.

Patient History

The patient reports a long history of neck pain dating back to a motor vehicle accident in college. The neck symptoms have come and gone over the years but had never limited her activities in any way. She noticed hand symptoms 4 years ago that included mild palm discomfort with occasional tingling that became severe for a brief period of time and has since been variable depending on what kinds of activities she is performing. For the past 4 months, the patient has spent a lot more time working on the computer both at work and at home and has noticed a steady increase in both pain and tingling. The past 4 weeks have been much more severe, requiring her to monitor activity. Her physician ordered radiographs and an NCV, which demonstrated slowing across both wrists. When questioned, she reports that she occasionally stumbles when she walks.

Mechanism: *No mechanism of injury (MOI) pain has been chronic for 4 weeks.*

Concordant Sign: *Concordant signs include seated position working over a computer, driving a car, riding a stationary bike, and gripping weights at the gym.*

Nature of the Condition; *The condition has made her discontinue many activities and has become a near constant pain with tingling. She takes 400 mg of Ibuprofen to get through the day.*

Behavior of the Symptoms: *The pain worsens with keyboard work as well as weight lifting and weight bearing on the hands. Her pain is relieved by general movement and shaking the hands.*

Endnotes

1. Levine DW, Simmons BP, Koris MJ, Daltroy LH, Hohl GG, Fossel AH, et al. A self-administered questionnaire for the assessment of severity of symptoms and functional status in carpal tunnel syndrome. J Bone Joint Surg Am. 1993;75:1585–92.

CASE 30

Setting: *Outpatient Orthopedics*
Date: *Present Day*
Medical Diagnosis: *Elbow Pain*

Charted Data

Name:	*Lawrence Ryder*	New Injury:	*Yes*
Age:	*42 years*	General Health:	*Good*
MRN:	*70602*	Amount of Exercise:	*30 minutes/day, 1 day/week*
Home Address:	*412 Stony Ridge Lane, Yankton, South Dakota*	Occupation:	*Swing set assembly*
		Household:	*Single, lives alone*
Date of Injury:	*3 months ago*	Hand Dominance:	*Right*
		Race	*African American*

Please fill in the location of your pain with a pencil.

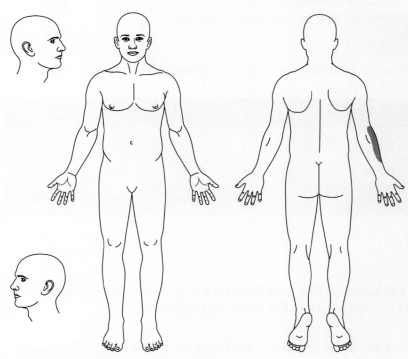

R Front L   L Back R

Pain Intensity Scale	
0	No Pain
1	Low-level pain, able to perform regular activities
2	
3	
4	Moderate-level pain, use of pain medication, activity limited but functional
(5)	
6	
7	High-level pain, use of pain medication, activity very limited—decreased function
8	
9	
10	Emergency Situation

Imaging Results

This patient has not had imaging studies done on his elbow.

Medications

Ibuprofen (PRN)

Past Medical History (Please check any items that apply to you.)

Unremarkable

Musculoskeletal:
- ○ Osteoarthritis
- ○ Rheumatoid Arthritis
- ○ Lupus/SLE
- ○ Fibromyalgia
- ○ Osteoporosis
- ○ Headaches

Musculoskeletal (continued)
- ○ Bulging Disc
- ○ Leg Cramps
- ○ Restless Legs
- ○ Jaw Pain/TMJ
- ○ History of Falling
- ○ Use of Cane or Walker

Musculoskeletal (continued)
- ○ Gout
- ○ Double Jointed
Other:_____

Neurological:
- ○ Stroke/TIA
- ○ Dementia

Neurological (continued)	Endocrine (continued)	Cardiopulmonary (continued)
o Polio	o Bladder Dysfunction	o High Blood Pressure
o Parkinson's Disease	o Liver Dysfunction	o Asthma
o Multiple Sclerosis	o Thyroid Dysfunction	o Shortness of Breath
o Epilepsy/Seizures	Other:_____	o COPD
o Concussion		o HIV/AIDS
o Numbness	**Cardiopulmonary:**	Other:_____
o Tingling	o Congestive Heart Failure	
Other:_____	o Heart Arrhythmia	**Other:**
	o Pacemaker	o Anxiety
Endocrine:	o High Cholesterol	o Depression
o Diabetes	o Blood Clots	o Cancer
o Kidney Dysfunction	o Anemia	

Chief Complaint: *Right forearm/elbow pain*
Goals for Therapy: *To work and play drums without pain.*
In the last week, how many days have you had pain? *5*
Pain worst: *When using screwdriver and other hand tools*

SANE Functional Rating

Please rate your **ability** to use your injured area on a 0 to 100% scale with **0%** being unable to use the injured area and **100%** being normal use of injured area in your daily activity: _____ *85%*

Also, if you exercise or have a sport activity or a job that requires special demands please rate your activity on the 0 to 100% scale: _____ *60%*

Patient-Specific Functional Scale

Please list 3 activities that you find are difficult because of this problem and circle the number that corresponds with your ability to perform the activity.

	Unable								No limitations	
1. Using screwdriver	1	2	(3)	4	5	6	7	8	9	10
2. Using the computer	1	2	3	4	5	6	(7)	8	9	10
3. Playing drums	1	2	3	(4)	5	6	7	8	9	10

Unique Outcomes Measures
Quick DASH = 31.8

Observation
The patient is 6 feet 3 inches and weighs 150 pounds (BMI = 18.0). He is tall and thin, stands with slouched upper thoracic posture and excessive extension in the lower cervical spine.

Patient History
The patient reports elbow ache began about 4 months ago, after starting a new job in which he assembles playground equipment.

Mechanism: *Symptoms began after about a month at the patient's new job. Discomfort began as an ache in the lateral elbow, and progressed over the past month into a burning pain in the dorsal and lateral forearm.*

Concordant Sign: *Symptoms worsened when the patient used a screwdriver or other small hand tools. Elbow pain also comes on after playing drums for about an hour. Previously the patient played 4 hours at local dances without pain.*

Nature of the Condition: *The 5/10 pain the patient reports occurs after working for half a day or drumming for about an hour. Pain during computer use is more of a nuisance in nature, but he states he does not usually spend too much time on the computer.*

Behavior of the Symptoms: *The patient's symptoms worsen during activities requiring gripping or forearm movements. Once aggravated, the pain subsides after 30 minutes of resting the arm. He has no difficulty sleeping.*

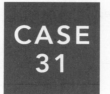

CASE 31

Setting: *Skilled Nursing Facility*

Date: *Present Day*

Medical Diagnosis: *Thoracic Strain*

Charted Data

Name:	*Lilly McClean*	General Health:	*Poor*
Age:	*84 years*	Amount of Exercise:	*0 hours/day, 0 days/week*
MRN:	*50522*	Occupation:	*Retired*
Home Address:	*134 West Street, Wilmington, North Carolina*	Household:	*Resident in skilled nursing facility*
Date of Injury:	*10 days*	Hand Dominance:	*Right*
New Injury:	*Yes*	Race:	*White*

Please fill in the location of your pain with a pencil.

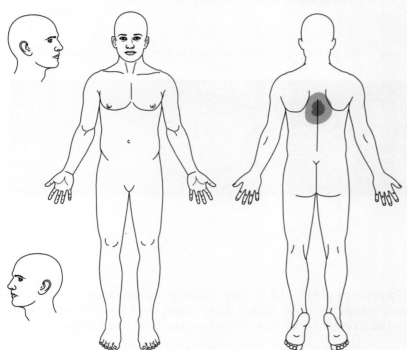

R Front L   L Back R

Pain Intensity Scale	
0	No Pain
1	Low level pain, able to perform regular activities
2	
3	
4	Moderate level pain, use of pain medication, activity limited but functional
5	
6	
(7)	High level pain, use of pain medication, activity very limited— decreased function
8	
9	
10	Emergency Situation

Imaging Results
The patient received no imaging.

Medications:
Acetaminophen and iron supplements

Past Medical History (Please check any items that apply to you.

Musculoskeletal:
- ☒ Osteoarthritis
- ○ Rheumatoid Arthritis
- ○ Lupus/SLE
- ○ Fibromyalgia
- ☒ Osteoporosis
- ○ Headaches

Musculoskeletal (continued)
- ○ Bulging Disc
- ○ Leg Cramps
- ○ Restless Legs
- ○ Jaw Pain/TMJ
- ○ History of Falling
- ○ Use of Cane or Walker

Musculoskeletal (continued)
- ○ Gout
- ○ Double Jointed

Other:_____

Neurological:
- ○ Stroke/TIA
- ○ Dementia

Neurological (continued)

o Polio
o Parkinson's Disease
o Multiple Sclerosis
o Epilepsy/Seizures
o Concussion
o Numbness
o Tingling
Other:_____

Endocrine:

o Diabetes
o Kidney Dysfunction

Endocrine (continued)

⊛ Bladder Dysfunction
o Liver Dysfunction
o Thyroid Dysfunction
Other:_____

Cardiopulmonary:

o Congestive Heart Failure
o Heart Arrhythmia
o Pacemaker
o High Cholesterol
o Blood Clots
⊛ Anemia

Cardiopulmonary (continued)

o High Blood Pressure
o Asthma
o Shortness of Breath
o COPD
o HIV/AIDS
Other:_____

Other:

o Anxiety
o Depression
o Cancer

Chief Complaint: *Mid-thoracic pain*
Goals for Therapy: *To reduce the pain enough to allow her to sleep.*
In the last week, how many days have you had pain? *7*
Pain worst: *Evening and during sleep*

SANE Functional Rating

Please rate your **ability** to use your injured area on a 0 to 100% scale with **0%** being unable to use the injured area and **100%** being normal use of injured area in your daily activity: _____ *25%*

Also. if you exercise or have a sport activity or a job that requires special demands please rate your activity on the 0 to 100% scale: _____ *N/A*

Patient-Specific Functional Scale

Please list 3 activities that you find are difficult because of this problem and circle the number that corresponds with your ability to perform the activity.

	Unable								No limitations	
1. Walking	1	2	3	4	5	6	7	(8)	9	10
2. Sitting	1	2	3	(4)	5	6	7	8	9	10
3. Bending over	1	2	3	4	(5)	6	7	8	9	10

Unique Outcomes Measures

Short Form 36 (SF-36) score = 26

Mini Mental State Examination score = 21

Observation

The patient is 5 feet 3 inches and weighs 106 pounds (BMI = 18.8). She exhibits excessive kyphosis and is relatively unhealthy in appearance. She uses a walker to move about. She is independent with her walker for ambulation and basic transfers but is unable to walk far or fast ever since her back pain began.

Patient History

The patient indicates a recent onset within the last 10 days. The pain initiated after she attempted to move a dresser at the facility (she dropped her glasses behind the dresser). She immediately felt pain and had difficulty finding positions of comfort after the incident.

Mechanism: *The pain initiated immediately after the patient attempted to lift the dresser.*

Concordant Sign: *Extension is sharp and painful, whereas flexion causes a dull ache.*

Nature of the Condition *The condition is very debilitating. The patient cannot sleep and is forced to try to sleep in a chair because lying back is too painful. Once the pain truly manifests itself, she can do nothing without significant discomfort.*

Behavior of the Symptoms: *The patient's worsens during lifting, carrying objects, and especially when she is in long-term positions, particularly when sitting.*

CASE 32

Setting: *Outpatient Orthopedics*
Date: *Present Day*
Medical Diagnosis: *Lumbar Radiculopathy*

Charted Data

Name:	*Mark Fontaine*	New Injury:	*Yes*
Age:	*49 years*	General Health:	*Good*
MRN:	*50507*	Amount of Exercise:	*0 hours/day, 0 days/week*
Home Address:	*123 Becks Street, Durham, North Carolina*	Occupation:	*Cable installer*
		Household:	*Lives with family*
		Hand Dominance:	*Right*
Date of Injury:	*2 months prior*	Race:	*White*

Please fill in the location of your pain with a pencil.

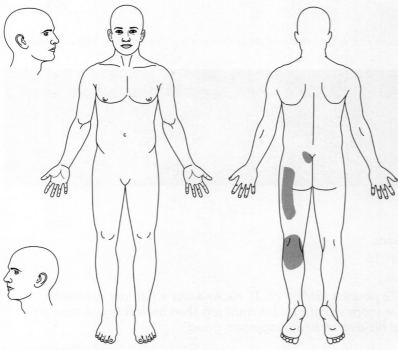

R Front L   L Back R

Pain Intensity Scale	
0	No Pain
1	Low-level pain, able to perform regular activities
2	
3	
4	Moderate-level pain, use of pain medication, activity limited but functional
(5)	
6	
7	High-level pain, use of pain medication, activity very limited—decreased function
8	
9	
10	Emergency Situation

Imaging Results
A radiograph was negative for a fracture of the low back. The patient has received no other imaging.

Medications
Over-the-counter Hyland's Leg Cramps, Ibuprofen

Past Medical History (Please check any items that apply to you.)

Musculoskeletal:
- ○ Osteoarthritis
- ○ Rheumatoid Arthritis
- ○ Lupus/SLE
- ○ Fibromyalgia
- ○ Osteoporosis
- ○ Headaches

Musculoskeletal (continued)
- ○ Bulging Disc
- ⊗ Leg Cramps
- ○ Restless Legs
- ○ Jaw Pain/TMJ
- ○ History of Falling
- ○ Use of Cane or Walker

Musculoskeletal (continued)
- ○ Gout
- ○ Double Jointed
Other:_____

Neurological:
- ○ Stroke/TIA
- ○ Dementia

Neurological (continued)	Endocrine (continued)	Cardiopulmonary (continued)

Neurological (continued)
- o Polio
- o Parkinson's Disease
- o Multiple Sclerosis
- o Epilepsy/Seizures
- o Concussion
- o Numbness
- o Tingling

Other:_____

Endocrine:
- o Diabetes
- o Kidney Dysfunction

Endocrine (continued)
- o Bladder Dysfunction
- o Liver Dysfunction
- o Thyroid Dysfunction

Other:_____

Cardiopulmonary:
- o Congestive Heart Failure
- o Heart Arrhythmia
- o Pacemaker
- o High Cholesterol
- o Blood Clots
- o Anemia

Cardiopulmonary (continued)
- o High Blood Pressure
- o Asthma
- o Shortness of Breath
- o COPD
- o HIV/AIDS

Other:_____

Other:
- o Anxiety
- o Depression
- o Cancer

Chief Complaint: *Left leg pain*
Goals for Therapy: *To get rid of the left leg pain.*
In the last week, how many days have you had pain? **7**
Pain worst: *Morning*

SANE Functional Rating

Please rate your **ability** to use your injured area on a 0 to 100% scale with **0%** being unable to use the injured area and **100%** being normal use of injured area in your daily activity: ___75%___

Also, if you exercise or have a sport activity or a job that requires special demands please rate your activity on the 0 to 100% scale: ___60%___

Patient-Specific Functional Scale

Please list 3 activities that you find are difficult because of this problem and circle the number that corresponds with your ability to perform the activity.

	Unable									No limitations
1. Walking	1	2	3	4	5	6	7	(8)	9	10
2. Sitting	1	2	3	(4)	5	6	7	8	9	10
3. Bending over	1	2	3	4	(5)	6	7	8	9	10

Unique Outcomes Measures

Oswestry disability index = 32%

Negative on both depression screen questions

Fear avoidance beliefs questionnaire score = 16

Observation

The patient is 5 feet 8 inches and weighs 172 pounds (BMI = 26.1). He exhibits a flat low back with a slight shift to the right. He appears to bear more weight on his right leg than his left leg. Although slightly deconditioned, he looks his age and his overall health appears good.

Patient History

He reports a gradual increase in leg symptoms over the last 2 months. The symptoms coincide with an increase in the hours he works as a cable installer, which he enjoys. He indicates he spends a great deal of the day driving or bent over running cable through homes.

Mechanism: *He cannot identify a specific incident that triggered his pain but he does know that it coincides with his increase in hours.*

Concordant Sign: *His worst pain occurs after long-term sitting. He reports left-sided leg pain to the calf. He can reproduce his left leg pain by reaching downward toward the floor (lumbar flexion).*

Nature of the Condition: *The patient indicates that the condition has greatly affected his work as a cable installer. He also notes that it takes several hours for his condition to decrease once it is irritated. At night, he takes a number of pain pills to decrease the pain in the leg.*

Behavior of the Symptoms: *The low back hurts nearly all the time but the leg pain appears worse after bouts of sitting or bending over.*

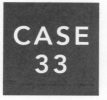

CASE 33

Setting: *Outpatient Orthopedics*

Date: *Present Day*

Medical Diagnosis: *Lumbar Strain*

Charted Data

Name:	*Karen Lindel*	General Health:	*Good*
Age:	*42 years*	Amount of Exercise:	*1 hour/day, 2–3 days/week*
MRN:	*894332*	Occupation:	*Veterinary technician*
Home Address:	*4168 North Maple, Lexington, Kentucky*	Household:	*Divorced, lives with her 6 children*
Date of Injury:	*9 months ago*	Hand Dominance:	*Right*
New Injury:	*Yes*	Race:	*White*

Please fill in the location of your pain with a pencil.

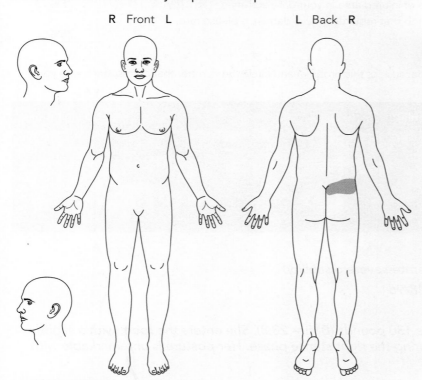

R Front L   L Back R

Pain Intensity Scale	
0	No Pain
1	Low-level pain, able to perform regular activities
2	
3	
(4)	Moderate-level pain, use of pain medication, activity limited but functional
5	
6	
7	High-level pain, use of pain medication, activity very limited— decreased function
8	
9	
10	Emergency Situation

Imaging Results

A radiograph of the thoracic and lumbar spines were unremarkable. Bilateral hips present with mild arthritic changes and joint space narrowing, left greater than right.

Medications

Zoloft, Lipitor, Insulin, Multi-vitamin with Iron, Ibuprofen (PRN)

Past Medical History (Please check any items that apply to you.)

Musculoskeletal:
- ○ Osteoarthritis
- ○ Rheumatoid Arthritis
- ○ Lupus/SLE
- ○ Fibromyalgia
- ○ Osteoporosis
- ○ Headaches

Musculoskeletal (continued)
- ○ Bulging Disc
- ○ Leg Cramps
- ○ Restless Legs
- ○ Jaw Pain/TMJ
- ○ History of Falling
- ○ Use of Cane or Walker

Musculoskeletal (continued)
- ○ Gout
- ○ Double Jointed
- Other:_____

Neurological:
- ○ Stroke/TIA
- ○ Dementia

Neurological (continued)

- ○ Polio
- ○ Parkinson's Disease
- ○ Multiple Sclerosis
- ○ Epilepsy/Seizures
- ○ Concussion
- ○ Numbness
- ○ Tingling

Other:_____

Endocrine:

- ⊗ Diabetes
- ○ Kidney Dysfunction

Endocrine (continued)

- ○ Bladder Dysfunction
- ○ Liver Dysfunction
- ○ Thyroid Dysfunction

Other:_____

Cardiopulmonary:

- ○ Congestive Heart Failure
- ○ Heart Arrhythmia
- ○ Pacemaker
- ⊗ High Cholesterol
- ○ Blood Clots
- ⊗ Anemia

Cardiopulmonary (continued)

- ⊗ High Blood Pressure
- ○ Asthma
- ○ Shortness of Breath
- ○ COPD
- ○ HIV/AIDS

Other:_____

Other:

- ⊗ Anxiety
- ⊗ Depression
- ○ Cancer

Chief Complaint: *Chronic low back pain*
Goals for Therapy: *To decrease back pain.*
In the last week, how many days have you had pain? *7*
Pain worst: *Lifting, twisting or going up stairs*

SANE Functional Rating

Please rate your **ability** to use your injured area on a 0 to 100% scale with **0%** being unable to use the injured area and **100%** being normal use of injured area in your daily activity: ___75%___

Also, if you exercise or have a sport activity or a job that requires special demands please rate your activity on the 0 to 100% scale: ___75%___

Patient-Specific Functional Scale

Please list 3 activities that you find are difficult because of this problem and circle the number that corresponds with your ability to perform the activity

	Unable									No limitations
1.Climb stairs	1	2	3	4	5	6	(7)	8	9	10
2. Sitting or standing for prolonged periods of time	1	2	3	(4)	5	6	7	8	9	10
3. Walking around the block	1	2	3	(4)	5	6	7	8	9	10

Unique Outcomes Measures

Oswestry disability index = 24/50 (moderate-severe disability)

Fear avoidance beliefs questionnaire = 48/96

Observation

The patient is 5 feet 2 inches and weighs 130 pounds (BMI = 23.8). She enters the room with a slightly antalgic gait and grimace on her face during the right stance phase. Her posture is unremarkable with slight increase in lumbar lordosis.

Patient History

The patient reports that her symptoms have not improved since onset. She states that the pain may have increased slightly since initial onset.

Mechanism: *The patient reports she was lifting a dog at work from the floor to a table beside her, when she heard a "pop" and felt immediate pain in her lower back and into her legs.*

Concordant Sign: *She indicates that she feels a dull, constant ache in her low back, and experiences an intermittent shooting, burning pain into her legs, more so in her left leg than right.*

Nature of the Condition: *The patient experiences 10/10 pain during activities such as stair negotiation and walking extended lengths. Her pain is currently 4/10.*

Behavior of the Symptoms: *Symptoms worsen during prolonged sitting or standing, and improve with heat or lying supine.*

CASE 34

Setting: *Outpatient Orthopedics*

Date: *Present Day*

Medical Diagnosis: *Lumbar Strain*

Charted Data

Name:	*Ella Patterson*	New Injury:	*Yes*
Age:	*36 years*	General Health:	*Good*
MRN:	*50501*	Amount of Exercise:	*Daily walks outside with dog and daughters*
Home Address:	*4072 Bair Road, Mount Clemens, Michigan*	Occupation:	*Stay-at-home mom*
Date of Injury:	*No specific onset, symptoms gradual over past 2 months*	Household:	*Married, lives with husband and 2 children*
		Hand Dominance:	*Right*
		Race:	*Black*

Please fill in the location of your pain with a pencil.

R Front L   L Back R

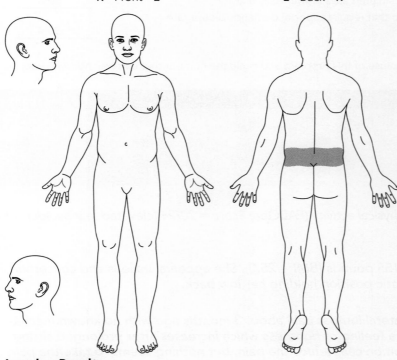

Pain Intensity Scale	
0	No Pain
1	Low-level pain, able to perform regular activities
2	
3	
4	Moderate-level pain, use of pain medication, activity limited but functional
5	
6	
7	High-level pain, use of pain medication, activity very limited— decreased function
8	
(9)	
10	Emergency Situation

Imaging Results

A radiograph of the lumbar spine yields no fractures, although osteophytes are present at the L4/L5 lumbar segment. Findings suggest normal age-related degenerative changes.

Medications

Naproxen (PRN), Ativan, Metoprolol

Past Medical History (Please check any items that apply to you)

Musculoskeletal:
- ○ Osteoarthritis
- ○ Rheumatoid Arthritis
- ○ Lupus/SLE
- ○ Fibromyalgia
- ○ Osteoporosis
- ○ Headaches

Musculoskeletal (continued)
- ○ Bulging Disc
- ○ Leg Cramps
- ○ Restless Legs
- ○ Jaw Pain/TMJ
- ○ History of Falling
- ○ Use of Cane or Walker

Musculoskeletal (continued)
- ○ Gout
- ⊗ Double Jointed
- Other: *Muscle Spasms*
  Back injury

Neurological:
- o Stroke/TIA
- o Dementia
- o Polio
- o Parkinson's Disease
- o Multiple Sclerosis
- o Epilepsy/Seizures
- o Concussion
- o Numbness
- o Tingling

Other:_____

Endocrine:
- o Diabetes
- o Kidney Dysfunction

Endocrine (continued)
- o Bladder Dysfunction
- o Liver Dysfunction
- o Thyroid Dysfunction

Other:_____

Cardiopulmonary:
- o Congestive Heart Failure
- o Heart Arrhythmia
- o Pacemaker
- o High Cholesterol
- o Blood Clots
- o Anemia
- ⊗ High Blood Pressure

Cardiopulmonary (continued)
- o Asthma
- o Shortness of Breath
- o COPD
- o HIV/AIDS

Other:_____

Other:
- ⊗ Anxiety
- ⊗ Depression
- o Cancer

Chief Complaint: *Bilateral low back pain*
Goals for Therapy: *To reduce pain in lower back so I can continue to take care of my family and do household activities.*
In the last week, how many days have you had pain? 7
Pain worst: *At the end of day after doing a lot of walking or standing*

SANE Functional Rating
Please rate your **ability** to use your injured area on a 0 to 100% scale with **0%** being unable to use the injured area and **100%** being normal use of injured area in your daily activity: _____50%_____

Also, if you exercise or have a sport activity or a job that requires special demands please rate your activity on the 0 to 100% scale: _____50%_____

Patient-Specific Functional Scale
Please list 3 activities that you find are difficult because of this problem and circle the number that corresponds with your ability to perform the activity.

	Unable								No limitations	
1. Walking	1	2	3	(4)	5	6	7	8	9	10
2. Standing	1	2	3	4	5	(6)	7	8	9	10
3. Sitting	1	2	(3)	4	5	6	7	8	9	10

Unique Outcomes Measures
Fear and avoidance beliefs questionnaire—physical activity (FABQpa) Score = 20/24 (elevated fear avoidance)
Oswestry disability index = 52/100

Observation
The patient is 5 feet 6 inches and weighs 155 pounds (BMI = 25.0). She appears anxious and concerned over her condition. She is seated in a lordotic position holding her low back.

Patient History
The patient reports a gradual onset of bilateral lumbar pain about 3 months ago with no known mechanism of injury. She reports that her pain is a feeling of tightness which increases after prolonged sitting and standing. At this time a change of position can reduce the pain, but nothing seems to take the pain away. She reports experiencing her spine "locking up" with sudden unexpected movements. The patient also reported that she was a gymnast from the ages of 8 to 18. She experienced an episode of low back pain when she was 14 when she landed awkwardly while dismounting the balance beam. She ignored the pain and continued with gymnastics once it resolved on its own.
Mechanism: *The patient could not identify any specific mechanism of injury to her spine.*
Concordant Sign: *She indicates that her pain is initiated after sitting at her computer desk or standing in one spot for long periods of time. She also reported that lying on her stomach produces her symptoms.*
Nature of the Condition: *The 9/10 pain that she reports occurs with stiffness or tightness in the lower back, and she experiences muscle spasms with long periods of standing or sitting.*
Behavior of the Symptoms: *The patient's symptoms worsen during long periods of sitting or standing in one position and lessen to a 4/10 pain when she changes positions. Pain medication and a moist-heat pack help reduce the pain at times. Symptoms seem to worsen around the time of her menstrual cycle.*

CASE 35

Setting: *Outpatient Orthopedics*

Date: *Present Day*

Medical Diagnosis: *Thoracic/Lumbar Strain*

Charted Data

Name:	*Alexis Johnson*	General Health:	*Fair*
Age:	*79 years*	Amount of Exercise:	*0—unable to exercise due to pain and weakness*
MRN:	*19023*		
Home Address:	*1417 Smith Avenue, Miami, Florida*	Occupation:	*Retired*
		Household:	*Married, lives with husband*
Date of Injury:	*6 to 8 months ago*	Hand Dominance:	*Left*
New Injury:	*Progressively worsening*	Race:	*White*

Please fill in the location of your pain with a pencil.

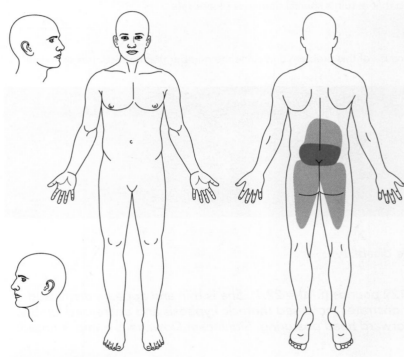

R Front L   L Back R

Pain Intensity Scale	
0	No Pain
1	Low-level pain, able to perform regular activities
2	
3	
(4)	Moderate-level pain, use of pain medication, activity limited but functional
5	
6	
7	High-level pain, use of pain medication, activity very limited— decreased function
8	
9	
10	Emergency Situation

Imaging Results

Radiograph results show decreased vertebral height in the anterior portion of the thoracic spine, suggesting new and old compression fractures.

Medications

Sectral, Naproxen, Ibuprofen PRN, Prednisone

Past Medical History (Please check any items that apply to you.)

Musculoskeletal:

- ⊗ Osteoarthritis
- ○ Rheumatoid Arthritis
- ○ Lupus/SLE
- ○ Fibromyalgia
- ⊗ Osteoporosis
- ○ Headaches

Musculoskeletal (continued)

- ○ Bulging Disc
- ○ Leg Cramps
- ○ Restless Legs
- ○ Jaw Pain/TMJ
- ⊗ History of Falling
- ⊗ Use of Cane or Walker

Musculoskeletal (continued)

- ○ Gout
- ○ Double Jointed

Other:_____

Neurological:

- ○ Stroke/TIA
- ○ Dementia

Neurological (continued)

- ○ Polio
- ○ Parkinson's Disease
- ○ Multiple Sclerosis
- ○ Epilepsy/Seizures
- ○ Concussion
- ○ Numbness
- ⊗ Tingling

Other:_____

Endocrine:

- ○ Diabetes
- ○ Kidney Dysfunction

Endocrine (continued)

- ○ Bladder Dysfunction
- ○ Liver Dysfunction
- ○ Thyroid Dysfunction

Other:_____

Cardiopulmonary:

- ○ Congestive Heart Failure
- ⊗ Heart Arrhythmia
- ○ Pacemaker
- ⊗ High Cholesterol
- ○ Blood Clots
- ○ Anemia

Cardiopulmonary (continued)

- ⊗ High Blood Pressure
- ○ Asthma
- ○ Shortness of Breath
- ○ COPD
- ○ HIV/AIDS

Other:_____

Other:

- ○ Anxiety
- ○ Depression
- ○ Cancer

Chief Complaint: *Low back pain*
Goals for Therapy: *To decrease pain and increase ability to be physically active.*
In the last week, how many days have you had pain? 7
Pain worst: *With activity or prolonged sitting/standing*

SANE Functional Rating

Please rate your **ability** to use your injured area on a 0 to 100% scale with **0%** being unable to use the injured area and **100%** being normal use of injured area in your daily activity: 75%

Also, if you exercise or have a sport activity or a job that requires special demands please rate your activity on the 0 to 100% scale: 75%

Patient-Specific Functional Scale

Please list 3 activities that you find are difficult because of this problem and circle the number that corresponds with your ability to perform the activity.

	Unable								No limitations	
1. Standing for long periods of time	1	2	(3)	4	5	6	7	8	9	10
2. Bending forward to reach items off ground	1	2	3	(4)	5	6	7	8	9	10
3. Walking to get mail	1	(2)	3	4	5	6	7	8	9	10

Unique Outcomes Measures

Oswestry disability index = 33% (moderate disability)

Observation

The patient is 5 feet 4 inches and weighs 129 pounds (BMI = 22.1). She is thin and appears distressed while seated during examination. She demonstrates increased thoracic kyphosis and decreased lumbar lordosis. She has rounded shoulders and forward head posturing. Significant Dowager's hump is noted.

Patient History

The patient reports progressive pain and alterations in bilateral lower extremity sensation. She cannot remember anything that caused these symptoms. Her back pain has been increasing slightly, since onset about 8 months ago, especially in the last 3 weeks. These changes have compromised her balance and contributed to a couple of recent falls.

Mechanism: *There was no specific incident that the patient was able to relate to the onset of these symptoms.*

Concordant Sign: *The patient indicates that her back pain increases with sitting or standing longer than 10 minutes. She states that this is typically when the tingling begins in her legs.*

Nature of the Condition: *The patient reports that her pain is worse with prolonged periods of sitting and standing, and that her pain decreases when she lies down.*

Behavior of the Symptoms: *Symptoms worsen during sitting or standing and lessen when she lies down or sleeps.*

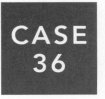

CASE 36

Setting: *Outpatient Orthopedics*

Date: *Present Day*

Medical Diagnosis: *Lumbar Spinal Stenosis*

Charted Data

Name:	*Lucy Williams*	General Health:	*Good*
Age:	*68 years*	Amount of Exercise:	*20 minutes /day, 3 days/week*
MRN:	*86259*	Occupation:	*Retired nurse but still works part time at local hospital*
Home Address:	*512 Brookview Lane, Baltimore, Maryland*	Household:	*Married, lives with husband*
Date of Injury:	*4 to 5 months ago*	Hand Dominance:	*Right*
New Injury:	*No*	Race:	*White*

Please fill in the location of your pain with a pencil.

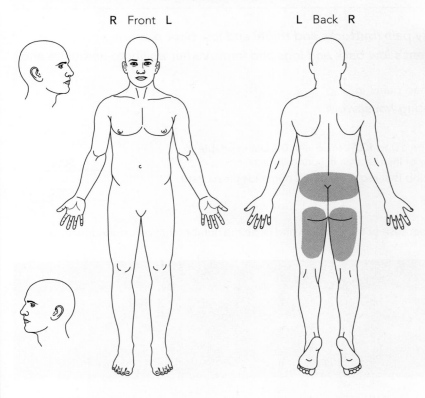

R   Front   L   L   Back   R

Pain Intesity Scale	
0	No Pain
1	Low-level pain, able to perform regular activities
2	
3	
4	Moderate-level pain, use of pain medication, activity limited but functional
5	
(6)	
7	High-level pain, use of pain medication, activity very limited—decreased function
8	
9	
10	Emergency Situation

Imaging Results

A radiograph of the lumbar spine yields no fractures and suggests moderate degenerative changes. The MRI demonstrates decreased disc height and minor disc bulging at L1–L3.

Medications

Fortical, Lopressor, Ibuprofen

Past Medical History (Please check any items that apply to you.)

Musculoskeletal:
- o Osteoarthritis
- o Rheumatoid Arthritis
- o Lupus/SLE
- o Fibromyalgia
- o Osteoporosis
- o Headaches
- o Bulging Disc
- o Leg Cramps
- o Restless Legs
- o Jaw Pain/TMJ
- o History of Falling
- o Use of Cane or Walker
- o Gout
- o Double Jointed

Other: **Osteopenia**

Neurological:
- o Stroke/TIA
- o Dementia

Neurological (continued)
- o Polio
- o Parkinson's Disease
- o Multiple Sclerosis
- o Epilepsy/Seizures
- o Concussion
- o Numbness
- o Tingling

Other:_____

Endocrine:
- o Diabetes
- o Kidney Dysfunction
- o Bladder Dysfunction
- o Liver Dysfunction
- o Thyroid Dysfunction

Other:_____

Cardiopulmonary:
- o Congestive Heart Failure
- o Heart Arrhythmia

Cardiopulmonary (continued)
- o Pacemaker
- o High Cholesterol
- o Blood Clots
- o Anemia
- ⊗ High Blood Pressure
- o Asthma
- o Shortness of Breath
- o COPD
- o HIV/AIDS

Other:_____

Other:
- ⊗ Anxiety
- o Depression
- o Cancer

Chief Complaint: *Bilateral lower extremity pain (buttocks and thigh) and low back pain*

Goals for Therapy: *To reduce pain in patient's low back and legs and improve her ability to ambulate and complete activities of daily living.*

In the last week, how many days have you had pain? *6*

Pain worst: *During work or while completing housework*

SANE Functional Rating

Please rate your **ability** to use your injured area on a 0 to 100% scale with **0%** being unable to use the injured area and **100%** being normal use of injured area in your daily activity: _____ 50%

Also, if you exercise or have a sport activity or a job that requires special demands please rate your activity on the 0 to 100% scale: _____ 50%

Patient-Specific Functional Scale

Please list 3 activities that you find are difficult because of this problem and circle the number that corresponds with your ability to perform the activity.

	Unable								No limitations	
1. Cooking	1	2	3	4	5	(6)	7	8	9	10
2. Standing at work	1	2	3	4	(5)	6	7	8	9	10
3. Walking outside for exercise	1	2	3	4	(5)	6	7	8	9	10

Unique Outcomes Measures

Oswestry disability index = 18/45 = 40% (moderate disability)

Fear avoidance beliefs questionnaire FABQpa = 15 and FABQw = 35; Total = 50 (high degree of fear and avoidance beliefs)

Observation

The patient is 5 feet 2 inches and weighs 135 pounds (BMI = 24.7). She appears to have a flattened lumbar lordosis and is somewhat hesitant to move, especially when standing in an erect posture. She ambulates with a wide-based gait, slow pace, and in a forward flexed position.

Patient History

The patient reports a history of back pain for over 20 years and has had a history of vertebral end plate fractures while working as a nurse. The pain has been manageable with a hot pack and use of ibuprofen but pain in both of her legs has increased in the last 4–5 months. She reports having difficulty with completing tasks at home, including cooking and cleaning; having difficulty with ambulating long distances and therefore requires sitting rest breaks; and states that she feels better when grocery shopping because she is able to lean on the shopping cart.

Mechanism: *There is no specific incident that the patient can recall but she has a long history of chronic back pain and a vertebral fracture.*

Concordant Sign: *The patient indicates that her lower back and lower extremity pain is initiated with standing for prolonged periods of time, walking, and when trying to correct her posture into an erect position.*

Nature of the Condition: *The 6/10 pain the patient reports occurs in her lower back and bilateral lower extremities, and she has difficulty completing standing tasks.*

Behavior of the Symptoms: *Symptoms worsen during standing and walking but lessen when she sits down or bends her trunk forward. Pain is variable throughout the day, depending on the activities she completes.*

CASE 37

Setting: *Outpatient Orthopedics*

Date: *Present Day*

Medical Diagnosis: *Lumbar Radiculopathy*

Charted Data

Name:	*Dave Shepplar*	General Health:	*Good*
Age:	*31 years*	Amount of Exercise:	*30 minutes/day, 3 days/ week*
MRN:	*66801*		
Home Address:	*628 Kimberly Circle, Dover, Maryland*	Occupation:	*Truck driver*
		Household:	*Married, lives with wife*
Date of Injury:	*2 years ago*	Hand Dominance:	*Right*
New Injury:	*No*	Race:	*White*

Please fill in the location of your pain with a pencil.

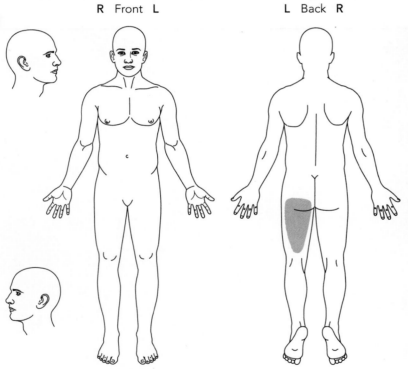

R Front L   L Back R

Pain Intensity Scale	
0	No Pain
1	Low-level pain, able to perform regular activities
2	
3	
(4)	Moderate-level pain, use of pain medication, activity limited but functional
5	
6	
7	High-level pain, use of pain medication, activity very limited—decreased function
8	
9	
10	Emergency Situation

Imaging Results

MRI (Magnetic Resonance Imaging) revealed a posterolateral disc protrusion at L4–L5, as well as age-related degenerative changes throughout the lumbar spine.

Medications

Hydrocodone (PRN), Cyclobenzaprine (PRN), Atorvastatin

Past Medical History (Please check any items that apply to you.)

Musculoskeletal:
- ○ Osteoarthritis
- ○ Rheumatoid Arthritis
- ○ Lupus/SLE
- ○ Fibromyalgia
- ○ Osteoporosis
- ○ Headaches
- ⊗ Bulging Disc
- ○ Leg Cramps
- ○ Restless Legs
- ○ Jaw Pain/TMJ
- ○ History of Falling
- ○ Use of Cane or Walker
- ○ Gout
- ○ Double Jointed

Other:_____

Neurological:
- ○ Stroke/TIA
- ○ Dementia

Neurological (continued)
- ○ Polio
- ○ Parkinson's Disease
- ○ Multiple Sclerosis
- ○ Epilepsy/Seizures
- ○ Concussion
- ○ Numbness
- ○ Tingling

Other:_____

Endocrine:
- ○ Diabetes
- ○ Kidney Dysfunction
- ○ Bladder Dysfunction
- ○ Liver Dysfunction
- ○ Thyroid Dysfunction

Other:_____

Cardiopulmonary:
- ○ Congestive Heart Failure
- ○ Heart Arrhythmia

Cardiopulmonary (continued)
- ○ Pacemaker
- ⊗ High Cholesterol
- ○ Blood Clots
- ○ Anemia
- ○ High Blood Pressure
- ○ Asthma
- ○ Shortness of Breath
- ○ COPD
- ○ HIV/AIDS

Other:_____

Other:
- ○ Anxiety
- ○ Depression
- ○ Cancer

Chief Complaint: *Left buttock pain and posterior thigh pain*

Goals for Therapy: *To reduce the pain so jogging can be resumed.*

In the last week, how many days have you had pain? *7*

Pain worst: *After sitting or driving in a car*

SANE Functional Rating

Please rate your **ability** to use your injured area on a 0 to 100% scale with **0%** being unable to use the injured area and **100%** being normal use of injured area in your daily activity: *85%*

Also, if you exercise or have a sport activity or a job that requires special demands please rate your activity on the 0 to 100% scale: *75%*

Patient-Specific Functional Scale

Please list 3 activities that you find are difficult because of this problem and circle the number that corresponds with your ability to perform the activity.

	Unable									No limitations
1. Driving	1	2	3	(4)	5	6	7	8	9	10
2. Jogging	1	2	3	4	5	(6)	7	8	9	10
3. Lifting weights	1	2	3	4	5	(6)	7	8	9	10

Unique Outcomes Measures

Lower extremity functional scale = 60/80 (25% moderate disability)

Observation

The patient is 5 feet 11 inches and weighs 175 pounds (BMI = 24.4). He is muscular and appears to be in excellent physical condition. He walks into the physical therapy gym with a slight limp and excessive out-toeing of the left lower extremity.

Patient History

The patient reports the onset of left buttock and posterior thigh pain about 2 years ago. He states that the pain began as an "annoying" dull ache in his buttock that he was able to ignore. Over the past 2 years it has traveled into his posterior thigh and the pain has become difficult to ignore. He likes to jog and lift weights, but he has been unable to jog or lift weights with his legs within the past month. He also indicates that he has been unable to drive a truck for more than 30 minutes at a time because of the pain. He reports that the pain is on the same side where his wallet is located in his back pocket. The patient decided to seek medical attention from his primary care physician, who indicated that his MRI showed a bulging disc in his lumbar spine that is causing his pain. The patient was referred to physical therapy before any surgical intervention.

Mechanism: *Although there was no specific incident, the patient did indicate that the first time he noticed the pain was after an 8-hour truck drive without any stops.*

Concordant Sign: *He indicates that his pain is initiated after driving or sitting for more than 30 minutes.*

Nature of the Condition: *The 5/10 pain the patient reports occurs as a dull ache while he is sitting. If he shifts his weight off that side or stands up and moves around, the pain reduces to a 3/10, but it does not completely resolve. Once the pain is initiated, he is unable to go for a jog or lift weights.*

Behavior of the Symptoms: *Symptoms worsen during sitting/driving and lessen when he takes pain medication or lies down flat on his back.*

CASE 38

Setting: *Superior Orthopedics*

Date: *Present Day*

Medical Diagnosis: *Latissimus Dorsi Strain*

Charted Data

Name:	*Joanna Phelps*	New Injury:	*Yes*
Age:	*61 years*	General Health:	*Decent*
MRN:	*59621*	Amount of Exercise:	*30 minutes/day, 3 days/week*
Home Address:	*745 Market Street, Westminster, Oregon*	Occupation:	*Retired*
		Household:	*Married, lives with husband*
Date of Injury:	*3 months ago*	Hand Dominance:	*Right*
		Race	*White*

Please fill in the location of your pain with a pencil.

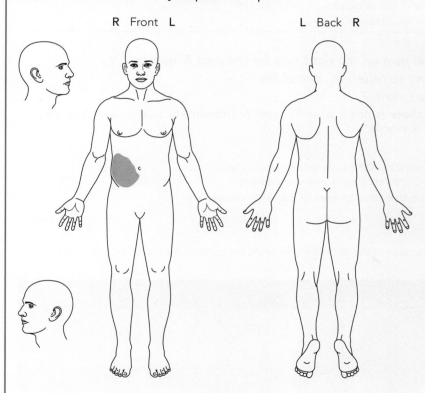

R Front L   L Back R

Pain Intensity Scale	
0	No Pain
1	Low-level pain, able to perform regular activities
2	
3	
4	Moderate-level pain, use of pain medication, activity limited but functional
(5)	
6	
7	High-level pain, use of pain medication, activity very limited—decreased function
8	
9	
10	Emergency Situation

Imaging Results

Radiographs of the chest and thoracic spine yielded no fractures and suggested only normal age-related degenerative changes. An abdominal CT scan as well as endoscopic retrograde cholangiopancreatography (ERCP) were performed and were all found to be normal.

Medications

Demerol by mouth

Past Medical History (Please check any items that apply to you.)

Musculoskeletal:
- ○ Osteoarthritis
- ○ Rheumatoid Arthritis
- ○ Lupus/SLE
- ○ Fibromyalgia
- ○ Osteoporosis
- ○ Headaches
- ○ Bulging Disc
- ○ Leg Cramps
- ○ Restless Legs
- ○ Jaw Pain/TMJ
- ○ History of Falling
- ○ Use of Cane or Walker
- ○ Gout
- ○ Double Jointed

Other:_____

Neurological:
- ○ Stroke/TIA
- ○ Dementia
- ○ Polio

Neurological (continued)
- ○ Parkinson's Disease
- ○ Multiple Sclerosis
- ○ Epilepsy/Seizures
- ○ Concussion
- ○ Numbness
- ○ Tingling

Other:_____

Endocrine:
- ○ Diabetes
- ○ Kidney Dysfunction
- ○ Bladder Dysfunction
- ○ Liver Dysfunction
- ○ Thyroid Dysfunction

Other:
- ⊗ Appendectomy
- ⊗ Abdominal Hysterectomy with single oophorectomy
- ⊗ Hiatal hernia repair
- ⊗ Cholecystectomy

Cardiopulmonary:
- ○ Congestive Heart Failure
- ○ Heart Arrhythmia
- ○ Pacemaker
- ○ High Cholesterol
- ○ Blood Clots
- ○ Anemia
- ○ High Blood Pressure
- ○ Asthma
- ○ Shortness of Breath
- ○ COPD
- ○ HIV/AIDS

Other:_____

Other:
- ○ Anxiety
- ○ Depression
- ○ Cancer

Chief Complaint: *Severe chronic abdominal pain on the right side for the past 3 months*

Goals for Therapy: *To decrease the pain and to return to normal life.*

In the last week, how many days have you had pain? 7

Pain worst: *The pain is near constant and there is not a specific time or movement that makes it worse; however, general activity seems to make it worse.*

SANE Functional Rating

Please rate your **ability** to use your injured area on a 0 to 100% scale with **0%** being unable to use the injured area and **100%** being normal use of injured area in your daily activity: *20%*

Also, if you exercise or have a sport activity or a job that requires special demands please rate your activity on the 0 to 100% scale: *10%*

Patient-Specific Functional Scale

Please list 3 activities that you find are difficult because of this problem and circle the number that corresponds with your ability to perform the activity.

	Unable								No limitations	
1. Yard work	(1)	2	3	4	5	6	7	8	9	10
2. Tucking my shirt in	1	(2)	3	4	5	6	7	8	9	10
3. Getting out of bed in the morning	1	2	3	(4)	5	6	7	8	9	10

Unique Outcomes Measures

There are no outcomes measures that are appropriate for this case.

Observation

The patient is 5 feet 4 inches and weighs 155 pounds (BMI = 26.6). She is a small, slightly stocky female who sits with a right lateral lean, forward head posture, and rounded shoulders. The patient tends to hold right side with hand and maintains a slouched posture while sitting and standing.

Patient History

The patient reports the pain beginning about 3 months ago and being similar to the pain she experienced prior to her cholecystectomy. The pain was not bad at first but began increasing about 2.5 months ago and turned into sharp shooting pain into the right upper quadrant with referral to the back. She notes a weight loss of 15 pounds over the last month. The patient does not recall a specific event but notes that the week prior to the pain she was in Las Vegas, playing the slot machines. The patient is very worried that there may be something seriously wrong even though testing reveals no sinister pathology.

Mechanism: *The patient does not recall a specific onset, but notes playing slot machines the week prior to her abdominal pain.*

Concordant Sign: *The patient indicates that her pain is increased with resisted glenohumeral extension, internal rotation, and adduction. Tenderness to palpation is also noted distal to the inferior angle of the right scapula eliciting her abdominal pain.*

Nature of the Condition: *The pain she reports occurs constantly throughout the day. It can be as high as 9/10 but usually stays around 5/10, depending on how active she is.*

Behavior of the Symptoms: *Symptoms are always present and are sharp and shooting into the right upper quadrant. The pain decreases slightly with splinting the right side.*

CASE 39

Setting: *Women's Health*

Date: *Present Day*

Medical Diagnosis: *Pubic Symphysis Diastasis*

Charted Data

Name:	*Polly Reading*	General Health:	*Good*
Age:	*37 years*	Amount of Exercise:	*45 minutes/day, 5 days/week*
MRN:	*76483*	Occupation:	*Homemaker*
Home Address:	*341 Wellburg Drive, Houston, Texas*	Household:	*Married, lives with husband and 3 children*
Date of Injury:	*3 weeks ago*	Hand Dominance:	*Right*
New Injury:	*Yes*	Race:	*White*

Please fill in the location of your pain with a pencil.

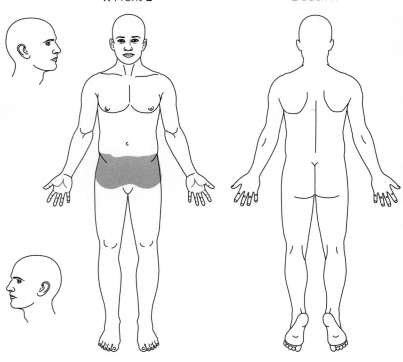

R Front L   L Back R

Pain Intensity Scale	
0	No Pain
1	Low-level pain, able to perform regular activities
2	
3	
4	Moderate-level pain, use of pain medication, activity limited but functional
5	
6	
7	High-level pain, use of pain medication, activity very limited—decreased function
8	
(9)	
10	Emergency Situation

Imaging Results

A Chamberlain's radiograph of the pelvis yields a 30mm separation of the pubic symphysis.

Medications

Prenatal vitamins and Tylenol (PRN)

Past Medical History (Please check any items that apply to you.)

Musculoskeletal:

- ○ Osteoarthritis
- ○ Rheumatoid Arthritis
- ○ Lupus/SLE
- ○ Fibromyalgia
- ○ Osteoporosis

Musculoskeletal (continued)

- ○ Headaches
- ⊗ Bulging Disc
- ○ Leg Cramps
- ○ Restless Legs
- ○ Jaw Pain/TMJ

Musculoskeletal (continued)

- ○ History of Falling
- ○ Use of Cane or Walker
- ○ Gout
- ○ Double Jointed
- Other:_____

Neurological:
- o Stroke/TIA
- o Dementia
- o Polio
- o Parkinson's Disease
- o Multiple Sclerosis
- o Epilepsy/Seizures
- o Concussion
- o Numbness
- o Tingling

Other:_____

Endocrine:
- o Diabetes

Endocrine (continued)
- o Kidney Dysfunction
- o Bladder Dysfunction
- o Liver Dysfunction
- o Thyroid Dysfunction

Other:_____

Cardiopulmonary:
- o Congestive Heart Failure
- o Heart Arrhythmia
- o Pacemaker
- o High Cholesterol
- o Blood Clots
- o Anemia

Cardiopulmonary (continued)
- o High Blood Pressure
- o Asthma
- o Shortness of Breath
- o COPD
- o HIV/AIDS

Other:_____

Other:
- o Anxiety
- o Depression
- o Cancer

Chief Complaint: *Bilateral hip and pelvic pain*

Goals for Therapy: *To be able to walk and take care of family*

In the last week, how many days have you had pain? *7*

Pain worst: *When standing and attempting to walk*

SANE Functional Rating

Please rate your **ability** to use your injured area on a 0 to 100% scale with **0%** being unable to use the injured area and **100%** being normal use of injured area in your daily activity: _10%_

Also, if you exercise or have a sport activity or a job that requires special demands please rate your activity on the 0 to 100% scale: _10%_

Patient-Specific Functional Scale

Please list **3 activities** that you find are difficult because of this problem and circle the number that corresponds with your ability to perform the activity.

	Unable									No limitations
1. Standing	1	2	(3)	4	5	6	7	8	9	10
2. Walking	1	(2)	3	4	5	6	7	8	9	10
3. Bending over to pick up kids	1	2	(3)	4	5	6	7	8	9	10

Unique Outcomes Measures

Lower extremity functional scale = 7/80, indicating she has significant difficulty with functional daily activities. The 7 points indicates very low function.

Observation

The patient is 5 feet 7 inches and weighs 145 pounds (BMI = 22.7). She is in good physical shape but demonstrates difficulty with standing and weight bearing. Patient is in physical distress.

Patient History

The patient reports that she gave birth to her daughter 3 weeks ago and that is when her symptoms began. Her physician advised her to remain on bed rest until her pain subsided.

Mechanism: *The birth of her third child seems to be her mechanism of injury, per patient and physician record.*

Concordant Sign: *The patient indicates that her pain presents upon weight bearing and ambulation. She has difficulty bending and lifting her children.*

Nature of the Condition: *The 9/10 pain she reports occurs when weight bearing. She attempts to deal with the pain to complete the task at hand and care for her children until she cannot handle the pain any longer.*

Behavior of the Symptoms: *The patient's symptoms worsen during standing, walking, and bending to pick up her children or items from the floor.*

CASE 40

Setting: *Outpatient Orthopedics*

Date: *Present Day*

Medical Diagnosis: *Groin pain*

Charted Data

Name: *Jenelle Hawthorne*

Age: *18 years*

MRN: *462789394*

Home Address: *7155 Greenhill Circle, Cincinnati, Ohio*

Date of Injury: *Insidious onset that started about 2 months ago*

New Injury: *Yes*

General Health: *Good*

Amount of Exercise: *90 minutes/day, 6 days/week*

Occupation: *High school student*

Household: *Lives with both parents and 2 younger siblings*

Hand Dominance: *Right*

Race: *Black*

Please fill in the location of your pain with a pencil.

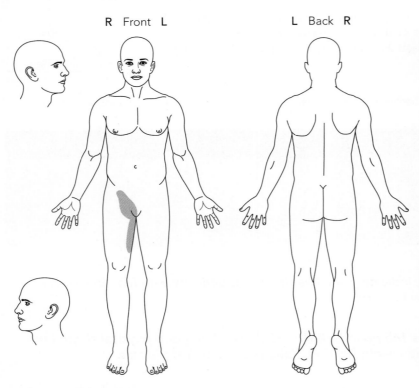

R Front L   L Back R

Pain Intesity Scale	
0	No Pain
1	Low-level pain, able to perform regular activities
2	
3	
4	Moderate-level pain, use of pain medication, activity limited but functional
⑤	
6	
7	High-level pain, use of pain medication, activity very limited— decreased function
8	
9	
10	Emergency Situation

Imaging Results
No imaging has been completed at this time.

Medications
Women's over-the-counter multivitamin, Ibuprofen

Past Medical History (Please check any items that apply to you.)

Musculoskeletal:
- ○ Osteoarthritis
- ○ Rheumatoid Arthritis
- ○ Lupus/SLE
- ○ Fibromyalgia
- ○ Osteoporosis

Musculoskeletal (continued)
- ⊗ Headaches
- ○ Bulging Disc
- ⊗ Leg Cramps
- ○ Restless Legs
- ○ Jaw Pain/TMJ

Musculoskeletal (continued)
- ○ History of Falling
- ○ Use of Cane or Walker
- ○ Gout
- ○ Double Jointed

Other:_____

Neurological:
- o Stroke/TIA
- o Dementia
- o Polio
- o Parkinson's Disease
- o Multiple Sclerosis
- o Epilepsy/Seizures
- o Concussion
- o Numbness
- o Tingling

Other:_____

Endocrine:
- o Diabetes
- o Kidney Dysfunction

Endocrine (continued)
- o Bladder Dysfunction
- o Liver Dysfunction
- o Thyroid Dysfunction

Other:_____

Cardiopulmonary:
- o Congestive Heart Failure
- o Heart Arrhythmia
- o Pacemaker
- o High Cholesterol
- o Blood Clots
- o Anemia
- o High Blood Pressure
- o Asthma

Cardiopulmonary (continued)
- o Shortness of Breath
- o COPD
- o HIV/AIDS

Other:_____

Other:
- ⊗ Anxiety
- o Depression
- o Cancer

Chief Complaint: *Pain along the right inguinal line that limits participation in sport*

Goals for Therapy: *To return to soccer without pain.*

In the last week, how many days have you had pain? *7*

Pain worst: *During soccer practice or soccer games*

SANE Functional Rating

Please rate your **ability** to use your injured area on a 0 to 100% scale with **0%** being unable to use the injured area and **100%** being normal use of injured area in your daily activity: 75%

Also, if you exercise or have a sport activity or a job that requires special demands please rate your activity on the 0 to 100% scale: 50%

Patient-Specific Functional Scale

Please list **3 activities** that you find are difficult because of this problem and circle the number that corresponds with your ability to perform the activity.

	Unable									No limitations
1. Playing soccer	1	2	3	(4)	5	6	7	8	9	10
2. Climbing stairs	1	2	3	4	(5)	6	7	8	9	10
3. Jogging	1	2	3	4	(5)	6	7	8	9	10

Unique Outcomes Measures

Lower Extremity Function Scale (LEFS) = 55/80

Observation

The patient is 5 feet 6 inches and weighs 120 pounds (BMI = 19.4). She is overall in good health and appears to be physically fit. The patient stands and ambulates with increased lumbar lordosis and mild antalgic gait.

Patient History

The patient reports groin pain localized to the right side and pain along her medial lower extremity. Over the past 2 months, she describes the pain as "burning" and general discomfort. She states the pain increases with coughing and sneezing. She is a high school student who has been playing soccer year round since she was 13 years old. She has strained her groin during soccer twice before, but reports the pain she is currently feeling is different from what she has experienced before. When the pain began about 2 months ago, she assumed it was another muscle strain so she decreased her practice frequency and intensity, but the pain never subsided. Therefore, she is now coming to see the physical therapist as a direct access patient.

Mechanism: *No specific incident correlates with the onset of pain.*

Concordant Sign: *The patient reports that soccer practice increases her pain, especially when she has to make sudden changes in directions.*

Nature of the Condition: *The pain began 2 months ago. Over the past week, the patient has not participated in soccer practice secondary to increased pain.*

Behavior of the Symptoms: *The pain is worse during soccer practices or games. The pain also increases whenever the patient sneezes or coughs. Her pain decreases with rest; however, her pain is never completely a 0/10. She reports she has at least 2/10 dull pain constantly.*

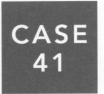

CASE 41

Setting: *Outpatient Orthopedics*

Date: *Present Day*

Medical Diagnosis: *Lumbar Strain*

Charted Data

Name:	*Allison Weaver*	Amount of Exercise:	*1 hour/day, 7 days/week*
Age:	*20 years*	Occupation:	*Forensic biology student, collegiate cross-country runner*
MRN:	*80902*		
Home Address:	*1874 Brockport Avenue, La Crosse, Wisconsin*	Household:	*Lives with four girls from the cross-country team*
Date of Injury:	*1 month ago*		
New Injury:	*Yes*	Hand Dominance:	*Right*
General Health:	*Good*	Race:	*White*

Please fill in the location of your pain with a pencil.

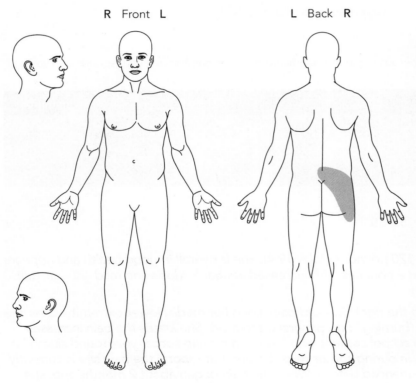

R Front L   L Back R

Pain Intensity Scale	
0	No Pain
1	Low-level pain, able to perform regular activities
2	
3	
4	Moderate-level pain, use of pain medication, activity limited but functional
5	
6	
7	High-level pain, use of pain medication, activity very limited— decreased function
(8)	
9	
10	Emergency Situation

Imaging Results
No imaging was performed.

Medications
Hydrocodone (PRN)

Past Medical History (Please check any items that apply to you.)

Musculoskeletal:

- ○ Osteoarthritis
- ○ Rheumatoid Arthritis
- ○ Lupus/SLE
- ○ Fibromyalgia
- ○ Osteoporosis
- ○ Headaches
- ○ Bulging Disc
- ○ Leg Cramps
- ○ Restless Legs
- ○ Jaw Pain/TMJ
- ○ History of Falling
- ○ Use of Cane or Walker
- ○ Gout
- ○ Double Jointed

Other: Stress fracture in tibia

Neurological:

- ○ Stroke/TIA
- ○ Dementia

Neurological (continued)

- ○ Polio
- ○ Parkinson's Disease
- ○ Multiple Sclerosis
- ○ Epilepsy/Seizures
- ○ Concussion
- ○ Numbness
- ○ Tingling

Other:_____

Endocrine:

- ○ Diabetes
- ○ Kidney Dysfunction
- ○ Bladder Dysfunction
- ○ Liver Dysfunction
- ○ Thyroid Dysfunction

Other:_____

Cardiopulmonary:

- ○ Congestive Heart Failure
- ○ Heart Arrhythmia

Cardiopulmonary (continued)

- ○ Pacemaker
- ○ High Cholesterol
- ○ Blood Clots
- ○ Anemia
- ○ High Blood Pressure
- ○ Asthma
- ○ Shortness of Breath
- ○ COPD
- ○ HIV/AIDS

Other:_____

Other:

- ○ Anxiety
- ○ Depression
- ○ Cancer
- ⊗ Amenorrhea

Chief Complaint: *Right-sided low back and buttock pain*

Goals for Therapy: *To reduce low back and buttock pain and return to running.*

In the last week, how many days have you had pain? *7*

Pain worst: *After running*

SANE Functional Rating

Please rate your **ability** to use your injured area on a 0 to 100% scale with **0%** being unable to use the injured area and **100%** being normal use of injured area in your daily activity: 75%

Also, if you exercise or have a sport activity or a job that requires special demands please rate your activity on the 0 to 100% scale: 65%

Patient-Specific Functional Scale

Please list **3 activities** that you find are difficult because of this problem and circle the number that corresponds with your ability to perform the activity.

	Unable								No limitations	
1. Running	1	2	3	(4)	5	6	7	8	9	10
2. Sitting to/from standing	1	2	3	4	5	6	(7)	8	9	10
3. Walking	1	2	3	4	5	6	(7)	8	9	10

Unique Outcomes Measures

Oswestry Disability Index = 40% (moderate disability with back pain)

Observation

The patient is 5 feet 6 inches and weighs 112 pounds (BMI = 18.1). She appears underweight and apprehensive over her condition. She sits in anterior pelvic tilt with an increased lordotic posture.

Patient History

Patient reports the onset of right-sided low back and buttock pain about 1 month ago during a 10-mile run the day after a cross-country meet. She reports that the onset of pain was around mile 4 of the run and continued to worsen throughout the run. Following the run she went to the team athletic trainer, who told her she strained the muscles in her back and to take a few days of rest. She took two days of rest, the pain seemed to disappear, and she returned to running again. The pain returned a mile into her run and became unbearable, requiring her to stop. The athletic trainer (ATC) recommended she see her physician. She reported that she did not present with numbness/tingling or bowel/bladder changes, so her physician did not order imaging because he told her it was a lumbar strain. He recommended that she should take 2 weeks off from running and wrote a prescription for physical therapy.

Mechanism: Although there was no specific incident, the patient did indicate that her coach recently increased her weekly mileage from 45 to 60 miles per week for the last two months, and her racing times have become slower than normal.

Concordant Sign: The patient indicates that her low back and buttock pain is initiated after running, walking, and standing up from a seated position.

Nature of the Condition: The 8/10 pain reported by the patient occurs as a sharp pain while she is running, walking, or sitting to/from a standing position. When the pain occurs during walking or running it is too severe for her to continue.

Behavior of the Symptoms: Symptoms worsen during running or walking and lessen once she sits down or lies down and rests.

CASE 42	Setting: *Outpatient Orthopedics*
	Date: *Present Day*
	Medical Diagnosis: *Costochondritis*

Charted Data

Name:	Marie Perez	New Injury:	No
Age:	32 years	General Health:	Good
MRN:	50543	Amount of Exercise:	1 hour/day, 2 days/week
Home Address:	1550 Plum Drive, Urban, Missouri	Occupation:	Preschool teacher
		Household:	Married, 2 children
Date of Injury:	4 days ago	Hand Dominance:	Right

Please fill in the location of your pain with a pencil.

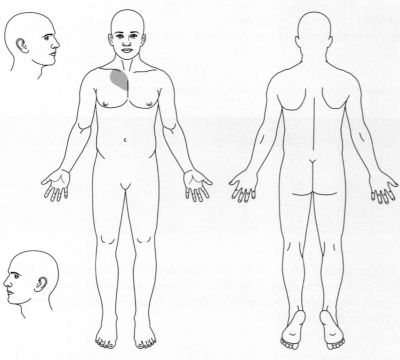

R Front L   L Back R

Pain Intensity Scale	
0	No Pain
1	Low-level pain, able to perform regular activities
2	
3	
4	Moderate-level pain, use of pain medication, activity limited but functional
5	
6	
(7)	High-level pain, use of pain medication, activity very limited— decreased function
8	
9	
10	Emergency Situation

Imaging Results
Plain film radiograph of the chest reveals no fractures and suggests normal findings.

Medications
Ibuprofen (PRN)

Past Medical History (Please check any items that apply to you.)
Unremarkable

Musculoskeletal:
- ○ Osteoarthritis
- ○ Rheumatoid Arthritis
- ○ Lupus/SLE
- ○ Fibromyalgia
- ○ Osteoporosis
- ○ Headaches

Musculoskeletal (continued)
- ○ Bulging Disc
- ○ Leg Cramps
- ○ Restless Legs
- ○ Jaw Pain/TMJ
- ○ History of Falling
- ○ Use of Cane or Walker

Musculoskeletal (continued)
- ○ Gout
- ○ Double Jointed
- Other:_____

Neurological:

- Stroke/TIA
- Dementia
- Polio
- Parkinson's Disease
- Multiple Sclerosis
- Epilepsy/Seizures
- Concussion
- Numbness
- Tingling

Other:_____

Endocrine:

- Diabetes
- Kidney Dysfunction

Endocrine (continued)

- Bladder Dysfunction
- Liver Dysfunction
- Thyroid Dysfunction

Other:_____

Cardiopulmonary:

- Congestive Heart Failure
- Heart Arrhythmia
- Pacemaker
- High Cholesterol
- Blood Clots
- Anemia
- High Blood Pressure
- Asthma

Cardiopulmonary (continued)

- Shortness of Breath
- COPD
- HIV/AIDS

Other:_____

Other:

- Anxiety
- Depression
- Cancer

Chief Complaint: *Chest pain*
Goals for Therapy: *To return to work and recreational activities without pain.*
In the last week, how many days have you had pain? *4*
Pain worst: *During lifting and exercise*

SANE Functional Rating

Please rate your **ability** to use your injured area on a 0 to 100% scale with **0%** being unable to use the injured area and **100%** being normal use of injured area in your daily activity: ___ *80%* ___

Also, if you exercise or have a sport activity or a job that requires special demands please rate your activity on the 0 to 100% scale: ___ *40%* ___

Patient-Specific Functional Scale

Please list 3 activities that you find are difficult because of this problem and circle the number that corresponds with your ability to perform the activity.

	Unable								No limitations	
1. Lifting children	1	2	3	(4)	5	6	7	8	9	10
2. Push-ups	1	2	(3)	4	5	6	7	8	9	10
3. Tae-kwon-do hand techniques	1	2	3	4	5	6	(7)	8	9	10

Observation

The patient is 5 feet 9 inches and weighs 163 pounds (BMI = 24.1). She stands with a slightly flexed forward posture, which she is able to correct with verbal cues. She demonstrates excessive thoracic kyphosis in the mid- and upper-thoracic region, her right shoulder is internally rotated compared to the left, and her right scapula is slightly protracted compared to left.

Patient History

The patient reports a localized pain in the right upper chest region anteriorly.

Mechanism: *Symptoms started as a sharp pain about 3 months ago when the patient lifted a 2-year-old child who was kicking during a temper tantrum. Symptoms subsided over a few days but were reaggravated 4 days ago after sparring in a tae-kwon-do tournament. In addition to the anterior pain, the patient complains of upper back stiffness on the right.*

Concordant Sign: *She indicates sharp pain comes on with lifting or use of the right upper extremity.*

Nature of the Condition: *A localized dull ache is present at rest, which increases to a sharp pain rated as 7/10 with lifting toddlers at work and with performing push-ups for tae-kwon-do. The patient notices the upper back stiffness when twisting, such as when checking traffic while driving.*

Behavior of the Symptoms: *Symptoms increase in intensity with lifting and worsen with repeated lifting or lifting heavier weights. During tae-kwon-do, using the right upper extremity for punching or blocking increases sharp pain; this decreases to an ache after the activity. Pain also increases when inhaling a deep breath.*

Setting: *Outpatient Orthopedics*

Date: *Present Day*

Medical Diagnosis: *Back Strain*

Charted Data

Name:	*Cameron David*	General Health:	*Good*
Age:	*29 years*	Amount of Exercise:	*1 hour/day, 3 days/week*
MRN:	*40301*	Occupation:	*Inventory manager, Computer and Home Electronics Warehouse*
Home Address:	*841 134th Court, Urban, Idaho*	Household:	*Single, lives alone in a second-floor apartment*
Date of Injury:	*1 day ago*	Hand Dominance:	*Right*
New Injury:	*Yes*		

Please fill in the location of your pain with a pencil.

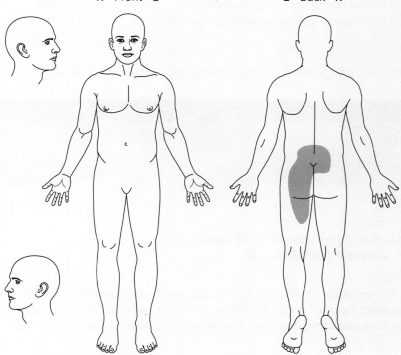

R   Front   L   L   Back   R

Pain Intensity Scale	
0	No Pain
1	Low-level pain, able to perform regular activities
2	
3	
4	Moderate-level pain, use of pain medication, activity limited but functional
(5)	
6	
7	High-level pain, use of pain medication, activity very limited— decreased function
8	
9	
10	Emergency Situation

Imaging Results

Plain film radiographs were taken last night after the incident and revealed no fractures.

Medications

Ibuprofen

Past Medical History (Please check any items that apply to you.)

Musculoskeletal:

- o Osteoarthritis
- o Rheumatoid Arthritis
- o Lupus/SLE
- o Fibromyalgia
- o Osteoporosis

Musculoskeletal (continued)

- o Headaches
- o Bulging Disc
- o Leg Cramps
- o Restless Legs
- o Jaw Pain/TMJ

Musculoskeletal (continued)

- o History of Falling
- o Use of Cane or Walker
- o Gout
- o Double Jointed

Other:_____

Neurological:	Endocrine (continued)	Cardiopulmonary (continued)
○ Stroke/TIA	⊗ Bladder Dysfunction	○ Shortness of Breath
○ Dementia	○ Liver Dysfunction	○ COPD
○ Polio	○ Thyroid Dysfunction	○ HIV/AIDS
○ Parkinson's Disease	Other:_____	Other:_____
○ Multiple Sclerosis		
○ Epilepsy/Seizures	**Cardiopulmonary:**	**Other:**
○ Concussion	○ Congestive Heart Failure	⊗ Anxiety
⊗ Numbness	○ Heart Arrhythmia	○ Depression
○ Tingling	○ Pacemaker	○ Cancer
Other:_____	○ High Cholesterol	
	○ Blood Clots	
Endocrine:	○ Anemia	
○ Diabetes	○ High Blood Pressure	
○ Kidney Dysfunction	○ Asthma	

Chief Complaint: *Low back pain (LBP)*
Goals for Therapy: *To reduce LBP.*
In the last week, how many days have you had pain? *1*
Pain worst: *Sitting and standing*

SANE Functional Rating

Please rate your **ability** to use your injured area on a 0 to 100% scale with **0%** being unable to use the injured area and **100%** being normal use of injured area in your daily activity: _____ *30%*

Also, if you exercise or have a sport activity or a job that requires special demands please rate your activity on the 0 to 100% scale: _____ *0%*

Patient-Specific Functional Scale

Please list **3 activities** that you find are difficult because of this problem and circle the number that corresponds with your ability to perform the activity.

	Unable								No limitations	
1. Sitting	1	2	③	4	5	6	7	8	9	10
2. Walking	1	2	3	4	5	⑥	7	8	9	10
3. Work	①	2	3	4	5	6	7	8	9	10

Unique Outcomes Measures

Oswestry Disability Index = 34/50 × 100 = 68%
Fear avoidance beliefs questionnaire physical activity subscale (FABQpa) = 20
Fear avoidance beliefs questionnaire work subscale (FABQw) = 32

Observation

The patient is 5 feet 8 inches and weighs 160 pounds (BMI = 24.3). He sits in the waiting room at the edge of his chair with shoulders leaning against back of chair; he slides to a half-kneel position on the floor and uses the arms of the chair to rise to a standing position. He moves in a slow, guarded manner when transitioning on and off the plinth.

Patient History

The patient reports that symptoms began yesterday evening when working in a warehouse. He has no previous history of LBP.

Mechanism: *The patient was on a platform getting a personal computer box off a high shelf when two such boxes began to fall. He states he moved quickly to prevent the boxes from falling when he noticed sudden LBP and left leg pain.*

Concordant Sign: *He indicates that the LBP and leg pain have been constantly present since onset and are worst with sitting, bending, or transitioning between positions.*

Nature of the Condition: *The 7/10 pain he reports in the low back and left leg began suddenly. The patient states he began to notice slight numbness in the saddle area a few hours after the incident. This morning he noticed difficulty emptying his bladder when sitting.*

Behavior of the Symptoms: *The pain increases as described above. The patient feels best when lying down. The numbness does not change with position changes.*

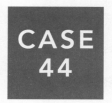

CASE 44

Setting: *Outpatient Orthopedics*

Date: *Present Day*

Medical Diagnosis: *Back Strain*

Charted Data

Name:	*Arvin Cheda*	General Health:	*Good*
Age:	*61 years*	Amount of Exercise:	*30 minutes/day, 3 days/week*
MRN:	*50602*	Occupation:	*Cook in high school cafeteria*
Home Address:	*917 Clarke Court, Tuttle, Oklahoma*	Household:	*Married; grown children live out of town*
Date of Injury:	*2 months ago*	Hand Dominance:	*Right*
New Injury:	*Yes*	Race	*Black*

Please fill in the location of your pain with a pencil.

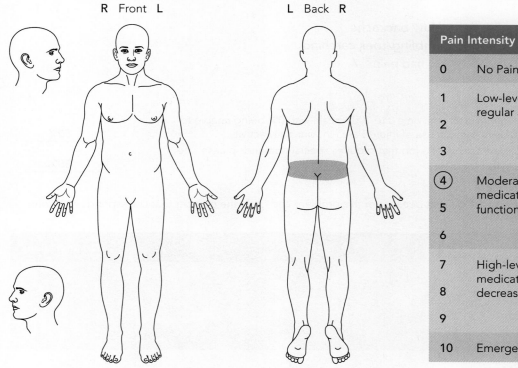

R Front L   L Back R

Pain Intensity Scale	
0	No Pain
1	Low-level pain, able to perform regular activities
2	
3	
④	Moderate-level pain, use of pain medication, activity limited but functional
5	
6	
7	High-level pain, use of pain medication, activity very limited— decreased function
8	
9	
10	Emergency Situation

Imaging Results

MR imaging of the lumbar spine suggests degenerative changes with mild central canal stenosis at L4/L5 and L5/S1.

Medications

Lopressor

Past Medical History (Please check any items that apply to you.)

Musculoskeletal:

- ○ Osteoarthritis
- ○ Rheumatoid Arthritis
- ○ Lupus/SLE
- ○ Fibromyalgia
- ○ Osteoporosis
- ○ Headaches
- ○ Bulging Disc
- ○ Leg Cramps
- ○ Restless Legs
- ○ Jaw Pain/TMJ
- ○ History of Falling
- ○ Use of Cane or Walker
- ○ Gout
- ○ Double Jointed

Other:_____

Neurological:

- ○ Stroke/TIA
- ○ Dementia
- ○ Polio

Neurological (continued)

- ○ Parkinson's Disease
- ○ Multiple Sclerosis
- ○ Epilepsy/Seizures
- ○ Concussion
- ○ Numbness
- ○ Tingling

Other:_____

Endocrine:

- ○ Diabetes
- ○ Kidney Dysfunction
- ○ Bladder Dysfunction
- ○ Liver Dysfunction
- ○ Thyroid Dysfunction

Other:_____

Cardiopulmonary:

- ○ Congestive Heart Failure
- ○ Heart Arrhythmia
- ○ Pacemaker

Cardiopulmonary (continued)

- ⊛ High Cholesterol
- ○ Blood Clots
- ○ Anemia
- ⊛ High Blood Pressure
- ○ Asthma
- ○ Shortness of Breath
- ○ COPD
- ○ HIV/AIDS

Other:_____

Other:

- ⊛ Anxiety
- ○ Depression
- ○ Cancer

Chief Complaint: *Ankle weakness and low backache*

Goals for Therapy: *To walk without stumbling/toes catching.*

In the last week, how many days have you had pain? *7*

Pain worst: *Standing at work*

SANE Functional Rating

Please rate your **ability** to use your injured area on a 0 to 100% scale with **0%** being unable to use the injured area and **100%** being normal use of injured area in your daily activity: *50%*

Also, if you exercise or have a sport activity or a job that requires special demands please rate your activity on the 0 to 100% scale: *30%*

Patient-Specific Functional Scale

Please list 3 activities that you find are difficult because of this problem and circle the number that corresponds with your ability to perform the activity.

	Unable								No limitations	
1. Standing at work	1	2	(3)	4	5	6	7	8	9	10
2. Walking	1	2	3	(4)	5	6	7	8	9	10
3. Bending	1	2	3	4	5	6	(7)	8	9	10

Unique Outcomes Measures

Oswestry disability index = 20/50 × 100 = 40% (moderate disability)

Fear avoidance beliefs questionnaire work subscale (FABQw) = 26

Observation

The patient is 5 feet 6 inches and weighs 180 pounds (BMI = 29) and is overweight. He expresses frustration in his short tolerance for standing and difficulty in ADLs and work activities. He demonstrates a flattened lumbar lordosis and reaches to countertop for support while standing in examination room.

Patient History

The patient complains of gradual onset of low backache over the past 1–2 months and his toes catching with walking over the past month. When the backache is more intense, his legs feel weaker and his toes catch on carpet and sometimes drag on the surface with walking.

Mechanism: *Backache and gait changes began gradually with insidious onset; however, the patient started back to work for the school-year about the same time the backache began. The job is a 4.5-hour shift that involves standing to prepare and serve food as well as cleaning the kitchen after the shift.*

Concordant Sign: *He indicates that his backache begins after being at work about 30 minutes and progressively worsens the longer he is standing or walking. The changes in walking are most noticeable after being at work 1–2 hours. He can't do yard work or go shopping after work because of difficulty walking and backache.*

Nature of the Condition: *The ache the patient reports is across the low back on both sides. He feels this pain could be tolerable but he is concerned about his toes dragging and fears falling. He denies bowel or bladder changes and denies any numbness or tingling.*

Behavior of the Symptoms: *Symptoms worsen with standing and walking and are relieved when the patient sits. He finds that pushing lunch trays on a cart at work is more comfortable than carrying them.*

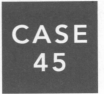

CASE 45

Setting: *Outpatient Orthopedic Clinic*

Date: *Present Day*

Medical Diagnosis: *Low Back Strain*

Charted Data

Name:	*Scott Liverpool*	New Injury:	*Yes*
Age:	*22 years*	General Health:	*Excellent*
MRN:	*50578*	Amount of Exercise:	*2 hours/day, 6 days/week*
Home Address:	*134 East Street, Atlanta, Georgia*	Occupation:	*Full-time student*
		Household:	*Resident in college dormitory*
Date of Injury:	*Progressive over 4 months*	Hand Dominance:	*Right*

Please fill in the location of your pain with a pencil.

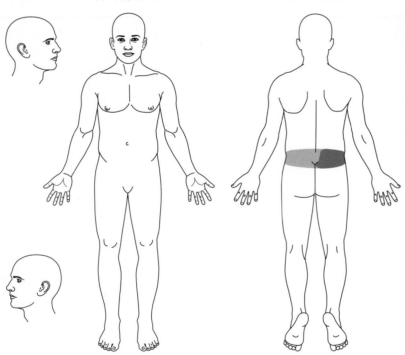

R Front L   L Back R

Pain Intensity Scale	
0	No Pain
1	Low-level pain, able to perform regular activities
2	
3	
4	Moderate-level pain, use of pain medication, activity limited but functional
5	
6	
⑦	High-level pain, use of pain medication, activity very limited— decreased function
8	
9	
10	Emergency Situation

Imaging Results
No imaging was performed prior to the initial examination.

Medications:
Ibuprofen 200-mg after playing racquetball

Past Medical History (Please check any items that apply to you.)
Unremarkable

Musculoskeletal:
- ○ Osteoarthritis
- ○ Rheumatoid Arthritis
- ○ Lupus/SLE
- ○ Fibromyalgia
- ○ Osteoporosis
- ○ Headaches
- ○ Bulging Disc
- ○ Leg Cramps
- ○ Restless Legs
- ○ Jaw Pain/TMJ
- ○ History of Falling
- ○ Use of Cane or Walker
- ○ Gout
- ○ Double Jointed

Other:_____

Neurological:
- ○ Stroke/TIA
- ○ Dementia

Neurological (continued)
- ○ Polio
- ○ Parkinson's Disease
- ○ Multiple Sclerosis
- ○ Epilepsy/Seizures
- ○ Concussion
- ○ Numbness
- ○ Tingling

Other:_____

Endocrine:
- ○ Diabetes
- ○ Kidney Dysfunction
- ○ Bladder Dysfunction
- ○ Liver Dysfunction
- ○ Thyroid Dysfunction

Other:_____

Cardiopulmonary:
- ○ Congestive Heart Failure
- ○ Heart Arrhythmia

Cardiopulmonary (continued)
- ○ Pacemaker
- ○ High Cholesterol
- ○ Blood Clots
- ○ Anemia
- ○ High Blood Pressure
- ○ Asthma
- ○ Shortness of Breath
- ○ COPD
- ○ HIV/AIDS

Other:_____

Other:
- ○ Anxiety
- ○ Depression
- ○ Cancer

Chief Complaint: *Daily intermittent low back pain (LBP) that was predominately right sided with occasional left-sided LBP*

Goals for Therapy: *To reduce the pain enough to allow athletic participation in racquetball.*

In the last week, how many days have you had pain? *7*

Pain worst: *After racquetball and prolonged sitting activities*

Numeric Pain Rating Scale (NPRS)[1,2]
The patient currently rates 4/10 but 7/10 at worst.

Visual Analog Scale (VAS)
This patient is currently at 43mm.

Patient-Specific Functional Scale
Please list 3 activities that you find are difficult because of this problem and circle the number that corresponds with your ability to perform the activity.

	Unable									No limitations
1. Prolonged sitting	1	2	3	(4)	5	6	7	8	9	10
2. Playing raquetball	1	2	(3)	4	5	6	7	8	9	10
3. Sleeping in LSL	1	2	3	4	(5)	6	7	8	9	10

Unique Outcome Measures
Oswestry disability index (ODI)[3] = 8/50 or 16% (minimal disability)

Observation

The patient is 181 cm and weighs 76.5 kg (BMI = 23.4). He presents with a minor lateral shift to the left in which his shoulders are positioned away from the more painful right side.

Patient History

The patient's LBP history consists of an initial episode 2.5 years prior to the current complaint that took place while playing racquetball. Since then, the patient has had episodic recurrences that are present less than half the days of the year. The current bout is of insidious onset and has been gradually progressing over the previous 4 months. Consistently, the back pain is exacerbated with playing racquetball. The patient has not received any medical care for his low back pain but does report use of ibuprofen after playing racquetball. The ibuprofen has become increasing less effective when his back pain is symptomatic.

Mechanism: *Flexion and rotation of the trunk to right or lateral bending of his trunk to the right.*

Concordant Sign: *The patient's concordant sign is playing racquetball, sitting in class, or driving.*

Nature of the Condition: *The patient's symptoms increased after 15 minutes of playing racquetball and lasted for 2–3 days after onset. He was able to sit during class or while driving for 30 minutes until symptoms began to increase. He scored a 16% on the ODI, indicating a minimal disability, and his current pain level on the NPRS is 4/10.*

Behavior of the Symptoms: *The pain worsens during racquetball, sitting, and sleeping with left side lying being most provocative. Standing and left side lying both reduce his symptoms.*

Endnotes

1. Roach KE, Brown MD, Dunigan KM, Kusek CL, Walas M. Test-retest reliability of patient reports of low back pain. J Orthop Sports Phys Ther. 1997;26:253–9.

2. Bolton JE. Accuracy of recall of usual pain intensity in back pain patients. Pain. 1999;83:533–9.

3. Fairbank JC, Couper J, Davies JB, O'Brien JP. The Oswestry low back pain disability questionnaire. Physiother. 1980;66:271–3.

CASE 46

Setting: *Outpatient Orthopedics*

Date: *Present Day*

Medical Diagnosis: *Upper Back Pain*

Charted Data

Name:	*Diane Pietzrach*	General Health:	*Good*
Age:	*52 years*	Amount of Exercise:	*15–30 minutes/day, 5 days/week (walking dog)*
MRN:	*77233*		
Home Address:	*540 153rd Street, Pike Rock, Minnesota*	Occupation:	*Baker*
		Household:	*Lives with husband*
Date of Injury:	*3 days ago*	Hand Dominance:	*Right*
New Injury:	*Yes*	Race	*Caucasian*

Please fill in the location of your pain with a pencil.

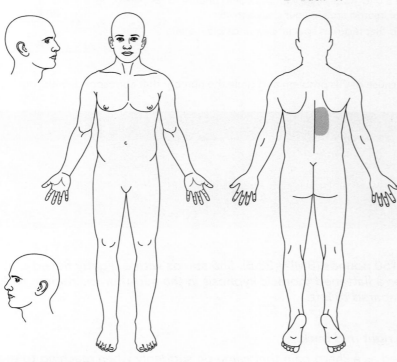

R Front L   L Back R

Pain Intensity Scale	
0	No Pain
1	Low-level pain, able to perform regular activities
2	
3	
4	Moderate-level pain, use of pain medication, activity limited but functional
(5)	
6	
7	High-level pain, use of pain medication, activity very limited—decreased function
8	
9	
10	Emergency Situation

Imaging Results

No imaging studies have been done on this patient.

Medications

Ibuprofen (PRN)

Past Medical History (Please check any items that apply to you.)

Musculoskeletal:
- ○ Osteoarthritis
- ○ Rheumatoid Arthritis
- ○ Lupus/SLE
- ○ Fibromyalgia
- ○ Osteoporosis

Musculoskeletal (continued)
- ⊗ Headaches
- ○ Bulging Disc
- ○ Leg Cramps
- ○ Restless Legs
- ○ Jaw Pain/TMJ

Musculoskeletal (continued)
- ○ History of Falling
- ○ Use of Cane or Walker
- ○ Gout
- ○ Double Jointed
- Other:_____

Neurological:
- o Stroke/TIA
- o Dementia
- o Polio
- o Parkinson's Disease
- o Multiple Sclerosis
- o Epilepsy/Seizures
- o Concussion
- o Numbness
- o Tingling

Other:_____

Endocrine:
- o Diabetes
- o Kidney Dysfunction

Endocrine (continued)
- o Bladder Dysfunction
- o Liver Dysfunction
- o Thyroid Dysfunction

Other:_____

Cardiopulmonary:
- o Congestive Heart Failure
- o Heart Arrhythmia
- o Pacemaker
- o High Cholesterol
- o Blood Clots
- o Anemia
- o High Blood Pressure
- o Asthma

Cardiopulmonary (continued)
- o Shortness of Breath
- o COPD
- o HIV/AIDS

Other:_____

Other:
- ⊗ Anxiety
- o Depression
- o Cancer

Chief Complaint: *Back pain*

Goals for Therapy: *To return to work and daily activities without pain.*

In the last week, how many days have you had pain? *3*

Pain worst: *Reaching overhead with right arm*

SANE Functional Rating

Please rate your **ability** to use your injured area on a 0 to 100% scale with **0%** being unable to use the injured area and **100%** being normal use of injured area in your daily activity: _____ *80%*

Also, if you exercise or have a sport activity or a job that requires special demands please rate your activity on the 0 to 100% scale: _____ *65%*

Patient-Specific Functional Scale

Please list 3 activities that you find are difficult because of this problem and circle the number that corresponds with your ability to perform the activity.

	Unable								No limitations	
1. Twisting to check traffic	1	2	(3)	4	5	6	7	8	9	10
2. Reaching with right arm	1	2	3	(4)	5	6	7	8	9	10
3. Breathing deeply	1	2	3	(4)	5	6	7	8	9	10

Observation

The patient is 5 feet 7 inches and weighs 150 pounds (BMI = 23.5). She stands with a slightly flexed cervicothoracic junction. She demonstrates a flattened thoracic kyphosis in the mid-thoracic region, and her right scapula is slightly protracted compared to left.

Patient History

The patient reports a localized pain in the right mid-back.

Mechanism: *The patient's symptoms started as a sharp pain that came on suddenly when reaching to the top shelf of a linen closet to place a blanket on an over-head shelf.*

Concordant Sign: *She indicates that a sudden sharp pain is present in the right upper back with over-head reaching or twisting her spine (especially while driving).*

Nature of the Condition: *The patient indicates that the sharp pain is accompanied by a sensation of a brief muscle spasm present in the same location. A deep ache is present in the same location when attempting to inhale deeply.*

Behavior of the Symptoms: *Once the sharp pain/spasm is present, the patient states that she gets relief from bending her trunk to the right and holding her right arm to her side. Pain also increases when taking a deep breath in or with resisted use of the right upper extremity, such as mixing batter or icing for cakes.*

Setting: *Outpatient Orthopedic Office*

Date: *Present Day*

Medical Diagnosis: *Lumbar Radiculopathy with Drop Foot (Right)*

Charted Data

Name:	*Tina Holland*	General Health:	*Poor*
Age:	*38 years*	Amount of Exercise:	*30 minutes/day, 2 days/ week*
MRN:	*34028*		
Home Address:	*978 Westchester Place, Kansas City, Missouri*	Occupation:	*Stay-at-home mother*
		Household:	*Married with 2 teenage daughters*
Date of Injury:	*1.5 months ago*		
New Injury:	*Insidious onset of low back pain with radicular symptoms and progressive development of right foot numbness and weakness*	Hand Dominance:	*Right*
		Race:	*Caucasian*

Please fill in the location of your pain with a pencil.

R Front L   L Back R

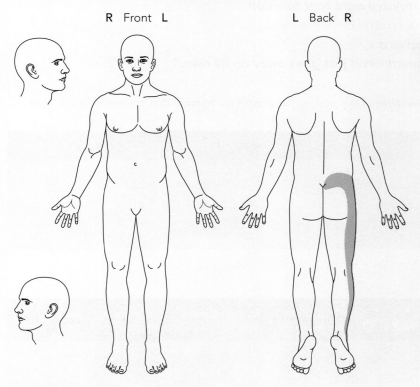

Pain Intensity Scale	
0	No Pain
1	Low-level pain, able to perform regular activities
2	
3	
4	Moderate-level pain, use of pain medication, activity limited but functional
⑤	
6	
7	High-level pain, use of pain medication, activity very limited— decreased function
8	
9	
10	Emergency Situation

Imaging Results

The patient had a MRI of her lumbar spine. The impression indicates abnormal fluid extending from the right-sided L4–5 and L5–S1 disc space posteriorly and just lateral to the spinous process. The etiology of this is uncertain. Abnormal signal previously noted in S1 and L5 has increased, but there is no evidence of a pathologic fracture or collapse of either of these vertebral bodies. This may represent neoplasia or post treatment changes.

Medications

10mg Lisinopril, 20mg Prilosec, 20mg Celexa

Past Medical History (Please check any items that apply to you.)

Musculoskeletal:
- ⊗ Osteoarthritis
- ○ Rheumatoid Arthritis
- ○ Lupus/SLE
- ○ Fibromyalgia
- ○ Osteoporosis
- ○ Headaches
- ○ Bulging Disc
- ○ Leg Cramps
- ○ Restless Legs
- ○ Jaw Pain/TMJ
- ○ History of Falling
- ○ Use of Cane or Walker
- ○ Gout
- ○ Double Jointed

Other:_____

Neurological:
- ○ Stroke/TIA
- ○ Dementia

Neurological (continued)
- ○ Polio
- ○ Parkinson's Disease
- ○ Multiple Sclerosis
- ○ Epilepsy/Seizures
- ○ Concussion
- ⊗ Numbness
- ○ Tingling

Other: _Drop foot_

Endocrine:
- ○ Diabetes
- ○ Kidney Dysfunction
- ○ Bladder Dysfunction
- ○ Liver Dysfunction
- ○ Thyroid Dysfunction

Other:_____

Cardiopulmonary:
- ○ Congestive Heart Failure
- ○ Heart Arrhythmia

Cardiopulmonary (continued)
- ○ Pacemaker
- ○ High Cholesterol
- ○ Blood Clots
- ○ Anemia
- ⊗ High Blood Pressure
- ○ Asthma
- ○ Shortness of Breath
- ○ COPD
- ○ HIV/AIDS

Other: _Chronic Ankle Swelling_

Other:
- ○ Anxiety
- ⊗ Depression
- ⊗ Cancer: Non-Hodgkins Lymphoma
- ○ Bipolar Disorder

Chief Complaint: _Low back pain (LBP) that causes sharp pains down the posterior right leg to the foot. Right foot numbness and significant weakness/clumsiness._

Goals for Therapy: _To decrease LBP and improve right foot function._

In the last week, how many days have you had pain? _7_

Pain worst: _When driving and bending forward_

Pain best: _When she "shakes it out"; "Sometimes it just goes away on its own."_

Patient-Specific Functional Scale

Please list 3 activities that you find are difficult because of this problem and circle the number that corresponds with your ability to perform the activity.

	Unable								No limitations	
1. Driving	①	2	3	4	5	6	7	8	9	10
2. Sitting activities	1	2	③	4	5	6	7	8	9	10
3. Standing activities	1	②	3	4	5	6	7	8	9	10

Unique Outcomes Measures
Pain Catastrophizing Scale

	Not at all	To a slight degree	To a moderate degree	To a great degree	All the time
I worry all the time about whether the pain will end.	0	1	2	③	4
I feel I can't go on.	⓪	1	2	3	4
It's terrible and I think it's never going to get any better.	0	1	②	3	4
It's awful and I feel that it overwhelms me.	0	①	2	3	4
I feel I can't stand it anymore.	0	①	2	3	4

	Not at all	To a slight degree	To a moderate degree	To a great degree	All the time
I become afraid that the pain will get worse.	0	(1)	2	3	4
I keep thinking of other painful events.	0	(1)	2	3	4
I anxiously want the pain to go away.	0	1	2	(3)	4
I can't seem to keep it out of my mind.	0	(1)	2	3	4
I keep thinking about how much it hurts.	0	(1)	2	3	4
I keep thinking about how badly I want the pain to stop.	0	(1)	2	3	4
There's nothing I can do to reduce the intensity of the pain.	0	(1)	2	3	4
I wonder whether something serious may happen.	(0)	1	2	3	4

Observation

The patient is 6 feet 2 inches and weighs 240 pounds (BMI = 30.8). She is seated with a left lateral lean in a standard chair.

Patient History

The patient reports that she noticed an insidious onset of low back and radicular pain approximately 1.5 months ago. She reports she has a history of low back pain and didn't think anything of this current episode. She thought she just threw something out of place. A week later she became more concerned when her right foot became "clumsy." She reports that she began to trip over "everything" and that activities such as prolonged driving would cause this foot to become "numb." When asked about her safety concerns while driving, she responded that her husband does not have a license and this is her only way to get around. She reports that driving and static positions make the numbness worse and that shaking her foot will help "wake it." The patient states that her physician ordered an MRI and wanted her to consult with a neurosurgeon, but she does not want to consider surgery at this time.

Mechanism: *Insidious onset. It is probable that direct tensioning and irritation of lower lumbar nerve roots could have resulted in the onset of symptoms.*

Concordant Sign: *The patient experiences a reproduction of pain along with sensory changes (numbness) of her right foot when placed into a "slump test" position.*

Nature of the Condition: *The symptoms appear to be acute in nature and are experienced by this patient when placed into a "slump test" position and resolve when she moves into extension. Her right foot weakness is constant.*

Behavior of the Symptoms: *This patient's symptoms would be classified in the category of "peripheral neuropathic" pain according to the "mechanism-based" classification system of pain.[1]*
  History of nerve injury, pathology or mechanical compromise
  Pain in a dermatomal or cutaneous distribution
  Pain/symptoms provocation with movement tests that move or compress neural tissue (ex. Straight Leg Raise)

Endnotes

1. Smart KM, Blake C, Staines A, et al. Self-reported pain severity, quality of life, disability, anxiety and depression in patients classified with nociceptive, peripheral neuropathic and central sensitisation pain. The discriminant validity of mechanism-based classification of low back (+-leg) pain. Man Ther. 2012;17:119–25.

CASE 48

Setting: *Acute Care Facility*

Date: *Present Day*

Medical Diagnosis: *Left Hip Osteoarthritis Status Post Total Hip Arthroplasty*

Charted Data

Name:	*Melinda Murray*
Age:	*57 years*
MRN:	*885678*
Home Address:	*21 Spring Street, Springfield, Massachusetts*
Date of Injury:	*1 day post-op*
New Injury:	*No, elective surgery*
General Health:	*Poor*
Amount of Exercise:	*0 hours/day, 0 days/week*
Occupation:	*Lunch lady*
Household:	*Married with 2 adult children living out of state*
Hand Dominance:	*Right*
Race:	*White*

20 pack-year smoking history, with multiple unsuccessful attempts to quit. She lives in a 1-story house with 5 steps to enter/exit her home. Patient was functionally independent prior to surgery at home and in the community using a straight cane

Current MD orders are for patient to be out of bed as tolerated with progressive activity in preparation for discharge. Patient can be weight bearing as tolerated (WBAT) on the left lower extremity (LLE).

Please fill in the location of your pain with a pencil.

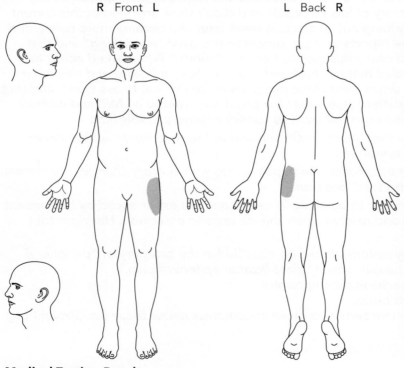

R Front L   L Back R

Pain Intensity Scale	
0	No Pain
1	Low-level pain, able to perform regular activities
2	
3	
④	Moderate-level pain, use of pain medication, activity limited but functional
5	
6	
7	High-level pain, use of pain medication, activity very limited— decreased function
8	
9	
10	Emergency Situation

Medical Testing Results

Prothrombin time/international normalized ratio (PT/INR) 2.5 (reference 0.9–1.1)[1]

- *Hemoglobin 11 (reference 12–16 g/100 ml)[1]*
- *Hematocrit 35 (reference 36%–47%)[1]*

Medications

Percocet, Lopressor, Vitamin D and Calcium supplements, Lovenox

Past Medical History (Please check any items that apply to you.)

Musculoskeletal:

- ⊗ Osteoarthritis
- ○ Rheumatoid Arthritis
- ○ Lupus/SLE
- ○ Fibromyalgia
- ⊗ Osteoporosis
- ○ Headaches
- ○ Bulging Disc
- ○ Leg Cramps
- ○ Restless Legs
- ○ Jaw Pain/TMJ
- ○ History of Falling
- ○ Use of Cane or Walker
- ○ Gout
- ○ Double Jointed

Other: *Carpal Tunnel Syndrome bilaterally*

Neurological:

- ○ Stroke/TIA
- ○ Dementia

Neurological (continued)

- ○ Polio
- ○ Parkinson's Disease
- ○ Multiple Sclerosis
- ○ Epilepsy/Seizures
- ○ Concussion
- ○ Numbness
- ○ Tingling

Other:_____

Endocrine:

- ○ Diabetes
- ○ Kidney Dysfunction
- ○ Bladder Dysfunction
- ○ Liver Dysfunction
- ○ Thyroid Dysfunction

Other:_____

Cardiopulmonary:

- ⊗ Hypertension
- ○ Coronary Artery Disease

Cardiopulmonary (continued)

- ○ Congestive Heart Failure
- ○ Heart Arrhythmia
- ○ Pacemaker
- ⊗ High Cholesterol
- ○ Blood Clots
- ○ Anemia
- ○ High Blood Pressure
- ○ Asthma
- ○ Shortness of Breath
- ○ COPD
- ○ HIV/AIDS

Other:_____

Other:

- ○ Anxiety
- ○ Depression
- ○ Cancer

Patient Presentation in Surgical Ward

The patient is 5 feet 2 inches and weighs 155 pounds (BMI = 28.3). She is lying in bed with the following equipment in place: lines and tubes: peripheral IV in left wrist, Foley catheter in place. Integumentary: Surgical incisions dressed and intact over left hip

Chief Complaint: *" I feel like a truck hit me."*

Goals for Therapy: *To be able to walk to the bathroom.*

In the last week, how many days have you had pain? *"My hip was killing me before surgery and honestly it's pretty sore now."*

Pain worst: *When medication wears off*

SANE Functional Rating

Please rate your **ability** to use your injured area on a 0 to 100% scale with **0%** being unable to use the injured area and **100%** being normal use of injured area in your daily activity: *30%*

Also, if you exercise or have a sport activity or a job that requires special demands please rate your activity on the 0 to 100% scale: *N/A*

Patient-Specific Functional Scale

Please list 3 activities that you find are difficult because of this problem and circle the number that corresponds with your ability to perform the activity.

	Unable								No limitations	
1. Walking	1	2	(3)	4	5	6	7	8	9	10
2. Standing	1	2	3	(4)	5	6	7	8	9	10
3. Moving in bed	1	2	(3)	4	5	6	7	8	9	10

Standardized Tests

Oxford hip score[2]
  Preoperatively = 48 points
  Postoperatively = 28 points
Timed up and go test (TUG) = 35 seconds (requires standard walker and contact guard *1 with verbal cueing for gait sequencing)

Endnotes

1. Acute Care Section Lab Values Resource Update 2012, American Physical Therapy Association.

2. Guide to Physical Therapist Practice, 2nd ed. American Physical Therapy Association. 200. S251–S267, S307–S313, S475–S483, S587–96.

Setting: *Home Health*

Date: *Present Day*

Medical Diagnosis: *Hip Pain*

Charted Data

Name:	*Blanche Kirkpatrick*	New Injury:	*No*
Age:	*79 years*	General Health:	*Poor*
MRN:	*50522*	Amount of Exercise:	*0 hours/day, 0 days/week*
Home Address:	*23 Akron Avenue, Birmingham, Alabama*	Occupation:	*Retired*
		Household:	*Lives at home with husband*
Date of Injury:	*3 months ago*	Hand Dominance:	*Right*
		Race:	*White*

Please fill in the location of your pain with a pencil.

R Front L   L Back R

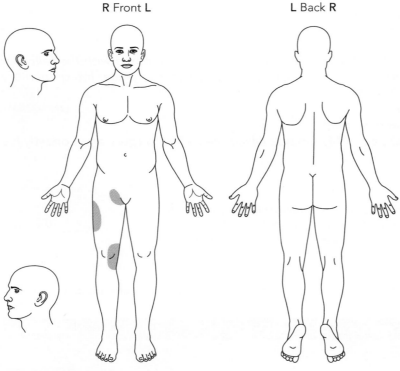

Pain Intensity Scale	
0	No Pain
1	Low-level pain, able to perform regular activities
2	
(3)	
4	Moderate-level pain, use of pain medication, activity limited but functional
5	
6	
7	High-level pain, use of pain medication, activity very limited—decreased function
8	
9	
10	Emergency Situation

Imaging Results

The patient has received radiographs of her right hip on two separate occasions, 9 months and 3 months ago. There were no fractures; however, there was reduced joint space in both her hips with subchondral bone sclerosis. The degeneration is worse in the right than left hip. Dexa exam indicates osteoporosis.

Past Medical History (Please check any items that apply to you.)

Musculoskeletal:

- ⊗ Osteoarthritis
- ○ Rheumatoid Arthritis
- ○ Lupus/SLE
- ○ Fibromyalgia
- ⊗ Osteoporosis
- ○ Headaches
- ○ Bulging Disc

Musculoskeletal (continued)

- ○ Leg Cramps
- ○ Restless Legs
- ○ Jaw Pain/TMJ
- ⊗ History of Falling
- ○ Use of Cane or Walker
- ○ Gout
- ○ Double Jointed

Other:_____

Neurological:

- ○ Stroke/TIA
- ○ Dementia
- ○ Polio
- ○ Parkinson's Disease
- ○ Multiple Sclerosis
- ○ Epilepsy/Seizures
- ○ Concussion
- ○ Numbness

Neurological (continued)

o Tingling

Other:_____

Endocrine:

o Diabetes
o Kidney Dysfunction
o Bladder Dysfunction
o Liver Dysfunction
o Thyroid Dysfunction

Other:_____

Cardiopulmonary:

o Congestive Heart Failure
o Heart Arrhythmia
o Pacemaker
o High Cholesterol
o Blood Clots
o Anemia
o High Blood Pressure
o Asthma
o Shortness of Breath

Cardiopulmonary (continued)

o COPD
o HIV/AIDS

Other:_____

Other:

o Anxiety
o Depression
o Cancer

Chief Complaint: *Difficulty walking*

Goals for Therapy: *To improve walking so that the patient is no longer house-bound.*

In the last week, how many days have you had pain? *7*

Pain worst: *During activity*

SANE Functional Rating

Please rate your **ability** to use your injured area on a 0 to 100% scale with **0%** being unable to use the injured area and **100%** being normal use of injured area in your daily activity: _____ 55% _____

Also, if you exercise or have a sport activity or a job that requires special demands please rate your activity on the 0 to 100% scale: _____ N/A _____

Patient-Specific Functional Scale

Please list 3 activities that you find are difficult because of this problem and circle the number that corresponds with your ability to perform the activity.

	Unable									No limitations
1. Walking	1	2	(3)	4	5	6	7	8	9	10
2. Stairs	1	2	3	(4)	5	6	7	8	9	10
3. Getting in the tub	1	2	3	4	(5)	6	7	8	9	10

Unique Outcomes Measures

Short form 36 (SF-36) = 32

Lower extremity functional scale (LEFS) = 28/80

Timed up and go (TUG) test (using a walker) = 18.4 seconds

Observation

The patient is 5 feet 5 inches and weighs 136 pounds (BMI = 22.6). Throughout the interview she does not walk and required assistance from sit to stand from her husband.

Patient History

The patient indicates a long-term decline in her health, which increased after experiencing a number of falls last year. There was no specific reason given for the falls but both the patient and her husband report that she just hasn't been herself and she loses her balance easily. Most falls occur while attempting to go to the bathroom during the night. The patient was institutionalized in a skilled nursing facility for short-term rehabilitation following a recent fall, but went home about 1 month ago. Since then, she hasn't walked on her own (except to the toilet) and has required help for all self-care activities from her husband.

Mechanism: *The patient indicates that she has some pain during standing but problems exist beyond this as well. She cannot identify a specific mechanism that caused the problem but did indicate bouts of dizziness about 1 year ago.*

Concordant Sign: *Full weight bearing on her right hip.*

Nature of the Condition: *Her condition is very debilitating. She can no longer care for herself nor can she prepare meals for her husband. She cannot bathe because of her inability to get into the bathtub.*

Behavior of the Symptoms: *The patient's condition has worsened since she has returned home. She improved some in the skilled nursing facility after receiving physical therapy.*

CASE 50

Setting: *Outpatient Orthopedics*

Date: *Present Day*

Medical Diagnosis: *Hip Pain*

Charted Data

Name:	*Hannah Robertson*	New Injury:	*Yes*
Age:	*28 years*	General Health:	*Good*
MRN:	*89345*	Amount of Exercise:	*1 hour/day, 4–5 days/week*
Home Address:	*1214 Oakcrest Street, Dublin, Georgia*	Occupation:	*Teacher*
		Household:	*Single*
Date of Injury:	*Insidious onset: 4 months ago*	Hand Dominance:	*Right*
		Race:	*White*

Please fill in the location of your pain with a pencil.

R Front L   L Back R

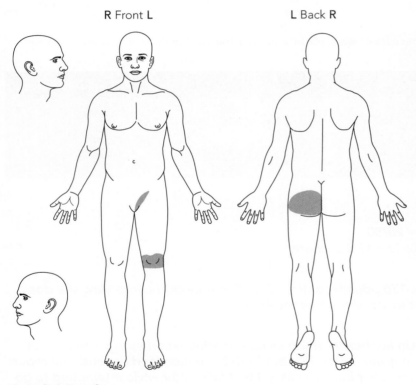

Pain Intensity Scale

0	No Pain
1	Low-level pain, able to perform regular activities
2	
3	
4	Moderate-level pain, use of pain medication, activity limited but functional
5	
6	
7	High-level pain, use of pain medication, activity very limited—decreased function
8	
(9)	
10	Emergency Situation

Imaging Results

A radiograph of the left hip indicated a cam-type lesion on the femoral head-neck junction with severe degeneration. An MRI will be performed if conservative physical therapy care proves ineffective.

Medications

Naproxen for pain relief

Past Medical History (Please check any items that apply to you.)

Musculoskeletal:

- ⊗ Osteoarthritis
- ○ Rheumatoid Arthritis
- ○ Lupus/SLE
- ○ Fibromyalgia
- ○ Osteoporosis
- ○ Headaches
- ⊗ Bulging Disc
- ○ Leg Cramps
- ○ Restless Legs
- ○ Jaw Pain/TMJ
- ○ History of Falling
- ○ Use of Cane or Walker
- ○ Gout
- ○ Double Jointed

Other: *ITB Syndrome, subluxing patella, ankle sprain*

Neurological:

- ○ Stroke/TIA
- ○ Dementia

Neurological (continued)

- ○ Polio
- ○ Parkinson's Disease
- ○ Multiple Sclerosis
- ○ Epilepsy/Seizures
- ○ Concussion
- ○ Numbness
- ○ Tingling

Other:_____

Endocrine:

- ○ Diabetes
- ○ Kidney Dysfunction
- ○ Bladder Dysfunction
- ○ Liver Dysfunction
- ○ Thyroid Dysfunction

Other:_____

Cardiopulmonary:

- ○ Congestive Heart Failure
- ○ Heart Arrhythmia

Cardiopulmonary (continued)

- ○ Pacemaker
- ○ High Cholesterol
- ○ Blood Clots
- ○ Anemia
- ○ High Blood Pressure
- ○ Asthma
- ○ Shortness of Breath
- ○ COPD
- ○ HIV/AIDS

Other:_____

Other:

- ○ Anxiety
- ○ Depression
- ○ Cancer

Chief Complaint: *Pain in the left buttock, groin, and distal quadriceps*

Goals for Therapy: *To continue workout regimen without pain.*

In the last week, how many days have you had pain? *7*

Pain worst: *With prolonged weight bearing*

SANE Functional Rating

Please rate your **ability** to use your injured area on a 0 to 100% scale with **0%** being unable to use the injured area and **100%** being normal use of injured area in your daily activity: ____*25%*____

Also, if you exercise or have a sport activity or a job that requires special demands please rate your activity on the 0 to 100% scale: ____*10%*____

Patient-Specific Functional Scale

Please list 3 activities that you find are difficult because of this problem and circle the number that corresponds with your ability to perform the activity.

	Unable									No limitations
1. Prolonged standing/walking	1	(2)	3	4	5	6	7	8	9	10
2. Climbing stairs	1	2	(3)	4	5	6	7	8	9	10
3. Aerobic exercise	1	(2)	3	4	5	6	7	8	9	10

Unique Outcomes Measures

Lower Extremity Functional Scale (LEFS) = 40/80

Observation

The patient is 5 feet 6 inches and weighs 169 pounds (BMI = 27.3), and she appears athletic. The patient ambulates with a mild antalgic gait, displays increased lumbar lordosis in standing, and displays bilateral pes planus.

Patient History

The patient reports a 4-month history of her pain that radiates from her buttock to her groin and distal quadriceps. She attributed the initial pain to a new workout regimen that included several repetitions of squats and lunges. However, the pain has persisted despite discontinuation of her workouts. She has seen a physical therapist that focused on flexibility and soft tissue mobilization, with no relief of symptoms. She has also seen several orthopedic surgeons who have recommended total hip arthroplasty (THA), but the patient would like to continue conservative treatment at this time. The patient is a full-time high school math teacher as well as a yoga instructor 3 nights a week.

Mechanism: *No specific mechanism of injury. The patient associates the initial pain with a new workout regimen.*

Concordant Sign: *The pain is described as a deep ache in the hip as well as burning and tightness in the buttocks and distal quadriceps.*

Nature of the Condition: *The patient indicates that rest and naproxen typically help to decrease the pain in all areas, but it worsens with prolonged weight bearing. Because the patient is a math teacher, she is often required to stand for long periods while instructing students. Thus, the pain is interfering with her performance as a teacher. She is also unable to work at her second job as a yoga instructor secondary to pain.*

Behavior of the Symptoms: *Any activity that requires prolonged weight bearing increases the patient's pain. This includes walking, jogging, and ascending and descending stairs. The pain decreases with rest but it never completely goes away.*

CASE 51

Setting: *Outpatient Orthopedics*

Date: *Present Day*

Medical Diagnosis: *Hamstring Cramps*

Charted Data

Name:	*Jack Hegden*	New Injury:	*Yes*
Age:	*27 years*	General Health:	*Good*
MRN:	*60187*	Amount of Exercise:	*90 minutes/day, 6 days/week*
Home Address:	*7563 Bruce Street, Fort Wayne, Indiana*	Occupation:	*Fireman*
		Household:	*Single, lives alone*
Date of Injury:	*Insidious onset about 1 year ago*	Hand Dominance:	*Right*
		Race:	*White*

Please fill in the location of your pain with a pencil.

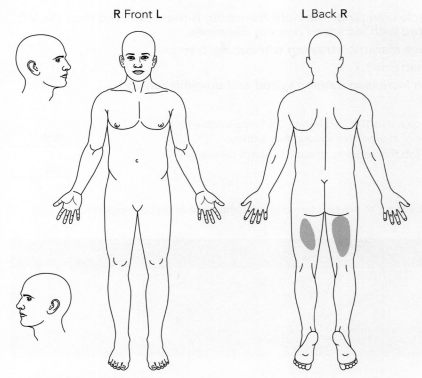

R Front L   L Back R

Pain Intensity Scale	
0	No Pain
1	Low-level pain, able to perform regular activities
2	
③	
4	Moderate-level pain, use of pain medication, activity limited but functional
5	
6	
7	High-level pain, use of pain medication, activity very limited—decreased function
8	
9	
10	Emergency Situation

Imaging Results
No imaging performed.

Medications
Ibuprofen (PRN), over-the-counter (OTC) multi-vitamins

Past Medical History (Please check any items that apply to you.)

Musculoskeletal:
- ○ Osteoarthritis
- ○ Rheumatoid Arthritis
- ○ Lupus/SLE
- ○ Fibromyalgia
- ○ Osteoporosis
- ○ Headaches
- ○ Bulging Disc
- ⊗ Leg Cramps
- ○ Restless Legs
- ○ Jaw Pain/TMJ
- ○ History of Falling
- ○ Use of Cane or Walker
- ○ Gout
- ○ Double Jointed

Other:_____

Neurological:
- ○ Stroke/TIA
- ○ Dementia

Neurological (continued)
- ○ Polio
- ○ Parkinson's Disease
- ○ Multiple Sclerosis
- ○ Epilepsy/Seizures
- ⊗ Concussion
- ○ Numbness
- ○ Tingling

Other:_____

Endocrine:
- ○ Diabetes
- ○ Kidney Dysfunction
- ○ Bladder Dysfunction
- ○ Liver Dysfunction
- ○ Thyroid Dysfunction

Other:_____

Cardiopulmonary:
- ○ Congestive Heart Failure
- ○ Heart Arrhythmia

Cardiopulmonary (continued)
- ○ Pacemaker
- ○ High Cholesterol
- ○ Blood Clots
- ○ Anemia
- ○ High Blood Pressure
- ○ Asthma
- ○ Shortness of Breath
- ○ COPD
- ○ HIV/AIDS

Other:_____

Other:
- ○ Anxiety
- ○ Depression
- ○ Cancer

Chief Complaint: *Bilateral hamstring muscle cramping. The right hamstring is more affected than the left hamstring. The symptoms are exacerbated with increased running distances.*

Goals for Therapy: *To return to competitive marathon training without leg cramps.*

In the last week, how many days have you had pain? *7*

Pain worst: *The pain reaches an 8/10 with increased running speed and downhill running.*

SANE Functional Rating

Please rate your **ability** to use your injured area on a 0 to 100% scale with **0%** being unable to use the injured area and **100%** being normal use of injured area in your daily activity: *70%*

Also, if you exercise or have a sport activity or a job that requires special demands please rate your activity on the 0 to 100% scale: *50%*

Patient-Specific Functional Scale

Please list 3 activities that you find are difficult because of this problem and circle the number that corresponds with your ability to perform the activity.

	Unable								No limitations	
1. Running	1	2	3	(4)	5	6	7	8	9	10
2. LE strength training	1	2	3	4	5	(6)	7	8	9	10
3. Going down stairs	1	2	3	4	5	6	(7)	8	9	10

Unique Outcomes Measures

Lower extremity functional scale (LEFS) = 56/80

Observation

The patient is 5 feet 11 inches and weighs 160 pounds (BMI = 22.3). He is overall in excellent health and in outstanding physical condition. The patient displays mild forward head and rounded shoulders. During gait, there is notable bilateral decreased knee extension in mid-stance and terminal swing.

Patient History

The patient has run several marathons over the past 10 years. He has been running competitively since he was 13 years old. He has experienced the hamstring cramping mainly in the right lower extremity during intense training periods. He saw a physical therapist after initial onset (about 1 year ago) who prescribed a general lower extremity flexibility program which he has continued to complete with no relief of symptoms. The patient also reports that he ensures maintenance of electrolyte levels during distance runs by supplementing with sports gels. When queried, the patient reports that the concussion is a very old work-related injury.

Mechanism: *There was no specific injury that precipitated the symptoms. The patient indicated only that increased training intensity brings his symptoms on.*

Concordant Sign: *The patient indicates that with downhill running and increased speed, he feels hamstring tightness begin, which develops into intense painful cramps.*

Nature of the Condition: *Once the hamstring cramps begin, they will typically escalate to an 8/10 pain and the patient has to discontinue running.*

Behavior of the Symptoms: *The symptoms worsen during running and other endurance training activities and subside once the patient discontinues activity and stretches.*

Setting: *Acute Care Hospital*

Date: *Present Day*

Medical Diagnosis: *Right Total Hip Arthroplasty*

Charted Data

Name:	*Michael Smith*	General Health:	*Good*
Age:	*68 years*	Amount of Exercise:	*30 minutes/day, 7 days/ week*
MRN:	*98954*		
Home Address:	*222 Jackson Street, Millersburg, Kentucky*	Occupation:	*Retired*
		Household:	*Single, lives alone*
Date of Injury:	*Surgery yesterday*	Hand Dominance:	*Right*
New Injury:	*Yes*	Race:	*White*

Please fill in the location of your pain with a pencil.

R Front L   L Back R

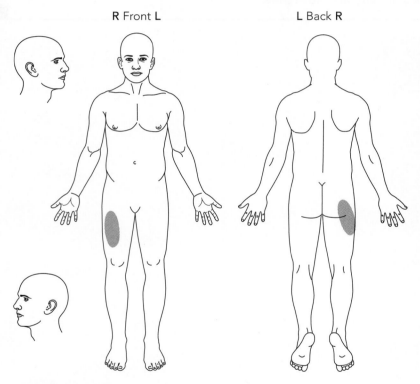

Pain Intensity Scale

0	No Pain
1 2 3	Low-level pain, able to perform regular activities
4 5 6	Moderate-level pain, use of pain medication, activity limited but functional
⑦ 8 9	High-level pain, use of pain medication, activity very limited—decreased function
10	Emergency Situation

Imaging Results

A radiograph of the right hip during surgery indicated proper alignment, no concerns noted.

Medications

Lipitor, Lopressor, and currently weaning off morphine for pain.

Past Medical History (Please check any items that apply to you.)

Musculoskeletal:
- ○ Osteoarthritis
- ○ Rheumatoid Arthritis
- ○ Lupus/SLE
- ○ Fibromyalgia
- ○ Osteoporosis

Musculoskeletal (continued)
- ○ Headaches
- ○ Bulging Disc
- ○ Leg Cramps
- ○ Restless Legs
- ○ Jaw Pain/TMJ

Musculoskeletal (continued)
- ○ History of Falling
- ○ Use of Cane or Walker
- ⊗ Gout
- ○ Double Jointed
- Other:_____

Neurological:
- ○ Stroke/TIA
- ○ Dementia
- ○ Polio
- ○ Parkinson's Disease
- ○ Multiple Sclerosis
- ○ Epilepsy/Seizures
- ○ Concussion
- ○ Numbness
- ○ Tingling

Other:_____

Endocrine:
- ○ Diabetes

Endocrine (continued)
- ○ Kidney Dysfunction
- ○ Bladder Dysfunction
- ○ Liver Dysfunction
- ○ Thyroid Dysfunction

Other:_____

Cardiopulmonary:
- ○ Congestive Heart Failure
- ○ Heart Arrhythmia
- ○ Pacemaker
- ⊗ High Cholesterol
- ○ Blood Clots
- ○ Anemia

Cardiopulmonary (continued)
- ⊗ High Blood Pressure
- ○ Asthma
- ○ Shortness of Breath
- ○ COPD
- ○ HIV/AIDS

Other:_____

Other:
- ○ Anxiety
- ○ Depression
- ⊗ Cancer-remission

Chief Complaint: *Right leg pain*

Goals for Therapy: *To return to normal activity.*

In the last week, how many days have you had pain? *7*

Pain worst: *End of the day prior to surgery; currently, everything hurts.*

SANE Functional Rating

Please rate your **ability** to use your injured area on a 0 to 100% scale with **0%** being unable to use the injured area and **100%** being normal use of injured area in your daily activity:

20%

Also, if you exercise or have a sport activity or a job that requires special demands please rate your activity on the 0 to 100% scale:

20% reported post-op

Patient-Specific Functional Scale

Please list 3 activities that you find are difficult because of this problem and circle the number that corresponds with your ability to perform the activity.

	Unable									No limitations
1. Getting out of bed	1	2	(3)	4	5	6	7	8	9	10
2. Walking	1	2	3	4	(5)	6	7	8	9	10
3. Going to the bathroom	1	2	3	(4)	5	6	7	8	9	10

Unique Outcomes Measures

Prior to Surgery: Oxford hip score = 10/48, indicating severe hip arthritis and may require surgical intervention
Lower extremity functional scale = 18/80

Observation

The patient is 6 feet 1 inch and weighs 176 pounds (BMI = 23.2). He appears to be a healthy male in decent physical condition. The patient is lying supine with the head of his bed minimally elevated with a wedge cushion in place. His entire right extremity is swollen and found to have about 2 cm of swelling in his right leg versus his left. The patient also has discoloration throughout the thigh of the right lower extremity.

Patient History

The patient's daughter reports that he is a very active retired firefighter. He walks 2 miles per day and lives alone but cares for himself without assistance. He also volunteers at a homeless shelter on a weekly basis. The patient began having increased hip pain about 3 years ago but did not want to have an operation and believed he could handle the pain.

Mechanism: *Although there was no specific incident that required this patient to have surgery, he noticed increased calf pain this morning.*

Concordant Sign: *The patient indicates that his pain is with any movement of his right lower extremity.*

Nature of the Condition: *The 7/10 pain he reports occurs throughout the day, but the calf pain is new.*

Behavior of the Symptoms: *Symptoms are worse in the morning since the surgery, and the patient reports beginning to experience stiffness in his legs as well as calf pain.*

CASE 53

Setting: *Outpatient Orthopedics*

Date: *Present Day*

Medical Diagnosis: *Anterior Knee Pain*

Charted Data

Name:	*Tiniqua Glasse*	General Health:	*Good*
Age:	*11 years*	Amount of Exercise:	*30 minutes/day, 2 days/week*
MRN:	*892812394*	Occupation:	*Student*
Home Address:	*92 Elm Street, Provo, Utah*	Household:	*Lives with both parents*
Date of Injury:	*Unknown*	Hand Dominance:	*Right*
New Injury:	*No; progressive*	Race:	*African American*

Please fill in the location of you pain with a pencil.

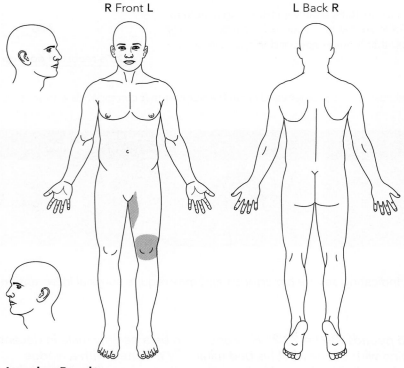

R Front L   L Back R

Pain Intensity Scale	
0	No Pain
1	Low- level pain, able to perform regular activities
2	
3	
4	Moderate-level pain, use of pain medication, activity limited but functional
5	
(6)	
7	High-level pain, use of pain medication, activity very limited—decreased function
8	
9	
10	Emergency Situation

Imaging Results

A radiograph of the knee yielded no bony abnormalities and proper alignment.

Medications

None prescribed. Occasionally takes Tylenol after gym class if exercise was very strenuous.

Past Medical History (Please check any items that apply to you.)

Unremarkable

Musculoskeletal:
- Osteoarthritis
- Rheumatoid Arthritis
- Lupus/SLE
- Fibromyalgia
- Osteoporosis
- Headaches

Musculoskeletal (continued)
- Bulging Disc
- Leg Cramps
- Restless Legs
- Jaw Pain/TMJ
- History of Falling
- Use of Cane or Walker

Musculoskeletal (continued)
- Gout
- Double Jointed

Other:_____

Neurological:
- Stroke/TIA

Neurological (continued)

- o Dementia
- o Polio
- o Parkinson's Disease
- o Multiple Sclerosis
- o Epilepsy/Seizures
- o Concussion
- o Numbness
- o Tingling

Other:_____

Endocrine:

- o Diabetes

Endocrine (continued)

- o Kidney Dysfunction
- o Bladder Dysfunction
- o Liver Dysfunction
- o Thyroid Dysfunction

Other:_____

Cardiopulmonary:

- o Congestive Heart Failure
- o Heart Arrhythmia
- o Pacemaker
- o High Cholesterol
- o Blood Clots

Cardiopulmonary (continued)

- o Anemia
- o High Blood Pressure
- o Asthma
- o Shortness of Breath
- o COPD
- o HIV/AIDS

Other:_____

Other:

- o Anxiety
- o Depression
- o Cancer

Chief Complaint: *Anterior knee pain that has been getting worse for several months*

Goals for Therapy: *To become pain free and be able to try out for team sports next year.*

In the last week, how many days have you had pain? *7*

Pain worst: *When walking and running*

SANE Functional Rating

Please rate your **ability** to use your injured area on a 0 to 100% scale with **0%** being unable to use the injured area and **100%** being normal use of injured area in your daily activity: *85%*

Also, if you exercise or have a sport activity or a job that requires special demands please rate your activity on the 0 to 100% scale: *75%*

Patient-Specific Functional Scale

Please list 3 activities that you find are difficult because of this problem and circle the number that corresponds with your ability to perform the activity.

	Unable								No limitations	
1. Playing basketball	1	2	3	4	(5)	6	7	8	9	10
2. Playing volleyball	1	2	3	4	(5)	6	7	8	9	10
3. Walking family dog	1	2	3	4	5	(6)	7	8	9	10

Unique Outcomes Measures

Lower extremity functional scale = 55/80

Observation

The patient is 4 feet 5 inches weighing 120 pounds (BMI = 30.0). She has a forward protruding abdomen and presents wearing well-fitted athletic shoes. In standing, she has reduced weight bearing on left lower extremity with foot forward and hip externally rotated. During ambulation she has decreased step length on the right, and left lateral trunk lean with single limb support on the left and the foot is held in an externally rotated position.

Patient History

The patient reports she has been having pain of an unspecified cause for several months; however, onset of pain did occur while wearing "shape-up" style athletic shoes. She reports she no longer wears those shoes, but does continue to have the knee pain, especially when involved in athletics at school. She enjoys playing basketball and volleyball in gym class but has concerns of feeling her leg will "give out" during running. The patient's mother stated that her daughter can no longer walk the family dog because her limp worsens with extended ambulation.

Mechanism: *Unknown*

Concordant Sign: *Running reproduces left anterior knee pain and left anteromedial hip pain.*

Nature of the Condition: *The patient has generalized weakness of left lower extremity and increased pain with physical activity.*

Behavior of the Symptoms; *The patient's symptoms of dull, aching pain at knee worsen with ambulation up to 6/10. Upon more vigorous activity, such as running or jumping, she has severe sharp groin pain of 8/10. Upon laying supine, she has relief of acute symptoms, but still feels a slight ache.*

CASE 54

Setting: *Outpatient Orthopedics*
Date: *Present Day*
Medical Diagnosis: *Right Hip Pain*

Charted Data

Name:	*Michael Dawson*	New Injury:	*Yes*
Age:	*55 years*	General Health:	*Good*
MRN:	*95943*	Amount of Exercise:	*15 minutes/day, 4 days/week*
Home Address:	*234 Miller Road, Bethlehem, Pennsylvania*	Occupation:	*Manual laborer*
		Household:	*Married*
		Hand Dominance:	*Left*
Date of Injury:	*4 months ago*	Race:	*White*

Please fill in the location of your pain with a pencil.

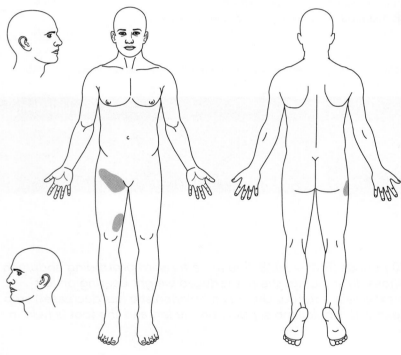

R Front L   L Back R

Pain Intensity Scale	
0	No Pain
1	Low-level pain, able to perform regular activities
2	
3	
(4)	Moderate-level pain, use of pain medication, activity limited but functional
5	
6	
7	High-level pain, use of pain medication, activity very limited—decreased function
8	
9	
10	Emergency Situation

Imaging Results

A radiograph of the right hip showed right hip joint space narrowing. The patient was then referred to physical therapy.

Medications:

Acetaminophen (PRN)

Past Medical History (Please check any items that apply to you.)

Musculoskeletal:
- ☒ Osteoarthritis
- ○ Rheumatoid Arthritis
- ○ Lupus/SLE
- ○ Fibromyalgia
- ○ Osteoporosis
- ○ Headaches

Musculoskeletal (continued)
- ○ Bulging Disc
- ○ Leg Cramps
- ○ Restless Legs
- ○ Jaw Pain/TMJ
- ○ History of Falling
- ○ Use of Cane or Walker

Musculoskeletal (continued)
- ○ Gout
- ○ Double Jointed
- Other:_____

Neurological:
- ○ Stroke/TIA
- ○ Dementia

Musculoskeletal (continued)

- ○ Polio
- ○ Parkinson's Disease
- ○ Multiple Sclerosis
- ○ Epilepsy/Seizures
- ○ Concussion
- ○ Numbness
- ○ Tingling

Other:_____

Endocrine:

- ○ Diabetes
- ○ Kidney Dysfunction

Endocrine (continued)

- ○ Bladder Dysfunction
- ○ Liver Dysfunction
- ○ Thyroid Dysfunction

Other:_____

Cardiopulmonary:

- ○ Congestive Heart Failure
- ○ Heart Arrhythmia
- ○ Pacemaker
- ⊗ High Cholesterol
- ○ Blood Clots
- ○ Anemia

Cardiopulmonary (continued)

- ○ High Blood Pressure
- ○ Asthma
- ○ Shortness of Breath
- ○ COPD
- ○ HIV/AIDS

Other:_____

Other:

- ⊗ Anxiety
- ○ Depression
- ○ Cancer

Chief Complaint: *Right hip pain*

Goals for Therapy: *To reduce hip pain.*

In the last week, how many days have you had pain? *7*

Pain worst: *Prolonged periods of standing and walking*

SANE Functional Rating

Please rate your **ability** to use your injured area on a 0 to 100% scale with **0%** being unable to use the injured area and **100%** being normal use of injured area in your daily activity: _75%_

Also, if you exercise or have a sport activity or a job that requires special demands please rate your activity on the 0 to 100% scale: _75%_

Patient-Specific Functional Scale

Please list 3 activities that you find are difficult because of this problem and circle the number that corresponds with your ability to perform the activity.

	Unable									No limitations
1. Walking	1	2	3	4	5	(6)	7	8	9	10
2. Stair negotiation	1	2	3	4	(5)	6	7	8	9	10
3. Sleeping	1	2	3	4	5	6	(7)	8	9	10

Unique Outcomes Measures

Western Ontario and McMaster Universities Arthritis Index (WOMAC) = 50/96

Harris hip score (HHS) = 52/100

Observation

The patient is 6 feet 1 inch and weighs 245 pounds (BMI = 32.3) and is considered obese. He ambulates with a cane and has a pronounced antalgic gait. There is a positive Trendelenburg's sign on the right hip observed. He has a shorter stride length and stance phase on the right lower extremity.

Patient History

The patient was unable to recall any specific mechanism of injury. He has been unable to attend his usual aerobic exercise classes for the last 2 months due to pain. His usual on-the-job walking has also decreased over the past 2 months as his pain has increased. There are no reports of clicking or popping in the right hip. The patient went to his primary care physician and radiographs were taken; the radiographs demonstrated joint space narrowing in the right hip. The patient reports he is a manual laborer at a local steel mill. He reports pain in right groin area, radiating into the right anterior thigh.

Mechanism: *No specific mechanism of injury was reported by the patient. There was an insidious onset.*

Concordant Sign: *The patient indicates hip pain increases with standing for prolonged periods, walking, rising and sitting into a chair, and when negotiating stairs.*

Nature of the Condition: *The 4/10 pain he reports is constant. He reports that pain levels increase at the end of the day, and that morning stiffness in right hip resolves within an hour of being up.*

Behavior of the Symptoms: *The patient's symptoms worsen during prolonged standing and walking. His pain is relieved by lying supine or sitting.*

Setting: *Inpatient Orthopedics*

Date: *Present Day*

Medical Diagnosis: *Open Reduction Internal Fixation of Right Proximal Femur*

Charted Data

Name:	*Della Dalmus*	General Health:	*Good*
Age:	*72 years*	Amount of Exercise:	*30 minutes/day, 2–3 days/ week*
MRN:	*51104*	Occupation:	*Retired, volunteers at her church*
Home Address:	*1112 South Forest Beach Drive, Hilton Head Island, South Carolina*	Household:	*Widowed, lives alone at home*
Date of Injury:	*4 days ago*	Hand Dominance:	*Right*
New Injury:	*Yes*	Race:	*Black*

Please fill in the location of your pain with a pencil.

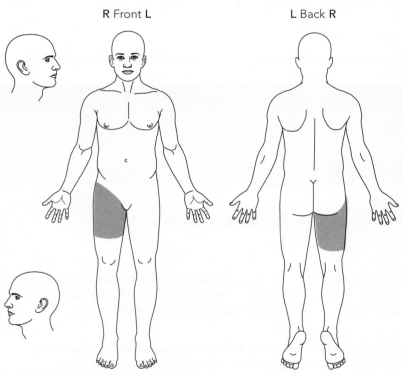

R Front L   L Back R

Pain Intensity Scale

0	No Pain
1	Low-level pain, able to perform regular activities
2	
3	
4	Moderate-level pain, use of pain medication, activity limited but functional
(5)	
6	
7	High-level pain, use of pain medication, activity very limited—decreased function
8	
9	
10	Emergency Situation

Imaging Results

Radiograph of the right hip joint and femur yields a facture in the right femoral neck, with an intramedullary rod to stabilize the bone, as well as presence of osteoarthritic and osteoporotic age-related changes.

Surgical Results

Open reduction internal fixation to right femoral neck using an intramedullary rod. No surgical complications noted.

Postsurgical Precautions

Weight bearing as tolerated on right lower extremity.

Medications

Hydrocodone (PRN), donepezil, warfarin

Past Medical History (Please check any items that apply to you.)

Musculoskeletal:

- ⊗ Osteoarthritis
- ○ Rheumatoid Arthritis
- ○ Lupus/SLE
- ○ Fibromyalgia
- ⊗ Osteoporosis
- ○ Headaches
- ○ Bulging Disc
- ○ Leg Cramps
- ○ Restless Legs
- ○ Jaw Pain/TMJ
- ⊗ History of Falling
- ⊗ Use of Cane or Walker
- ○ Gout
- ○ Double Jointed

Other:_____

Neurological:

- ○ Stroke/TIA
- ⊗ Dementia

Neurological (continued)

- ○ Polio
- ○ Parkinson's Disease
- ○ Multiple Sclerosis
- ○ Epilepsy/Seizures
- ○ Concussion
- ○ Numbness
- ○ Tingling

Other:_____

Endocrine:

- ○ Diabetes
- ○ Kidney Dysfunction
- ○ Bladder Dysfunction
- ○ Liver Dysfunction
- ○ Thyroid Dysfunction

Other:_____

Cardiopulmonary:

- ○ Congestive Heart Failure

Cardiopulmonary (continued)

- ○ Heart Arrhythmia
- ○ Pacemaker
- ○ High Cholesterol
- ⊗ Blood Clots
- ○ Anemia
- ○ High Blood Pressure
- ○ Asthma
- ○ Shortness of Breath
- ○ COPD
- ○ HIV/AIDS

Other:_____

Other:

- ○ Anxiety
- ○ Depression
- ○ Cancer

Chief Complaint: *Right hip pain from the right hip open reduction internal fixation (ORIF) after tripping on a rug and falling at home.*

Goals for Therapy: *To reduce hip pain and to be able to walk and get around at home (12 stairs).*

In the last week, how many days have you had pain? *7*

Pain worst: *All movements of the hip*

SANE Functional Rating

Please rate your **ability** to use your injured area on a 0 to 100% scale with **0%** being unable to use the injured area and **100%** being normal use of injured area in your daily activity: _____ *0%*

Patient-Specific Functional Scale

Please list 3 activities that you find are difficult because of this problem and circle the number that corresponds with your ability to perform the activity.

	Unable									No limitations
1. Walk	(1)	2	3	4	5	6	7	8	9	10
2. Rolling in bed	1	2	(3)	4	5	6	7	8	9	10
3. Transferring	(1)	2	3	4	5	6	7	8	9	10

Unique Outcomes Measures

Functional independence measure (FIM) = A score of 2 on all physical therapy scoring sections (maximal assistance: patient can perform 25% to 49% of task).

Observation

The patient is 5 feet 2 inches and weighs 115 pounds (BMI = 21). She is petite, has moderate thoracic kyphosis, and is anxious with any right hip movement secondary to pain.

Patient History

The patient reports increasing discomfort in her bilateral hip joints over the past several years. She states that she tripped over a rug in her kitchen and fell at home 4 days ago. She was unable to get up off the floor so she hit her Life Alert button. She was taken to the local hospital by ambulance and was attended to in the emergency department. Radiographs were taken and showed a right femoral neck fracture. The next day the patient underwent an ORIF of the right femur. The patient has mild dementia at this point and occasional memory loss and gets confused when she is asked to follow multi-step commands. Family members have confirmed that she can get slightly agitated when she realizes that she is having difficulty with memory.

Mechanism: *Fracture from falling on right hip.*

Concordant Sign: *The patient indicates that her pain is initiated after any movement of the hip.*

Nature of the Condition: *She reports 7–8/10 pain with movement and 4/10 pain at rest.*

Behavior of the Symptoms: *She indicates that her pain is increased after any movement of the hip and the pain worsens throughout the day or when pain medication wears off. Her symptoms lessen with rest in the supine position and with pain medication.*

CASE 56

Setting: *Outpatient Orthopedic Office*

Date: *Present Day*

Medical Diagnosis: *Chronic Low Back, Buttock, Hip, and Thigh Pain*

Charted Data

Name:	*Stephanie Wu*	New Injury:	*Pain increased 6 weeks ago*
Age:	*20 years*	General Health:	*Excellent*
MRN:	*32089*	Amount of Exercise:	*2–3 hours/day, 7 days/ week*
Home Address:	*213 Amethyst Cr., Sedona, Arizona*	Occupation:	*Student*
Date of Injury:	*No specific injury date, progressive onset over 2 years*	Household:	*Lives with two roommates in a 2nd-floor flat*
		Hand Dominance:	*Right*
		Race:	*Asian*

Please fill in the location of your pain with a pencil.

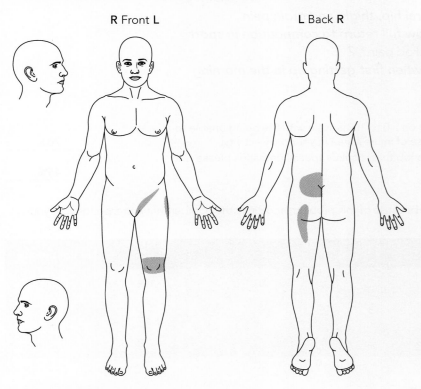

R Front L   L Back R

Pain Intensity Scale

0	No Pain
1	Low-level pain, able to perform regular activities
2	
3	
4	Moderate-level pain, use of pain medication, activity limited but functional
5	
6	
(7)	High-level pain, use of pain medication, activity very limited—decreased function
8	
9	
10	Emergency Situation

Imaging Results

Radiographs were negative for pathology in the hip. Lumbar spine imaging revealed mild degenerative changes.

Medications

Aspirin (PRN), Xanax

Past Medical History (Please check any items that apply to you.)

Musculoskeletal:
- ○ Osteoarthritis
- ○ Rheumatoid Arthritis
- ○ Lupus/SLE
- ○ Fibromyalgia
- ○ Osteoporosis
- ⊗ Headaches
- ○ Bulging Disc
- ○ Leg Cramps
- ○ Restless Legs
- ○ Jaw Pain/TMJ
- ○ History of Falling
- ○ Use of Cane or Walker
- ○ Gout
- ○ Double Jointed

Other:_____

Neurological:
- ○ Stroke/TIA
- ○ Dementia

Neurological (continued)
- ○ Polio
- ○ Parkinson's Disease
- ○ Multiple Sclerosis
- ○ Epilepsy/Seizures
- ○ Concussion
- ○ Numbness
- ○ Tingling

Other:_____

Endocrine:
- ○ Diabetes
- ○ Kidney Dysfunction
- ○ Bladder Dysfunction
- ○ Liver Dysfunction
- ○ Thyroid Dysfunction

Other:_____

Cardiopulmonary:
- ○ Congestive Heart Failure

Cardiopulmonary (continued)
- ○ Heart Arrhythmia
- ○ Pacemaker
- ○ High Cholesterol
- ○ Blood Clots
- ○ Anemia
- ○ High Blood Pressure
- ○ Asthma
- ○ Shortness of Breath
- ○ COPD
- ○ HIV/AIDS

Other:_____

Other:
- ⊗ Anxiety
- ○ Depression
- ○ Cancer
- ○ Bipolar Disorder

Chief Complaint: *Chronic low back, lateral hip, thigh, and groin pain*

Goals for Therapy: *To reduce pain to allow full return to competition in sport*

In the last week, how many days have you had pain? *7*

Pain worst: *During training, sometimes when first getting up in the morning*

Pain best: *During periods of rest*

SANE Functional Rating

Please rate your **ability** to use your injured area on a 0 to 100% scale with **0%** being unable to use the injured area and **100%** being normal use of injured area in your daily activity: 70%

Also, if you exercise or have a sport activity or a job that requires special demands please rate your activity on the 0 to 100% scale: 45%

Patient-Specific Functional Scale

Please list 3 activities that you find are difficult because of this problem and circle the number that corresponds with your ability to perform the activity.

	Unable								No limitations	
1. Running	1	2	③	4	5	6	7	8	9	10
2. Cross-training	1	2	3	4	⑤	6	7	8	9	10
3. Climbing stairs	1	2	3	④	5	6	7	8	9	10

Unique Outcomes Measures

Lower extremity functional scale = 59/80

Observation

The patient is 5 feet 3 inches and weighs 103 pounds (BMI = 18.2). She is very thin but has an athletic build with excellent lower body tone and a very skinny upper body. She appears in excellent condition and is seated in a slouched runner's posture.

Patient History

The patient indicates she has a history of low back pain that started a couple of years ago but it has been very manageable. She states that she has had numerous running injuries over the years and reports that whenever her weekly mileage is over 110 she usually experiences some form of physical breakdown. She has had shin splints, plantar fasciitis, hip pain, and anterior knee pain, but she can usually manage the problems with rest and conservative care. This time, the pain has been more significant and she has not been able to bring it down with rest and NSAIDS. Her physician ordered radiographs and referred her to this clinic. She reports a snapping sensation in the front of her hip that is painful in the groin region. During the subjective examination, when asked about her eating habits, she stated that she eats regularly and enough. When questioned, she reported menstrual cycle disturbances and that she currently has amenorrhea.

Mechanism: *This new pain been present for 6 weeks and is aggravated by running long distances, climbing stairs, and other weight-bearing activities. The exact mechanism is yet to be determined.*

Concordant Sign: *Repetitive weight-bearing activities. The longer she performs them, the worse the pain gets.*

Nature of the Condition: *This condition is worse than a nuisance but not really disabling, since the patient is limited to less than half her usual mileage, but she is able to perform normal activities of daily living. However, the symptoms are getting worse and weight bearing is gradually getting very limited.*

Behavior of the Symptoms: *Symptoms can be bad in the morning with first weight bearing but generally ease a little before increasing as the day's activities increase. The behavior of the symptoms has increased from unpleasant to very painful and almost constant.*

CASE 57

Setting: *Inpatient Orthopedics*

Date: *Present Day*

Medical Diagnosis: *Recurrent Hamstring Pulls*

Charted Data

Name:	*Pedro Rodriguez*	General Health:	*Excellent*
Age:	*26 years*	Amount of Exercise:	*2 hours/day, 6–7 days/ week*
MRN:	*91629*	Occupation:	*Semi-professional baseball player*
Home Address:	*2966 West Main Street, Fort Lauderdale, Florida*	Household:	*Lives alone in a 2nd-floor apartment*
Date of Injury:	*9 days ago*	Hand Dominance:	*Right*
New Injury:	*No, fourth episode in 2 years*	Race:	*Hispanic*

Please fill in the location of your pain with a pencil.

R Front L   L Back R

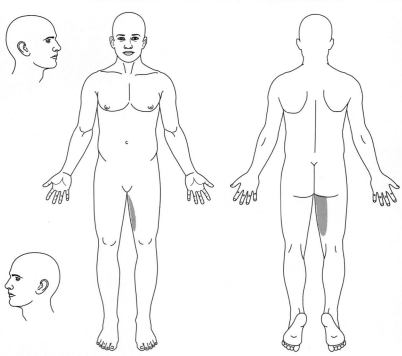

Pain Intensity Scale	
0	No Pain
1	Low-level pain, able to perform regular activities
2	
3	
4	Moderate-level pain, use of pain medication, activity limited but functional
(5)	
6	
7	High-level pain, use of pain medication, activity very limited— decreased function
8	
9	
10	Emergency Situation

Imaging Results
None performed.

Medications
Aleve PRN

Past Medical History (Please check any items that apply to you.)

Musculoskeletal:
- ○ Osteoarthritis
- ○ Rheumatoid Arthritis
- ○ Lupus/SLE
- ○ Fibromyalgia
- ○ Osteoporosis

Musculoskeletal (continued)
- ○ Headaches
- ○ Bulging Disc
- ○ Leg Cramps
- ○ Restless Legs
- ○ Jaw Pain/TMJ

Musculoskeletal (continued)
- ○ History of Falling
- ○ Use of Cane or Walker
- ○ Gout
- ○ Double Jointed

Other: *ankle sprains*

Neurological:
- o Stroke/TIA
- o Dementia
- o Polio
- o Parkinson's Disease
- o Multiple Sclerosis
- o Epilepsy/Seizures
- o Concussion
- o Numbness
- o Tingling

Other:_____

Endocrine:
- o Diabetes
- o Kidney Dysfunction

Endocrine (continued)
- o Bladder Dysfunction
- o Liver Dysfunction
- o Thyroid Dysfunction

Other:_____

Cardiopulmonary:
- o Congestive Heart Failure
- o Heart Arrhythmia
- o Pacemaker
- o High Cholesterol
- o Blood Clots
- o Anemia
- o High Blood Pressure
- o Asthma

Cardiopulmonary (continued)
- o Shortness of Breath
- o COPD
- o HIV/AIDS

Other:_____

Other:
- o Anxiety
- o Depression
- o Cancer

Chief Complaint: *Pain in the posterior right thigh that is easily exacerbated by sprinting*

Goals for Therapy: *To reduce posterior right thigh pain and return to sprinting and weight-lifting activities without difficulty.*

In the last week, how many days have you had pain? *5*

Pain worst: *The day after heavy weight lifting like squatting and/or sprinting*

SANE Functional Rating

Please rate your **ability** to use your injured area on a 0 to 100% scale with **0%** being unable to use the injured area and **100%** being normal use of injured area in your daily activity: 85%

Also, if you exercise or have a sport activity or a job that requires special demands please rate your activity on the 0 to 100% scale: 40%

Patient-Specific Functional Scale

Please list 3 activities that you find are difficult because of this problem and circle the number that corresponds with your ability to perform the activity.

	Unable									No limitations
1. Sprinting	1	2	3	4	5	6	(7)	8	9	10
2. Heavy squatting	1	2	3	(4)	5	6	7	8	9	10
3. Playing baseball	1	2	3	4	5	6	(7)	8	9	10

Unique Outcomes Measures:

Lower extremity functional scale = 70/80

Observation

The patient is 6 feet 1 inch and weighs 215 pounds (BMI = 28.4). He is a very fit and muscular man who does not at all appear overweight, as the BMI score would imply since his body fat percentage would appear to be <10%.

Patient History

The patient reports a 2-year history of repeated right hamstring injuries that began with a pull during outfield practice. The original injury mostly healed but he continued to have some posterior thigh aching with weight lifting and/or sprints. Subsequently, the hamstring has been reinjured 4–5 times. Currently, the posterior thigh aches with heavy squatting and the ache also includes the medial thigh and results in delayed onset muscle soreness that lasts 1–2 days post exercise, making it very difficult to get daily training accomplished.

Mechanism: *Sprinting*

Concordant Sign: *Pain is increased with any activity that either maximally stretches the hamstrings or requires very strong muscular contractions repetitively, especially eccentric contractions.*

Nature of the Condition: *The patient reports 5/10 pain with aggravating activities, especially on the following day, but can be 0/10 most of the time.*

Behavior of the Symptoms: *Symptoms are highly dependent on the amount of activity that is required and how hard the patient pushes himself physically. Any deep squatting can give him symptoms, and as he increases the resistance, the symptoms get worse.*

CASE 58

Setting: *Outpatient Orthopedic Office*

Date: *Present Day*

Medical Diagnosis: *Lateral Hip and Thigh Pain*

Charted Data

Name:	*Monica Smith*	New Injury:	*Pain increased 1 month ago*
Age:	*22 years*	General Health:	*Excellent*
MRN:	*34891*	Amount of Exercise:	*90 minutes/day, 6 days/week*
Home Address:	*717 Baseline Road, Lincoln, Nebraska*	Occupation:	*Student*
		Household:	*Lives in dormitory with a roommate*
Date of Injury:	*No specific injury date, progressive onset 1.5 years*	Hand Dominance:	*Right*
		Race:	*Caucasian*

Please fill in the location of your pain with a pencil.

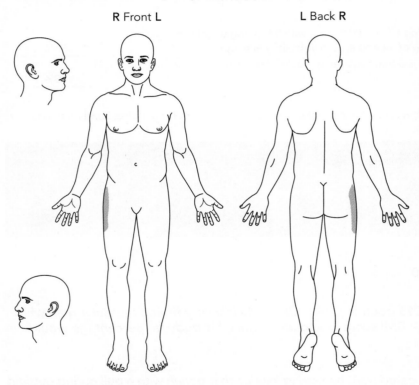

R Front L   L Back R

Pain Intensity Scale	
0	No Pain
1	Low-level pain, able to perform regular activities
2	
3	
4	Moderate-level pain, use of pain medication, activity limited but functional
5	
⑥	
7	High-level pain, use of pain medication, activity very limited—decreased function
8	
9	
10	Emergency Situation

Imaging Results

Radiographs were negative for significant pathology in the hip but the patient was told that there is some evidence of mild degenerative disc changes in her lower lumbar spine.

Medications

Aleve (PRN)

Past Medical History (Please check any items that apply to you.)
Unremarkable

Musculoskeletal:
- ○ Osteoarthritis
- ○ Rheumatoid Arthritis
- ○ Lupus/SLE
- ○ Fibromyalgia
- ○ Osteoporosis
- ○ Headaches
- ○ Bulging Disc
- ○ Leg Cramps
- ○ Restless Legs
- ○ Jaw Pain/TMJ
- ○ History of Falling
- ○ Use of Cane or Walker
- ○ Gout
- ○ Double Jointed

Other:_____

Neurological:
- ○ Stroke/TIA
- ○ Dementia

Neurological (continued)
- ○ Polio
- ○ Parkinson's Disease
- ○ Multiple Sclerosis
- ○ Epilepsy/Seizures
- ○ Concussion
- ○ Numbness
- ○ Tingling

Other:_____

Endocrine:
- ○ Diabetes
- ○ Kidney Dysfunction
- ○ Bladder Dysfunction
- ○ Liver Dysfunction
- ○ Thyroid Dysfunction

Other:_____

Cardiopulmonary:
- ○ Congestive Heart Failure
- ○ Heart Arrhythmia

- ○ Pacemaker
- ○ High Cholesterol
- ○ Blood Clots
- ○ Anemia
- ○ High Blood Pressure
- ○ Asthma
- ○ Shortness of Breath
- ○ COPD
- ○ HIV/AIDS

Other:_____

Other:
- ○ Anxiety
- ○ Depression
- ○ Cancer
- ○ Bipolar Disorder

Chief Complaint: *Lateral hip and thigh pain*

Goals for Therapy: *To reduce pain to allow full participation in sport.*

In the last week, how many days have you had pain? *7*

Pain worst: *During training or when lying on the involved hip*

Pain best: *During periods of rest*

SANE Functional Rating
Please rate your **ability** to use your injured area on a 0 to 100% scale with **0%** being unable to use the injured area and **100%** being normal use of injured area in your daily activity: _*80%*_

Also, if you exercise or have a sport activity or a job that requires special demands please rate your activity on the 0 to 100% scale: _*50%*_

Patient-Specific Functional Scale
Please list 3 activities that you find are difficult because of this problem and circle the number that corresponds with your ability to perform the activity.

	Unable									No limitations
1. Running	1	2	3	4	5	6	(7)	8	9	10
2. Jumping	1	2	3	4	(5)	6	7	8	9	10
3. Lying on the hip	1	(2)	3	4	5	6	7	8	9	10

Unique Outcomes Measures
Lower extremity functional scale = 68/80

Observation
The patient is 5 feet 6 inches and weighs 133 pounds (BMI = 21.5). She appears very athletic and in excellent condition and is seated on the treatment table in a slouched posture.

Patient History

The patient indicates she has a history of low back pain but this has not been a problem nor has it limited her daily participation in sport. She states that 5 years ago, she injured her back playing in a soccer match when she cut to her right and had a collision with a defender and landed awkwardly. She missed 3 weeks of games and training but quickly recovered. Since that time, she experiences intermittent back pain that does not limit her activity but causes some lasting discomfort.

During the last 1.5 years, she has experienced a gradual increase in lateral thigh and hip pain. It began suddenly, following a week-long summer soccer training camp, and has progressively worsened to the point, during the past 2 months, where participation can be difficult and it does limit her performance in games and participation in practice and training. When the symptoms are at their worst, the patient also experiences a funny tingling sensation in her lateral thigh as well.

Mechanism: *The pain is long-standing. The only physical mechanism of injury appears to be potential soft tissue damage possibly associated with overuse in sport and training. The patient has identified activities that make the pain worse, including running (some pain), jumping (more pain), and squatting (the worst pain).*

Concordant Sign: *The patient's symptoms are reproduced when the lateral hip is palpated.*

Nature of the Condition: *When the pain is mild, it is a nuisance, but when it is inflamed after a good deal of activity or lying on the hip for too long, it can limit activity and motion.*

Behavior of the Symptoms: *The patient has a mild to moderate amount of irritability and symptoms appear to be simply movement specific.*

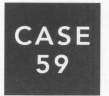

CASE 59

Setting: *Acute Rehabilitation Facility*

Date: *Present Day*

Medical Diagnosis: *Left Total Knee Arthroplasty*

Charted Data

Name:	*Roberta Hood*	Amount of Exercise:	*"Not too much 'cause my knees really hurt"*
Age:	*63 years*		
MRN:	*2568903*	Occupation:	*Retired bus driver*
Home Address:	*15 Foxmore Lane, Schenectady, New York*	Household:	*Single; lives in a 1-bedroom apartment on the 2nd floor with no elevator*
Date of Injury:	*Surgery 4 days ago*		
New Injury:	*Yes*	Hand Dominance:	*Right*
General Health:	*Fair*	Race:	*Black*

Current MD orders are for the patient to be out of bed as tolerated with progressive activity. Patient can be WBAT on LLE.

Please fill in the location of your pain with a pencil.

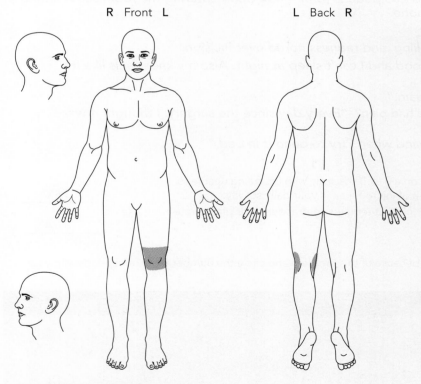

R Front L   L Back R

Pain Intensity Scale	
0	No Pain
1	Low-level pain, able to perform regular activities
2	
3	
4	Moderate-level pain, use of pain medication, activity limited but functional
5	
6	
7	High-level pain, use of pain medication, activity very limited— decreased function
(8)	
9	
10	Emergency Situation

Medical Testing Results

Hemoglobin 13 (reference 12–16 g/100 ml)

Hematocrit 40 (reference 36%–47%)[1]

White blood cell (WBC) count 15,000 (reference 3,900–10,700)

Medications

Lopressor, Micronase, Synthroid, Coumadin, Extra-strength Tylenol, Mevacor, Ativan PRN

Past Medical History (Please check any items that apply to you.)

Musculoskeletal:
- ⊗ Osteoarthritis
- ○ Rheumatoid Arthritis
- ○ Lupus/SLE
- ○ Fibromyalgia
- ○ Osteoporosis
- ○ Headaches
- ○ Bulging Disc
- ○ Leg Cramps
- ○ Restless Legs
- ○ Jaw Pain/TMJ
- ○ History of Falling
- ○ Use of Cane or Walker
- ○ Gout
- ○ Double Jointed

Neurological:
- ○ Stroke/TIA
- ○ Dementia
- ○ Polio

Neurological (continued)
- ○ Parkinson's Disease
- ○ Multiple Sclerosis
- ○ Epilepsy/Seizures
- ○ Concussion
- ○ Numbness
- ○ Tingling
Other:_____

Endocrine:
- ⊗ Diabetes
- ○ Kidney Dysfunction
- ○ Bladder Dysfunction
- ○ Liver Dysfunction
- ⊗ Thyroid Dysfunction
Other:_____

Cardiopulmonary:
- ⊗ Hypertension
- ⊗ Coronary Artery Disease

Cardiopulmonary (continued)
- ○ Congestive Heart Failure
- ○ Heart Arrhythmia
- ○ Pacemaker
- ⊗ High Cholesterol
- ○ Blood Clots
- ○ Anemia
- ○ High Blood Pressure
- ○ Asthma
- ○ Shortness of Breath
- ○ COPD
- ○ HIV/AIDS
Other:_____

Other:
- ⊗ Anxiety
- ○ Depression
- ○ Cancer

Patient Presentation

Observation
The patient is 5 feet 2 inches and weighs 235 pounds (BMI = 43). Upon entering the room she is sitting up in the recliner chair talking on the phone.

Integumentary
Surgical incisions sutured. Warmth, swelling, and redness noted over incision.

Chief Complaint: *"The food here is no good and I can't sleep at night. Also my knee feels like it's burning up."*

Goals for Therapy: *"To get rid of all my pain."*

In the last week, how many days have you had pain? *"Every day since the surgery. I thought it was supposed to feel better but it doesn't."*

Pain worst: *"When I step on the left leg and when I try to bend it in bed."*

SANE Functional Rating

Please rate your **ability** to use your injured area on a 0 to 100% scale with **0%** being unable to use the injured area and **100%** being normal use of injured area in your daily activity: _____ 25%

Also, if you exercise or have a sport activity or a job that requires special demands please rate your activity on the 0 to 100% scale: _____ N/A

Patient-Specific Functional Scale

Please list **3 activities** that you find are difficult because of this problem and circle the number that corresponds with your ability to perform the activity,

	Unable								No limitations	
1. Walking	1	②	3	4	5	6	7	8	9	10
2. Standing	1	2	③	4	5	6	7	8	9	10
3. Moving in bed	①	2	3	4	5	6	7	8	9	10

Standardized Tests
Functional independence measure (FIM) mobility subscale 32 points/91 points

Endnotes

1. Acute Care Section Lab Values Resource Update 2012, American Physical Therapy Association.

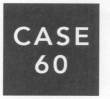

CASE 60

Setting: *Outpatient Orthopedic Facility*

Date: *Present Day*

Medical Diagnosis: *Anterior Knee Pain*

Charted Data

Name:	*Terry Knead*	General Health:	*Very good*
Age:	*38 years*	Amount of Exercise:	*An active jogger/runner*
MRN:	*21121*	Occupation:	*Lawyer*
Home Address:	*213 West 2nd street, Ontario, New Jersey*	Household:	*Married with 2 daughters, ages 11 and 15*
Date of Injury:	*3 weeks prior*	Hand Dominance:	*Left*
New Injury:	*Yes*	Race:	*White*

Please fill in the location of your pain with a pencil.

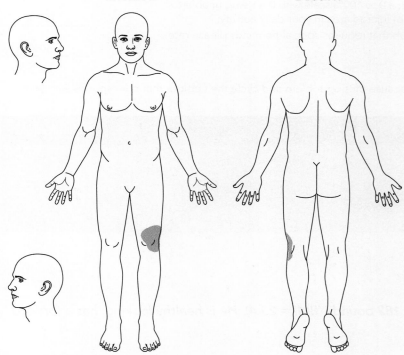

R Front L   L Back R

Pain Intensity Scale	
0	No Pain
1	Low-level pain, able to perform regular activities
2	
3	
(4)	Moderate-level pain, use of pain medication, activity limited but functional
5	
6	
7	High-level pain, use of pain medication, activity very limited—decreased function
8	
9	
10	Emergency Situation

Imaging Results
No imaging was performed.

Medications
Aspirin daily, Ibuprofen PRN

Past Medical History (Please check any items that apply to you.)

Musculoskeletal:
- ○ Osteoarthritis
- ○ Rheumatoid Arthritis
- ○ Lupus/SLE
- ○ Fibromyalgia
- ○ Osteoporosis

Musculoskeletal (continued)
- ○ Headaches
- ○ Bulging Disc
- ○ Leg Cramps
- ○ Restless Legs
- ○ Jaw Pain/TMJ

Musculoskeletal (continued)
- ○ History of Falling
- ○ Use of Cane or Walker
- ○ Gout
- ○ Double Jointed

Neurological:
- ○ Stroke/TIA
- ○ Dementia
- ○ Polio
- ○ Parkinson's Disease
- ○ Multiple Sclerosis
- ○ Epilepsy/Seizures
- ○ Concussion
- ○ Numbness
- ○ Tingling

Other:_____

Endocrine:
- ○ Diabetes

Endocrine (continued)
- ○ Kidney Dysfunction
- ○ Bladder Dysfunction
- ○ Liver Dysfunction
- ○ Thyroid Dysfunction

Other:_____

Cardiopulmonary:
- ○ Hypertension
- ○ Coronary Artery Disease
- ○ Congestive Heart Failure
- ○ Heart Arrhythmia
- ○ Pacemaker
- ⊛ High Cholesterol

Cardiopulmonary (continued)
- ○ Blood Clots
- ○ Anemia
- ○ High Blood Pressure
- ○ Asthma
- ○ Shortness of Breath
- ○ COPD
- ○ HIV/AIDS

Other:_____

Other:
- ○ Anxiety
- ○ Depression
- ○ Cancer

Chief Complaint: *"Left knee pain. I get anterior knee pain when I run over 3 miles."* The condition worsens in hilly terrain.

Goals for Therapy: *"Get rid of all my pain."*

In the last week, how many days have you had pain? *"The pain occurs only when I run. I run to control my cholesterol and to keep my weight down thus I don't want to sacrifice running."*

SANE Functional Rating

Please rate your **ability** to use your injured area on a 0 to 100% scale with **0%** being unable to use the injured area and **100%** being normal use of injured area in your daily activity: _____ 100%

Also, if you exercise or have a sport activity or a job that requires special demands please rate your activity on the 0 to 100% scale: _____ 60%

Patient-Specific Functional Scale

Please list 3 activities that you find are difficult because of this problem and circle the number that corresponds with your ability to perform the activity.

	Unable								No limitations	
1. Squatting	1	2	3	4	5	6	7	(8)	9	10
2. Running	1	2	3	4	(5)	6	7	8	9	10
3. Leg extension exercises	1	2	3	4	5	6	(7)	8	9	10

Unique Outcomes Measures
Lower extremity functional scale = 60/80

Observation
The patient is 6 feet 2 inches and weighs 182 pounds (BMI = 23.4). He is healthy looking, has a forward head posture, and is alert and eager.

Patient History
The patient reports a long-term history of running. He has had progressive knee aches over the last several years but overall has never had the problems that he has now.

Mechanism: *Insidious onset*

Concordant Sign: *Running*

Nature of the Condition: *Worsens with longer running*

Behavior of the Symptoms: *"The pain is worse when I run. It starts at 3 miles and worsens as I go further."*

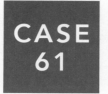

CASE 61

Setting: *Outpatient Orthopedics*

Date: *Present Day*

Medical Diagnosis: *Right Knee Pain*

Charted Data

Name:	*Tim Franklin*	General Health:	*Good*
Age:	*58 years*	Amount of Exercise:	*30 minutes/day, 3 days/ week*
MRN:	*50672*		
Home Address:	*317 Eden Court, Trenton, New Jersey*	Occupation:	*Computer repair technician*
		Household:	*Married, lives in 2-story home*
Date of Injury:	*No specific injury, onset of pain 8 months ago*	Hand Dominance:	*Left*
New Injury:	*No*	Race:	*White*

Please fill in the location of your pain with a pencil.

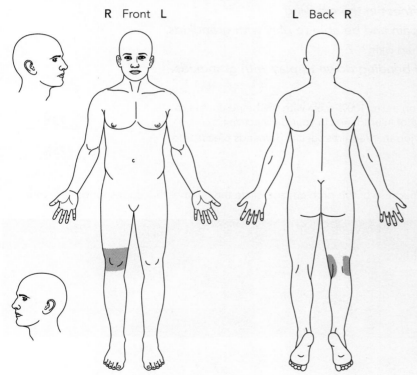

R Front L   L Back R

Pain Intensity Scale	
0	No Pain
1	Low-level pain, able to perform regular activities
2	
3	
④	Moderate-level pain, use of pain medication, activity limited but functional
5	
6	
7	High-level pain, use of pain medication, activity very limited— decreased function
8	
9	
10	Emergency Situation

Imaging Results
No images available.

Medications
Lipitor, Atenolol, Tylenol (PRN)

Past Medical History (Please check any items that apply to you.)

Musculoskeletal:
- o Osteoarthritis
- o Rheumatoid Arthritis
- o Lupus/SLE
- o Fibromyalgia
- o Osteoporosis
- o Headaches
- o Bulging Disc
- o Leg Cramps
- o Restless Legs
- o Jaw Pain/TMJ
- o History of Falling
- o Use of Cane or Walker
- o Gout
- o Double Jointed

Other:_____

Neurological:
- o Stroke/TIA
- o Dementia

Neurological (continued)
- o Polio
- o Parkinson's Disease
- o Multiple Sclerosis
- o Epilepsy/Seizures
- o Concussion
- o Numbness
- o Tingling

Other:_____

Endocrine:
- o Diabetes
- o Kidney Dysfunction
- o Bladder Dysfunction
- o Liver Dysfunction
- o Thyroid Dysfunction

Other:_____

Cardiopulmonary:
- o Congestive Heart Failure
- o Heart Arrhythmia

- o Pacemaker
- ⊗ High Cholesterol
- o Blood Clots
- o Anemia
- ⊗ High Blood Pressure
- o Asthma
- o Shortness of Breath
- o COPD
- o HIV/AIDS

Other:_____

Other:
- o Anxiety
- o Depression
- o Cancer

Chief Complaint: *Right knee pain and stiffness in the morning*

Goals for Therapy: *To reduce right knee pain and be able to play with grandkids.*

In the last week, how many days have you had pain? *7*

Pain worst: *When climbing the stairs and bending down to play with grandkids.*

SANE Functional Rating

Please rate your **ability** to use your injured area on a 0 to 100% scale with **0%** being unable to use the injured area and **100%** being normal use of injured area in your daily activity: _____ *75%* _____

Also, if you exercise or have a sport activity or a job that requires special demands please rate your activity on the 0 to 100% scale: _____ *75%* _____

Patient-Specific Functional Scale

Please list 3 activities that you find are difficult because of this problem and circle the number that corresponds with your ability to perform the activity.

	Unable								No limitations	
1. Playing with grandkids	1	2	③	4	5	6	7	8	9	10
2. Climbing the stairs	1	2	3	4	⑤	6	7	8	9	10
3. Walking the dog	1	2	3	4	⑤	6	7	8	9	10

Unique Outcomes Measures

Lower extremity functional scale = 40/80

Berg balance scale = 50

Observation

The patient is 6 feet 1 inch and weighs 235 pounds (BMI = 31.0). He has a large frame with central obesity. He appears to guard his right knee when transitioning from sit to stand. There is mild swelling noted in the right knee.

Patient History

The patient reports right knee pain beginning about 8 months ago. He played football throughout high school and played on the weekends throughout adulthood until he was 45 years old. He reports having no previous injuries, other than a mild ankle and knee sprain.

Mechanism: There was no specific incident that caused his right knee pain. It came on insidiously with no trauma.

Concordant Sign: The patient indicates that his right knee pain increases when climbing the stairs or squatting down to play with his grandkids. He also feels the pain when transitioning from sit to stand. After walking his dogs for 15–20 minutes, the right knee pain begins to increase. He complains of a "creaking sensation" in his right knee when performing any movement at the knee.

Nature of the Condition: He awakes with 5/10 pain that decreases to 2/10 after being awake and moving for 20 minutes. Pain increases throughout the day with long walks, when sitting and standing from chairs, and ascending and descending the stairs.

Behavior of the Symptoms: His symptoms worsen with previously described weight-bearing activities and diminish with unloading.

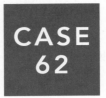

CASE 62

Setting: *Outpatient Orthopedics*

Date: *Present Day*

Medical Diagnosis: *Lateral Meniscus Tear and Surgical Repair*

Charted Data

Name:	*Jasmine Leonard*	General Health:	*Excellent, very fit*
Age:	*17 years*	Amount of Exercise:	*2 hours/day, 5–6 days/ week*
MRN:	*876002*		
Home Address:	*556 East Francis Ave, Swisher, Indiana*	Occupation:	*Student*
		Household:	*Single, lives with parents*
Date of Injury:	*2 weeks ago*	Hand Dominance:	*Right*
New Injury:	*Yes*	Race:	*African American*

Please fill in the location of your pain with a pencil.

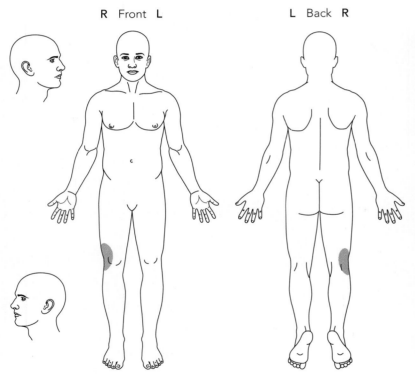

Pain Intensity Scale	
0	No Pain
1	Low-level pain, able to perform regular activities
2	
3	
4	Moderate-level pain, use of pain medication, activity limited but functional
(5)	
6	
7	High-level pain, use of pain medication, activity very limited— decreased function
8	
9	
10	Emergency Situation

Imaging Results

Radiograph was negative for knee pathology at initial emergency department visit. A magnetic resonance image 2 days later verified radial lateral meniscal tear to right knee, with no trauma to ligamentous tissue. No remarkable degenerative changes.

Medications

Ibuprofen (PRN)

Past Medical History (Please check any items that apply to you.)

Musculoskeletal:
- o Osteoarthritis
- o Rheumatoid Arthritis
- o Lupus/SLE
- o Fibromyalgia
- o Osteoporosis
- o Headaches
- o Bulging Disc
- o Leg Cramps
- o Restless Legs
- o Jaw Pain/TMJ
- o History of Falling
- o Use of Cane or Walker
- o Gout
- o Double Jointed

Other:_____

Neurological:
- o Stroke/TIA
- o Dementia

Neurological (continued)
- o Polio
- o Parkinson's Disease
- o Multiple Sclerosis
- o Epilepsy/Seizures
- o Concussion
- o Numbness
- o Tingling

Other:_____

Endocrine:
- o Diabetes
- o Kidney Dysfunction
- o Bladder Dysfunction
- o Liver Dysfunction
- o Thyroid Dysfunction

Other:_____

Cardiopulmonary:
- o Congestive Heart Failure
- o Heart Arrhythmia

Cardiopulmonary (continued)
- o Pacemaker
- o High Cholesterol
- ⊗ Blood Clots
- o Anemia
- o High Blood Pressure
- o Asthma
- o Shortness of Breath
- o COPD
- o HIV/AIDS

Other:_____

Other:
- o Anxiety
- o Depression
- o Cancer

Chief Complaint: *Right knee pain*

Goals for Therapy: *To return to prior level of function including sporting activities.*

In the last week, how many days have you had pain? *7*

Pain worst: *During ambulation*

SANE Functional Rating

Please rate your **ability** to use your injured area on a 0 to 100% scale with **0%** being unable to use the injured area and **100%** being normal use of injured area in your daily activity: _____ 0%_____

Also, if you exercise or have a sport activity or a job that requires special demands please rate your activity on the 0 to 100% scale: _____ 0%_____

Patient-Specific Functional Scale

Please list 3 activities that you find are difficult because of this problem and circle the number that corresponds with your ability to perform the activity.

	Unable								No limitations	
1. Walking	1	2	3	(4)	5	6	7	8	9	10
2. Basketball	(1)	2	3	4	5	6	7	8	9	10
3. Driving	(1)	2	3	4	5	6	7	8	9	10

Unique Outcomes Measures

Lower extremity functional scale = 25/80

Observation

Patient is 5 feet 7 inches tall and weighs 130 pounds (BMI = 20.4). She is thin but muscular and appears to be athletic. The patient ambulated into therapy office using axillary crutches and with knee extension brace locked in 0° extension. Inspection of right knee reveals well-healing surgical incisions with no concern for infection. There is slight ecchymosis and effusion surrounding the right knee.

Patient History

The patient reports that the initial injury occurred 3 weeks ago during basketball practice when she "twisted her knee" during a quick stop and change of direction down the court. She states that the pain was immediate and she was taken out of practice and cryotherapy was administered by an athletic trainer. The patient's father took her to the emergency department (ED) that evening with referral to an orthopedist after a negative radiograph.

The patient was treated by an orthopedist 2 days after the injury and was scheduled for surgical repair of lateral meniscus upon MRI results 1 week following the initial office visit. Outpatient surgery was performed with no complications and the patient was discharged to home that evening. She returned to ED 2 days following surgery with "excruciating pain" in her right calf with edema and diminished sensation in her right foot. Doppler screening revealed distal DVT and the patient was given anticoagulation therapy, admitted for monitoring, and released after a 2-day inpatient stay.

She is now at beginning of second week postsurgical repair of the right lateral meniscus. The orthopedist ordered partial weight bearing (20%) with use of axillary crutches, with all weight-bearing activities performed while wearing the knee extension brace.

Concordant Sign: *Pain is increased with knee range of motion, ambulation with crutches, and all weight bearing activities.*

Mechanism: *Change of direction on weight-bearing lower extremity during basketball practice*

Nature of the Condition: *The patient reports 7/10 pain at worst and 2/10 at best with aching and sharp sensations of pain with weight bearing through right lower extremity; her pain resolves when sitting.*

Behavior of the Symptoms: *The patient's pain symptoms increase during ambulation with crutches.*

CASE 63

Setting: *Outpatient Orthopedics*

Date: *Present Day*

Medical Diagnosis: *Anterior Cruciate Ligament Reconstruction*

Charted Data

Name:	*Nikki Moore*	Amount of Exercise:	*1–3 hours/day, 5–6 days/week*
Age:	*15 years*		
MRN:	*50523*	Occupation:	*High school student and basketball player*
Home Address:	*22 Tremont Drive, Zoar, Ohio*	Household:	*Lives at home with parents and twin sister*
Date of Injury:	*12 days ago*		
New Injury:	*Yes*	Hand Dominance:	*Right*
General Health:	*Good*	Race:	*White*

Please fill in the location of your pain with a pencil.

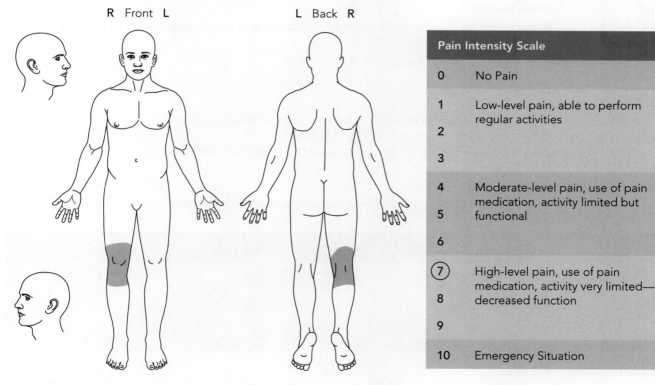

R Front L

L Back R

Pain Intensity Scale	
0	No Pain
1	Low-level pain, able to perform regular activities
2	
3	
4	Moderate-level pain, use of pain medication, activity limited but functional
5	
6	
⑦	High-level pain, use of pain medication, activity very limited—decreased function
8	
9	
10	Emergency Situation

Imaging Results

A magnetic resonance imaging (MRI) of the right knee yields a tear of the right anterior cruciate and medial collateral ligaments.

Surgical Results

Complete tear of the right anterior cruciate ligament and partial tear of the medial collateral ligament were discovered. The hamstring tendon autograft was used to reconstruct the anterior cruciate ligament. No surgical complications were noted at the time of hospital discharge.

Medications

Oxycodone (PRN), Albuterol (inhaler, PRN)

Past Medical History (Please check any items that apply to you.)

Musculoskeletal:
- ○ Osteoarthritis
- ○ Rheumatoid Arthritis
- ○ Lupus/SLE
- ○ Fibromyalgia
- ○ Osteoporosis
- ○ Headaches
- ○ Bulging Disc
- ○ Leg Cramps
- ○ Restless Legs
- ○ Jaw Pain/TMJ
- ○ History of Falling
- ○ Use of Cane or Walker
- ○ Gout
- ○ Double Jointed

Other:_____

Neurological:
- ○ Stroke/TIA
- ○ Dementia

Neurological (continued)
- ○ Polio
- ○ Parkinson's Disease
- ○ Multiple Sclerosis
- ○ Epilepsy/Seizures
- ○ Concussion
- ○ Numbness
- ○ Tingling

Other:_____

Endocrine:
- ○ Diabetes
- ○ Kidney Dysfunction
- ○ Bladder Dysfunction
- ○ Liver Dysfunction
- ○ Thyroid Dysfunction

Other:_____

Cardiopulmonary:
- ○ Congestive Heart Failure
- ○ Heart Arrhythmia

Cardiopulmonary (continued)
- ○ Pacemaker
- ○ High Cholesterol
- ○ Blood Clots
- ○ Anemia
- ○ High Blood Pressure
- ⊗ Asthma
- ○ Shortness of Breath
- ○ COPD
- ○ HIV/AIDS

Other:_____

Other:
- ○ Anxiety
- ○ Depression
- ○ Cancer

Chief Complaint: *Right knee pain*

Goals for Therapy: *To decrease knee pain, walk without crutches, and eventually return to playing basketball.*

In the last week, how many days have you had pain? *7*

Pain worst: *Any knee movements*

SANE Functional Rating

Please rate your **ability** to use your injured area on a 0 to 100% scale with **0%** being unable to use the injured area and **100%** being normal use of injured area in your daily activity: ___0%___

Also, if you exercise or have a sport activity or a job that requires special demands please rate your activity on the 0 to 100% scale: ___0%___

Patient-Specific Functional Scale

Please list 3 activities that you find are difficult because of this problem and circle the number that corresponds with your ability to perform the activity.

	Unable									No limitations
1. Standing	1	2	3	4	(5)	6	7	8	9	10
2. Walking	1	2	3	(4)	5	6	7	8	9	10
3. Playing basketball	(1)	2	3	4	5	6	7	8	9	10

Unique Outcomes Measures

Lower extremity functional scale (LEFS) = 16/80 (maximal disability)

Observation

The patient is 5 feet 10 inches and weighs 140 pounds (BMI = 20.1). She is thin but athletic. She is using bilateral axillary crutches as she is weight bearing as tolerated on her right lower extremity. She also is wearing a DonJoy knee brace on her right knee per her surgeon's orders. While attempting to sit on the examination table, she appears to be in moderate pain with slight knee movement per facial grimace.

Patient History

The patient reports right knee pain that began 12 days ago after an injury during a basketball game when she was guarding another player. She reports that she turned quickly on her right leg and suddenly her knee gave out and she fell to the ground. She reported that she was unable to stand and her right knee pain was unbearable. One week after her injury she underwent ACL reconstruction using a hamstring tendon autograft.

Mechanism: *Based on the patient's description, the mechanism of injury appears to be from a torsional force of the femur on the tibia during a basketball game.*

Concordant Sign: *Her pain is initiated with bending and straightening at the knee, as well as getting leg in and out of bed and weight bearing.*

Nature of the Condition: *She indicates that her knee pain at rest remains at 3/10. After completing knee ROM activities, her pain has increased to 8/10.*

Behavior of the Symptoms: *The patient's symptoms worsen during standing and walking activities. Her symptoms decrease when she rests her leg in a neutral position, with ice and with pain medication.*

CASE 64

Setting: *Outpatient Orthopedics*

Date: *Present Day*

Medical Diagnosis: *Quadriceps Tendinopathy*

Charted Data

Name:	*Billy McGraw*	Amount of Exercise:	*1–2 hours/day, 6 days/ week*
Age:	*15 years*	Occupation:	*High school student, basketball, soccer, and track athlete*
MRN:	*32587*		
Home Address:	*6530 Birchhaven Street, Dublin, Ohio*	Household:	*Single, lives with mom, dad, and brother*
Date of Injury:	*2 weeks ago*		
New Injury:	*Yes*	Hand Dominance:	*Right*
General Health:	*Good*	Race:	*White*

Please fill in the location of your pain with a pencil.

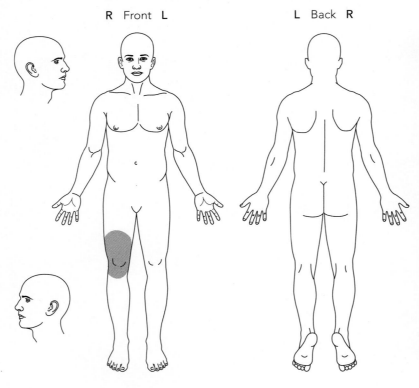

R Front L   L Back R

Pain Intensity Scale	
0	No Pain
1	Low-level pain, able to perform regular activities
2	
3	
4	Moderate-level pain, use of pain medication, activity limited but functional
5	
(6)	
7	High-level pain, use of pain medication, activity very limited—decreased function
8	
9	
10	Emergency Situation

Imaging Results

A radiograph of the knee yielded no evidence of a patellar fracture or significant edema and is otherwise unremarkable.

Medications

Atrovent, Advil

Past Medical History (Please check any items that apply to you.)

Musculoskeletal:

- o Osteoarthritis
- o Rheumatoid Arthritis
- o Lupus/SLE
- o Fibromyalgia
- o Osteoporosis
- o Headaches
- o Bulging Disc
- o Leg Cramps
- o Restless Legs
- o Jaw Pain/TMJ
- o History of Falling
- o Use of Cane or Walker
- o Gout
- o Double Jointed

Other: _Tendinitis of Right Knee_

Neurological:

- o Stroke/TIA
- o Dementia

Neurological (continued)

- o Polio
- o Parkinson's Disease
- o Multiple Sclerosis
- o Epilepsy/Seizures
- o Concussion
- o Numbness
- o Tingling

Other:_____

Endocrine:

- o Diabetes
- o Kidney Dysfunction
- o Bladder Dysfunction
- o Liver Dysfunction
- o Thyroid Dysfunction

Other:_____

Cardiopulmonary:

- o Congestive Heart Failure
- o Heart Arrhythmia

Cardiopulmonary (continued)

- o Pacemaker
- o High Cholesterol
- o Blood Clots
- o Anemia
- o High Blood Pressure
- ⊗ Asthma
- o Shortness of Breath
- o COPD
- o HIV/AIDS

Other:_____

Other:

- ⊗ Anxiety
- o Depression
- o Cancer

Chief Complaint: *Pain in right anterior thigh and superior border of patella*

Goals for Therapy: *To reduce the pain and be able to compete in high school basketball season.*

In the last week, how many days have you had pain? *5*

Pain worst: *During basketball conditioning*

SANE Functional Rating

Please rate your **ability** to use your injured area on a 0 to 100% scale with **0%** being unable to use the injured area and **100%** being normal use of injured area in your daily activity:

_70%_

Also, if you exercise or have a sport activity or a job that requires special demands please rate your activity on the 0 to 100% scale:

_60%_

Patient-Specific Functional Scale

Please list 3 activities that you find are difficult because of this problem and circle the number that corresponds with your ability to perform the activity.

	Unable									No limitations
1. Running	1	2	3	4	(5)	6	7	8	9	10
2. Jumping	1	2	3	4	5	(6)	7	8	9	10
3. Walking to school	1	2	3	4	5	6	7	(8)	9	10

Unique Outcomes Measures

Lower extremity functional scale (LEFS) = 50/80 (62.5% of maximal function)

Observation

The patient is 5 feet 9 inches and weighs 160 pounds (BMI = 23.6). No redness or swelling is noted surrounding the right knee. However, there is a mild contusion on his right anterior thigh with about a ¾-inch difference in girth at distal end of rectus femoris on right compared to his left. The patient has slight forward head and rounded shoulder posturing in standing. Also, he maintains a slightly flexed position of his right knee in standing. He presents with normal alignment of his lower extremities (no excessive rotation at the hips or tibial torsion and normal Q angle). The patient demonstrates a heel-toe pattern of gait with a normal base of support but a decreased stance phase is noted on his right lower extremity. The patient also demonstrates excessive pronation while standing and ambulating and does not have any orthotic devices.

Patient History

The patient reports that he has a history of tendonitis of his right knee that began approximately 2 years ago. He states that he saw his physician initially and followed the doctor's recommendations of ice and rest. The patient had not received prior physical therapy services for this condition. He is a multi-sport athlete (basketball and track) and is currently having difficulty making it through basketball conditioning. He reports that the top of his knee is tender when touched and he is icing his knee at home and taking Advil to assist with pain control, but it is not working as well as it had previously. He also states that his knee feels stiff the morning after his previous conditioning session.

Mechanism: The patient has a 2-year history of tendonitis of his right knee and has recently had a gradual onset of pain within the last 2 weeks. He has recently started conditioning for his basketball season, which accompanies his increase in symptoms. He also collided with another player while at practice 3 days ago and that has slightly increased his pain.

Concordant Sign: He indicates that his pain is initiated with running and jumping skills in basketball.

Nature of the Condition: The 6/10 pain he reports at the superior border of his patella begins shortly after running to warm up for conditioning, and it continues to progress throughout his conditioning session.

Behavior of Condition: The reports that his pain increases with running and repetitive jumping activities and lessens after he has finished his conditioning and is able to rest.

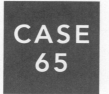

CASE 65

Setting: *Acute Inpatient*

Date: *Present Day*

Medical Diagnosis: *Acute Left Total Knee Arthroplasty (TKA)*

Charted Data

Name:	*Sally Turner*	General Health:	*Good*
Age:	*67 years*	Amount of Exercise:	*30 minutes to 1 hour/day, 4 days/week*
MRN:	*95560*		
Home Address:	*5275 Belmont Circle, Nashville, Tennessee*	Occupation:	*Retired teacher, babysits 2 grandchildren 3 days/week*
Date of Injury:	*Osteoarthritis (OA) for 10 years*	Household:	*Married, lives with husband*
New Injury:	*Total knee arthroplasty, yesterday*	Hand Dominance:	*Right*
		Race:	*White*

Please fill in the location of your pain with a pencil.

R Front L   L Back R

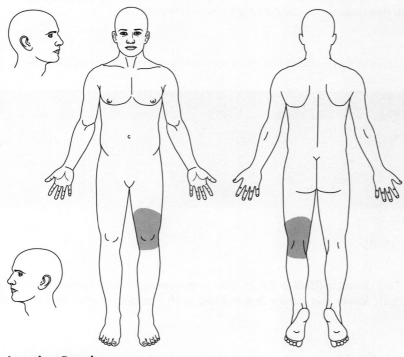

Pain Intensity Scale	
0	No Pain
1	Low-level pain, able to perform regular activities
2	
3	
4	Moderate-level pain, use of pain medication, activity limited but functional
5	
6	
7	High-level pain, use of pain medication, activity very limited— decreased function
(8)	
9	
10	Emergency Situation

Imaging Results

No post-op radiographs are available.

Medications

Albuterol (as needed), Fosamax, Tylenol 500 mg every 6 hours prior to surgery, Heparin, Codeine

Past Medical History (Please check any items that apply to you.)

Musculoskeletal:
- ⊗ Osteoarthritis
- ○ Rheumatoid Arthritis
- ○ Lupus/SLE
- ○ Fibromyalgia
- ○ Osteoporosis

Musculoskeletal (continued)
- ○ Headaches
- ○ Bulging Disc
- ○ Leg Cramps
- ○ Restless Legs
- ○ Jaw Pain/TMJ

Musculoskeletal (continued)
- ○ History of Falling
- ○ Use of Cane or Walker
- ○ Gout
- ○ Double Jointed
- Other: *Osteopenia*

Neurological:
- o Stroke/TIA
- o Dementia
- o Polio
- o Parkinson's disease
- o Multiple Sclerosis
- o Epilepsy/Seizures
- o Concussion
- o Numbness
- o Tingling

Other:_____

Endocrine:
- o Diabetes
- o Kidney Dysfunction

Endocrine (continued)
- o Bladder Dysfunction
- o Liver Dysfunction
- o Thyroid Dysfunction

Other: *Hysterectomy*

Cardiopulmonary:
- o Congestive Heart Failure
- o Heart Arrhythmia
- o Pacemaker
- o High Cholesterol
- o Blood Clots
- o Anemia
- o High Blood Pressure
- ⊛ Asthma

Cardiopulmonary (continued)
- o Shortness of Breath
- o COPD
- o HIV/AIDS

Other:_____

Other:
- o Anxiety
- o Depression
- o Cancer

Chief Complaint: *Left knee pain, swelling, loss of range of motion (ROM), and post-TKA*

Goals for Therapy: *To reduce swelling and pain, and return to walking.*

In the last week, how many days have you had pain? *7*

Pain worst: *Right now*

SANE Functional Rating

Please rate your **ability** to use your injured area on a 0 to 100% scale with **0%** being unable to use the injured area and **100%** being normal use of injured area in your daily activity: *75%*

Also, if you exercise or have a sport activity or a job that requires special demands please rate your activity on the 0 to 100% scale: *0%*

Patient-Specific Functional Scale

Please list **3 activities** that you find are difficult because of this problem and circle the number that corresponds with your ability to perform the activity.

	Unable								No limitations	
1. Laying in bed	1	2	3	(4)	5	6	7	8	9	10
2. Getting to the bathroom	(1)	2	3	4	5	6	7	8	9	10
3. Sitting	1	2	(3)	4	5	6	7	8	9	10

Unique Outcomes Measures

Lower extremity functional scale (LEFS) = 15/80

Observation

The patient is 5 feet 2 inches and weighs 160 pounds (BMI = 29.3). She is overweight and appears to be in significant pain while lying in bed. Her right lower extremity is elevated with bandages and an ice pack around her right knee.

Patient History

She reports right knee pain for 10 years. Prior to having this surgery she reported using cortisone shots, medications, physical therapy, and activity modification to control pain so that she could put off having surgery.

Mechanism: *The patient underwent total knee arthroplasty yesterday.*

Concordant Sign: *She indicates the pain she is experiencing is constant.*

Nature of the Condition: *The patient complains of an 8/10 pain at its worst and a 6/10 at its best since the surgery.*

Behavior of the Symptoms: *Her pain worsens when rolling or moving in bed, using a walker to get to the bathroom, and bending her knee. Pain decreases when her lower extremity is elevated while using cryotherapy.*

CASE 66

Setting: *Acute Care Hospital*

Date: *Present Day*

Medical Diagnosis: **Osteoarthritis** *of the Right Knee Status Post Total Knee Arthroplasty (TKA)*

Charted Data

Name:	*Sue Ellen Bauer*	General Health:	*Good*
Age:	*62 years*	Amount of Exercise:	*0 hours/day, 0 days/week*
MRN:	*50753*	Occupation:	*Transcriptionist for medical billing agency*
Home Address:	*234 Sunflower Drive, Raleigh, North Carolina*	Household:	*Lives independently with husband in one-story house*
Date of Injury:	*Surgery yesterday*		
New Injury:	*7 years chronic*	Hand Dominance:	*Right*

Please fill in the location of your pain with a pencil.

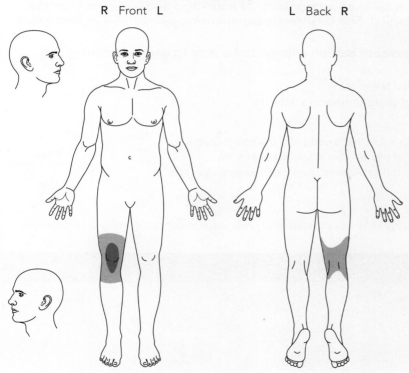

R Front L   L Back R

Pain Intensity Scale	
0	No Pain
1	Low-level pain, able to perform regular activities
2	
3	
4	Moderate-level pain, use of pain medication, activity limited but functional
5	
6	
⑦	High-level pain, use of pain medication, activity very limited—decreased function
8	
9	
10	Emergency Situation

Imaging Results

Presurgical radiograph and MRI revealed substantial deterioration of the articular surfaces of both the femur and the tibia. No fractures present.

Medications

160 mg Valsartan once daily,[1] 25 mg rofecoxib once daily,[1] 3.75 mg hydrocodone-acetaminophen twice daily[1]

Past Medical History (Please check any items that apply to you.)

Musculoskeletal:
- ⊗ Osteoarthritis
- ○ Rheumatoid Arthritis
- ○ Lupus/SLE
- ○ Fibromyalgia
- ○ Osteoporosis
- ○ Headaches
- ○ Bulging Disc
- ○ Leg Cramps
- ○ Restless Legs
- ○ Jaw Pain/TMJ
- ○ History of Falling
- ○ Use of Cane or Walker
- ○ Gout
- ○ Double Jointed

Other:_____

Neurological:
- ○ Stroke/TIA

Neurological (continued)
- ○ Dementia
- ○ Polio
- ○ Parkinson's Disease
- ○ Multiple Sclerosis
- ○ Epilepsy/Seizures
- ○ Concussion
- ○ Numbness
- ○ Tingling

Other:_____

Endocrine:
- ○ Diabetes
- ○ Kidney Dysfunction
- ○ Bladder Dysfunction
- ○ Liver Dysfunction
- ○ Thyroid Dysfunction

Other:_____

Cardiopulmonary:
- ○ Congestive Heart Failure
- ○ Heart Arrhythmia
- ○ Pacemaker
- ○ High Cholesterol
- ○ Blood Clots
- ○ Anemia
- ⊗ High Blood Pressure
- ○ Asthma
- ○ Shortness of Breath
- ○ COPD
- ○ HIV/AIDS

Other:_____

Other:
- ○ Anxiety
- ○ Depression
- ○ Cancer

Chief Complaint: *Patient underwent right total knee arthroplasty 24 hours ago and is currently on the medical-surgical floor of an acute care hospital. She is currently experiencing pain as well as decreased knee flexion and extension.*

Goals for Therapy: *To decrease pain and increase motion enough to be able to enjoy gardening and playing with her grandchildren.*

In the last week, how many days have you had pain? *7*

Pain worst: *Evening and during prolonged weight-bearing activity*

SANE Functional Rating

Please rate your **ability** to use your injured area on a 0 to 100% scale with **0%** being unable to use the injured area and **100%** being normal use of injured area in your daily activity: _____ *70%* _____

Also, if you exercise or have a sport activity or a job that requires special demands please rate your activity on the 0 to 100% scale: _____ *N/A* _____

Patient-Specific Functional Scale

Please list 3 activities that you find are difficult because of this problem and circle the number that corresponds with your ability to perform the activity.

	Unable								No limitations	
1. Prolonged standing	1	2	(3)	4	5	6	7	8	9	10
2. Kneeling	1	(2)	3	4	5	6	7	8	9	10
3. Stairs	1	2	3	4	(5)	6	7	8	9	10

Unique Outcomes Measures[1]

	Trial 1	Trial 2	Trial 3
6-Minute Walk Test	367.9 m	429.8 m	494.8 m
30-Second Sit to Stand	14 reps	21 reps	25 reps
WOMAC			
Pain	11	9	0

	Trial 1	Trial 2	Trial 3
Stiffness	6	4	3
Physical function impairment	37	31	1
Proprioception			
Angle of Reproduction (involved knee)	22	6	6
Threshold (involved knee)	3	3	2

Observation

The patient is 5 feet 4 inches and weighs 182 pounds (BMI = 31.2). She has a 6.5" incision over the anterior aspect of her knee. The incision is dressed with gauze and some red drainage is present. Her knee is swollen compared to the contralateral side but is not red or warm to the touch. The patient is lethargic but her skin color is normal. No fever or perspiration present.

Patient History

The patient is obese and there is no past medical history of depression or other mental illness. She denies participating in regular exercise but enjoys gardening and playing with her 2 young grandchildren at the local park. She has a history of high blood pressure that is controlled with medication.

Mechanism: *Seven years ago the patient was diagnosed with osteoarthritis (OA) of both knees. Her pain and functional limitation slowly increased in the right knee until finally a TKA was recommended by her orthopedic surgeon for her right lower extremity. Patient is 24 hours status/post (s/p) TKA and complains of pain with movement, especially knee flexion.*

Concordant Sign: *Before surgery, pain was a deep ache present within the knee joint itself. The patient now describes pain as a constant sharp pain of 2/10 that increases to 5/10 with continuous passive motion (CPM) flexion and extension of the knee.*

Nature of the Condition: *The patient's condition became debilitating enough for the orthopedic surgeon to recommend a TKA. Pain currently is controlled with analgesics.*

Behavior of the Symptoms: *Pain worsens with movement but the patient's joint becomes stiff with periods of rest.*

Endnotes

1. Jaggers J, Simpson C, Nyland J, et al. Prehabilitation before knee arthroplasty increases postsurgical function: a case study. J Strength Cond Res. May 2007;21(2):632–4. Accessed October 9, 2012.

Setting: *Outpatient Orthopedic Clinic*

Date: *Present Day*

Medical Diagnosis: *Patellofemoral Pain Syndrome (PFPS)*

Charted Data

		General Health:	*Good*
Name:	*Zoe Cunningham*	Amount of Exercise:	*90 minutes/day, 6 days/week*
Age:	*37 years*		
MRN:	*50590*	Occupation:	*Lawyer*
Home Address:	*2139 Jennifer Lane, Raleigh, North Carolina*	Household:	*Recently divorced, lives in single-story house*
Date of Injury:	*4 months ago*	Hand Dominance:	*Right*
New Injury:	*No*	Race:	*Caucasian*

Please fill in the location of your pain with a pencil.

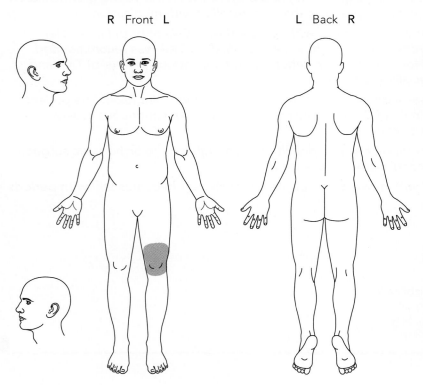

R Front L   L Back R

Pain Intensity Scale	
0	No Pain
1	Low-level pain, able to perform regular activities
2	
3	
4	Moderate-level pain, use of pain medication, activity limited but functional
5	
(6)	
7	High-level pain, use of pain medication, activity very limited—decreased function
8	
9	
10	Emergency Situation

Imaging Results

Radiograph and MRI results revealed normal findings. Imaging was negative for evidence of a fracture or moderate to severe ligamentous disruption.

Medications

Ibuprofen PRN

Past Medical History (Please check any items that apply to you.)

Musculoskeletal:
- ○ Osteoarthritis
- ○ Rheumatoid Arthritis
- ○ Lupus/SLE
- ○ Fibromyalgia
- ○ Osteoporosis
- ⊗ Headaches
- ○ Bulging Disc
- ○ Leg Cramps
- ○ Restless Legs
- ○ Jaw Pain/TMJ
- ○ History of Falling
- ○ Use of Cane or Walker
- ○ Gout
- ○ Double Jointed

Other:_____

Neurological:
- ○ Stroke/TIA
- ○ Dementia

Neurological (continued)
- ○ Polio
- ○ Parkinson's Disease
- ○ Multiple Sclerosis
- ○ Epilepsy/Seizures
- ○ Concussion
- ○ Numbness
- ○ Tingling

Other:_____

Endocrine:
- ○ Diabetes
- ○ Kidney Dysfunction
- ○ Bladder Dysfunction
- ○ Liver Dysfunction
- ○ Thyroid Dysfunction

Other:_____

Cardiopulmonary:
- ○ Congestive Heart Failure
- ○ Heart Arrhythmia

Cardiopulmonary (continued)
- ○ Pacemaker
- ○ High Cholesterol
- ○ Blood Clots
- ○ Anemia
- ○ High Blood Pressure
- ⊗ Asthma
- ○ Shortness of Breath
- ○ COPD
- ○ HIV/AIDS

Other:_____

Other:
- ○ Anxiety
- ○ Depression
- ○ Cancer

Chief Complaint: *Progressively worsening left anterior knee pain during prolonged activity*

Goals for Therapy: *To reduce or eliminate anterior knee pain during activity in order to resume triathlon training.*

In the last week, how many days have you had pain? *7*

Pain worst: *Running (more than 2 miles)*

SANE Functional Rating

Please rate your **ability** to use your injured area on a 0 to 100% scale with **0%** being unable to use the injured area and **100%** being normal use of injured area in your daily activity: _____ *70%* _____

Also, if you exercise or have a sport activity or a job that requires special demands please rate your activity on the 0 to 100% scale: _____ *25%* _____

Patient-Specific Functional Scale

Please list 3 activities that you find are difficult because of this problem and circle the number that corresponds with your ability to perform the activity.

	Unable									No limitations
1. Running	1	2	③	4	5	6	7	8	9	10
2. Climbing stairs	1	②	3	4	5	6	7	8	9	10
3. Squatting	1	②	3	4	5	6	7	8	9	10

Unique Outcomes Measures

Lower extremity functional scale (LEFS)[1] = 44/80

Functional index questionnaire (FIQ)[2] = 6

Observation

The patient is 5 feet 6 inches and weighs 135 pounds (BMI = 21.8). She presents as a well-conditioned female with bilateral lateral patella tracking and grade II crepitus in the left knee. Her posture is normal. During ambulation, she demonstrates decreased stance time on the left lower extremity. There is no visible edema or redness.

Patient History

The patient indicates onset of initial pain 4 months ago with progressively worsening symptoms. Her pain is worse when climbing stairs, squatting, and running, and with prolonged sitting. She is usually very physically active and has completed marathons in the past. Currently, she is attempting to train for a triathlon but has had to significantly decrease her training due to left anterior knee pain. The patient has a negative history for any prior knee injury or pain. She has no history of surgery of any kind.

Mechanism: *4 months of progressively worsening symptoms. No direct trauma.*

Concordant Sign: *Reproduction of pain with prolonged squatting (>20 sec.) and when climbing stairs (>5 stairs).*

Nature of the Condition: *The condition mildly limits the patient's daily activities such as room navigation and her work as a lawyer, but it severely limits running, squatting, stair navigation, and walking long distances.*

Behavior of the Symptoms: *Her pain worsens during activity, especially when the patellofemoral joint is placed in a compressed position for a prolonged period of time. Rest alleviates her pain.*

Endnotes

1. Binkley JM, Stratford PW, Lott SA, Riddle DL. The lower extremity functional scale (LEFS): Scale development, measurement, properties, and clinical application. Phys Ther. 1999;79(4):371–83.

2. Harrison E, Quinney H, Magee D, Sheppard M, McQuarrie A. Analysis of outcome measures used in the study of patellofemoral pain syndrome. Physiother Can. 1995;47(4):264–72.

CASE 68

Setting: *Outpatient Orthopedics*

Date: **Present Day**

Medical Diagnosis: *Knee Strain*

Charted Data

Name:	*Jacob Taylor*
Age:	*17 years*
MRN:	*51461*
Home Address:	*302 Court Street, Schleswig, Iowa*
Date of Injury:	*2 days ago*
New Injury:	*Yes*
General Health:	*Good*

Amount of Exercise:	*Plays football but season hasn't started. No other formal exercise. Helps grandparents with farm work about 2 hours/day 4 days/week*
Occupation:	*High school student*
Household:	*Lives with parents and younger sister*
Race:	*Caucasian*

Please fill in the location of your pain with a pencil.

R Front L   L Back R

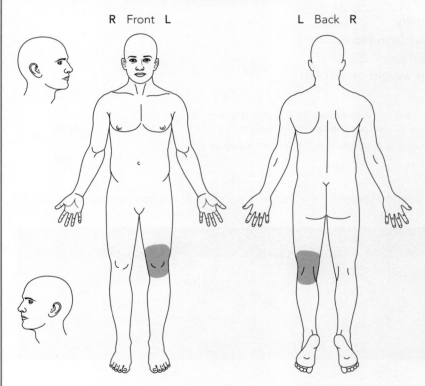

Pain Intensity Scale	
0	No Pain
1 2 3	Low-level pain, able to perform regular activities
(4) 5 6	Moderate-level pain, use of pain medication, activity limited but functional
7 8 9	High-level pain, use of pain medication, activity very limited—decreased function
10	Emergency Situation

Imaging Results

A radiograph of the knee yields no fractures.

Medications

Ibuprofen (PRN)

Past Medical History (Please check any items that apply to you.)

Musculoskeletal:
- ○ Osteoarthritis
- ○ Rheumatoid Arthritis
- ○ Lupus/SLE
- ○ Fibromyalgia
- ○ Osteoporosis
- ○ Headaches
- ○ Bulging Disc
- ○ Leg Cramps
- ○ Restless Legs
- ○ Jaw Pain/TMJ
- ○ History of Falling
- ○ Use of Cane or Walker
- ○ Gout
- ○ Double Jointed

Other:_____

Neurological:
- ○ Stroke/TIA
- ○ Dementia
- ○ Polio

Neurological (continued)
- ○ Parkinson's Disease
- ○ Multiple Sclerosis
- ○ Epilepsy/Seizures
- ○ Concussion
- ○ Numbness
- ○ Tingling

Other:_____

Endocrine:
- ○ Diabetes
- ○ Kidney Dysfunction
- ○ Bladder Dysfunction
- ○ Liver Dysfunction
- ○ Thyroid Dysfunction

Other:_____

Cardiopulmonary:
- ○ Congestive Heart Failure
- ○ Heart Arrhythmia
- ○ Pacemaker

Cardiopulmonary (continued)
- ○ High Cholesterol
- ○ Blood Clots
- ○ Anemia
- ○ High Blood Pressure
- ○ Asthma
- ○ Shortness of Breath
- ○ COPD
- ○ HIV/AIDS

Other:_____

Other:
- ⊗ Anxiety
- ○ Depression
- ○ Cancer

Chief Complaint: *Knee stiffness and instability*

Goals for Therapy: *To return to football and farm work.*

In the last week, how many days have you had pain? *2*

Pain worst: *Trying to bend left knee or put weight on left leg*

SANE Functional Rating

Please rate your **ability** to use your injured area on a 0 to 100% scale with **0%** being unable to use the injured area and **100%** being normal use of injured area in your daily activity: _____ 40%

Also, if you exercise or have a sport activity or a job that requires special demands please rate your activity on the 0 to 100% scale: _____ 0%

Patient-Specific Functional Scale

Please list 3 activities that you find are difficult because of this problem and circle the number that corresponds with your ability to perform the activity.

	Unable									No limitations
1. Walking	1	2	3	4	5	(6)	7	8	9	10
2. Stairs	1	2	3	(4)	5	6	7	8	9	10
3. Work with pigs on the farm	(1)	2	3	4	5	6	7	8	9	10

Unique Outcomes Measures

Lower extremity functional scale (LEFS) = 32/80 (40% of maximum function)[1]

Observation

The patient is 5 feet 11 inches and weighs 170 pounds (BMI = 23.7). Mild swelling is present in the anterior knee, especially along medial patellar border. Modified stroke test is graded as 1 + (bulge of fluid on the medial side of the knee during the test).[2] The patient walks without an assistive device with the knee held in slight flexion. Stance time on the left lower extremity is limited versus right.

Patient History

The patient reports injuring his knee 2 days ago. Since the injury, pain has decreased but he continues to have difficulty walking.

Mechanism: *The patient reports injuring his knee when loading pigs onto a trailer. He reports twisting his knee when he moved quickly to close a gate that a pig was trying to run through. The knee started to swell about an hour later.*

Concordant Sign: *Pain is in the knee with walking or with attempts at bending it.*

Nature of the Condition: *The 4/10 pain is an ache deep in the knee. The knee feels stiff yet unstable.*

Behavior of the Symptoms: *The patient states that the knee "gives out" while walking; it happens more when trying to go down stairs so the patient reports he has now modified the way he uses stairs (lowering himself to each step with the uninjured leg). The knee feels stiff if it remains in one position too long, such as after prolonged sitting.*

Endnotes

1. Binkley JM, Stratford PW, Lott SA, Riddle DL. The lower extremity functional scale (LEFS): scale development, measurement properties, and clinical application. North American Orthopaedic Rehabilitation Research Network. Phys Ther. 1999 Apr;79(4):371–83.

2. Sturgill LP, Snyder-Mackler L, Manal TJ, Axe MJ. Interrater reliability of a clinical scale to assess knee joint effusion. J Orthop Sports Phys Ther. 2009;39:845–9.

CASE 69

Setting: *Outpatient Orthopedics*

Date: *Present Day*

Medical Diagnosis: *Knee Strain*

Charted Data

Name:	*Nancy Stellar*	New Injury:	*Yes*
Age:	*23 years*	General Health:	*Excellent*
MRN:	*50505*	Amount of Exercise:	*45 minutes of running, 4–5 times /week*
Home Address:	*1543 Appleton Street, Maple Ridge, Vermont*	Occupation:	*Student*
		Household:	*Single*
Date of Injury:	*3-week history*	Race:	*Caucasian*

Please fill in the location of your pain with a pencil.

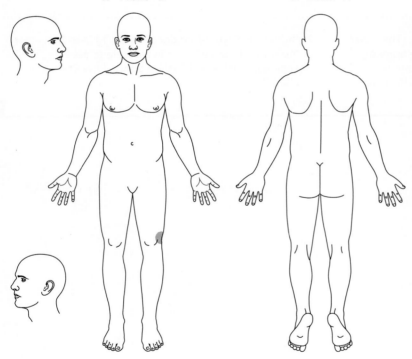

R Front L   L Back R

Pain Intensity Scale	
0	No Pain
1	Low-level pain, able to perform regular activities
2	
3	
(4)	Moderate-level pain, use of pain medication, activity limited but functional
5	
6	
7	High-level pain, use of pain medication, activity very limited—decreased function
8	
9	
10	Emergency Situation

Imaging Results
No imaging was performed.

Medications
Advil (PRN) decreased swelling and allowed additional movement of the knee

Past Medical History (Please check any items that apply to you.)

Musculoskeletal:

- o Osteoarthritis
- o Rheumatoid Arthritis
- o Lupus/SLE
- o Fibromyalgia
- o Osteoporosis
- o Headaches
- o Bulging Disc
- o Leg Cramps
- o Restless Legs
- o Jaw Pain/TMJ
- o History of Falling
- o Use of Cane or Walker
- o Gout
- o Double Jointed

Other: Sprain of her left knee MCL

Neurological:

- o Stroke/TIA
- o Dementia

Neurological (continued)

- o Polio
- o Parkinson's Disease
- o Multiple Sclerosis
- o Epilepsy/Seizures
- o Concussion
- o Numbness
- o Tingling

Other:_____

Endocrine:

- o Diabetes
- o Kidney Dysfunction
- o Bladder Dysfunction
- o Liver Dysfunction
- o Thyroid Dysfunction

Other:_____

Cardiopulmonary:

- o Congestive Heart Failure
- o Heart Arrhythmia

Cardiopulmonary (continued)

- o Pacemaker
- o High Cholesterol
- o Blood Clots
- o Anemia
- o High Blood Pressure
- o Asthma
- o Shortness of Breath
- o COPD
- o HIV/AIDS

Other:_____

Other:

- o Anxiety
- o Depression
- o Cancer

Chief Complaint: *Lateral/anterior Left knee pain*

Goals for Therapy: *To return to running and to be able to perform day-to-day activity without pain.*

In the last week, how many days have you had pain? *7*

Pain worst: *When attempting to straighten the knee or twist while weight bearing*

Numerical Pain Rating Scale (NPRS)

This patient noted a constant 3/10 pain that worsened to a 6/10 when she attempted to straighten the knee or while twisting in a weight-bearing position.

Unique Outcomes Measures

Lower extremity functional scale (LEFS)[2] = 43/80

Observation

The patient is 5 feet tall and weighs 165 pounds (BMI = 32.2). Her postural assessment shows apprehensiveness to weight bearing on her left lower extremity. Also, knee effusion and ecchymosis were observed around the knee and lateral calf.

Patient History

The patient reports a traumatic injury sustained while sled riding 19 days prior to the physical examination. She reports she propelled off of a ramp traveling at high speeds and landing primarily on her left lower extremity with her knee flexed underneath her body. She denies any popping or clicking sensation at the time of injury. Also, bystanders and friends denied seeing any boney misalignments.

Following the trauma, she was able to ambulate but with significant pain. Since the time of incident, she reports the status of her knee is improving but continues to have constant knee pain (3/10) that worsens with walking, stairs, straightening of her knee, and twisting on the knee during weight bearing (6/10). The patient states she is most comfortable with her knee slightly flexed with a pillow supporting the knee posteriorly.

Mechanism: *Traumatic flexion/rotation left knee injury that occurred while sled riding*

Concordant Sign: *Knee extension or weight bearing while twisting.*

Nature of the Condition: *The patient considers her condition somewhat disabling because she has had to stop running, walks and performs stairs with moderate difficulty, and is unable to find a position or movement that is pain free. Her lower extremity functional scale score of 43/80 places her in severe disability category.*

Behavior of the Symptoms: *Her symptoms are a constant 3/10 pain that worsen throughout the day since so many of her daily activities involve weight bearing and knee extension. The patient reports these activities are unavoidable. She is able to reduce the pain level in the evening by placing the knee in a comfortable and supported position but it generally takes about an hour for it to calm.*

Endnotes

1. Bolton JE. Accuracy of recall of usual pain intensity in back pain patients. Pain 1999;83:533–9.

2. Binkley, J. The lower extremity functional scale (LEFS): Scale development, measurement properties, and clinical application. Phys Ther. 1999;79:371–83.

CASE 70

Setting: *Outpatient Orthopedics*

Date: *Present Day*

Medical Diagnosis: *Knee Pain*

Charted Data

Name:	*William McClaskey*	New Injury:	*Yes*
Age:	*21 years*	General Health:	*Excellent*
MRN:	*96223*	Amount of Exercise:	*2 hours of mixed activity per day, 4–5 times /week*
Home Address:	*2289 Whispering Pines Lane, Boise, Idaho*	Occupation:	*Student*
		Household:	*Single*
Date of Injury:	*2 weeks ago*	Race:	*Caucasian*

Please fill in the location of your pain with a pencil.

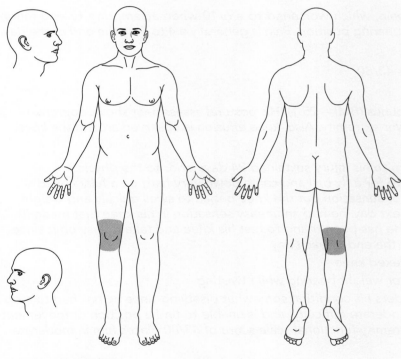

R Front L   L Back R

Pain Intesity Scale	
0	No Pain
1	Low-level pain, able to perform regular activities
2	
(3)	
4	Moderate-level pain, use of pain medication, activity limited but functional
5	
6	
7	High-level pain, use of pain medication, activity very limited—decreased function
8	
9	
10	Emergency Situation

Imaging Results
No imaging was performed.

Medications
Advil (PRN) decreased swelling that allowed additional movement of the knee

Past Medical History (Please check any items that apply to you.)

Musculoskeletal:
- o Osteoarthritis
- o Rheumatoid Arthritis
- o Lupus/SLE
- o Fibromyalgia
- o Osteoporosis
- o Headaches

Musculoskeletal (continued)
- o Bulging Disc
- o Leg Cramps
- o Restless Legs
- o Jaw Pain/TMJ
- o History of Falling
- o Use of Cane or Walker

Musculoskeletal (continued)
- o Gout
- o Double Jointed
- Other: *Sprain of her left knee MCL*

Neurological:
- o Stroke/TIA

Neurological (continued)

- o Dementia
- o Polio
- o Parkinson's Disease
- o Multiple Sclerosis
- o Epilepsy/Seizures
- o Concussion
- o Numbness
- o Tingling

Other:_____

Endocrine:

- o Diabetes

Endocrine (continued)

- o Kidney Dysfunction
- o Bladder Dysfunction
- o Liver Dysfunction
- o Thyroid Dysfunction

Other:_____

Cardiopulmonary:

- o Congestive Heart Failure
- o Heart Arrhythmia
- o Pacemaker
- o High Cholesterol
- o Blood Clots

Cardiopulmonary (continued)

- o Anemia
- o High Blood Pressure
- o Asthma
- o Shortness of Breath
- o COPD
- o HIV/AIDS

Other:_____

Other:

- o Anxiety
- o Depression
- o Cancer

Chief Complaint: *Right knee pain*

Goals for Therapy: *To return to running and training without pain.*

In the last week, how many days have you had pain? *7*

Pain worst: *When attempting to fully straighten or fully flex the knee. Twisting while weight bearing is also very painful. General activity throughout the day increases discomfort and swelling.*

Numerical Pain Rating Scale (NPRS)[1]

The patient noted a constant 1 to 2/10 pain, which worsened to a 6/10 when attempting to end-range knee motion or while twisting in a weight-bearing position. Pain is generally a 4 to 5 by the end of the day.

Unique Outcomes Measures

Lower extremity functional scale (LEFS)[2] = 43/80

Observation

The patient is 6 feet tall and weighs 185 pounds (BMI = 25.1). His postural assessment shows apprehensiveness to weight bearing on the right lower extremity. Also, knee effusion is observed around the knee.

Patient History

The patient reports a traumatic mechanism to his injury sustained 24 days prior to the physical examination while playing softball. He dove for a fly ball and came down very hard on a fully flexed knee. He experienced no popping sound or sensation but the knee began to swell quickly and weight bearing was painful immediately. By the next day, he had an uneasy sensation in his knee that made it feel loose—like it wanted to "give-way." He has been trying to rest his knee and take it easy on it since that time and is using ice and elevation at the end of each day.

Mechanism: *Traumatic landing on a fully flexed knee*

Concordant Sign: *End-range knee motion or weight bearing while twisting*

Nature of the Condition: *The patient considers his condition somewhat disabling since he has had to stop running, walks and performs stairs with moderate difficulty, and is unable to find a position or movement that is completely pain free. His lower extremity functional scale score of 43/80 places him in moderate to severe disability category.*

Behavior of the Symptoms: *The symptoms are a constant 1–2/10 pain that worsens throughout the day since so many of the patient's daily activities involve weight bearing and knee extension. These activities are reported to be unavoidable by the patient. He is able to reduce the pain level in the evening by elevating and supporting the knee in mid-range (40° of flexion), but it generally takes at least 30 minutes for it to calm down.*

Endnotes

1. Bolton JE. Accuracy of recall of usual pain intensity in back pain patients. Pain 1999;83:533–9.

2. Binkley JM, Stratford PW, Lott SA, Riddle DL. The lower extremity functional scale (LEFS): scale development, measurement properties, and clinical application. North American Orthopaedic Rehabilitation Research Network. Phys Ther. 1999;79:371–83.

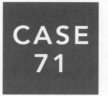

CASE 71

Setting: *Outpatient Orthopedics*

Date: *Present Day*

Medical Diagnosis: *Patellar Dislocation*

Charted Data

Name: *Steve Beaker*

Age: *18 years*

MRN: *83481*

Home Address: *515 Kensington Way, El Paso, Texas*

Date of Injury: *8 days ago*

New Injury: *Yes*

General Health: *Excellent*

Amount of Exercise: *1 hour of mixed activity per day, 7 days/week*

Occupation: *Student*

Household: *Single*

Race: *Caucasian*

Please fill in the location of your pain with a pencil.

R   Front   L   L   Back   R

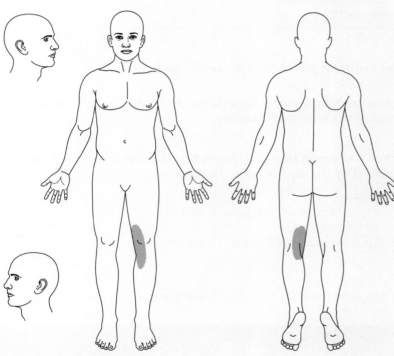

Pain Intensity Scale	
0	No Pain
1	Low-level pain, able to perform regular activities
2	
3	
4	Moderate-level pain, use of pain medication, activity limited but functional
5	
(6)	
7	High-level pain, use of pain medication, activity very limited—decreased function
8	
9	
10	Emergency Situation

Imaging Results
No imaging was performed.

Medications
Vicodin (PRN) or Advil (PRN)

Past Medical History (Please check any items that apply to you.)
Unremarkable

Musculoskeletal:
- ○ Osteoarthritis
- ○ Rheumatoid Arthritis
- ○ Lupus/SLE
- ○ Fibromyalgia
- ○ Osteoporosis
- ○ Headaches
- ○ Bulging Disc
- ○ Leg Cramps
- ○ Restless Legs
- ○ Jaw Pain/TMJ
- ○ History of Falling
- ○ Use of Cane or Walker
- ○ Gout
- ○ Double Jointed

Other:

Neurological:
- ○ Stroke/TIA
- ○ Dementia

Neurological (continued)
- ○ Polio
- ○ Parkinson's Disease
- ○ Multiple Sclerosis
- ○ Epilepsy/Seizures
- ○ Concussion
- ○ Numbness
- ○ Tingling

Other:_____

Endocrine:
- ○ Diabetes
- ○ Kidney Dysfunction
- ○ Bladder Dysfunction
- ○ Liver Dysfunction
- ○ Thyroid Dysfunction

Other:_____

Cardiopulmonary:
- ○ Congestive Heart Failure
- ○ Heart Arrhythmia

Cardiopulmonary (continued)
- ○ Pacemaker
- ○ High Cholesterol
- ○ Blood Clots
- ○ Anemia
- ○ High Blood Pressure
- ○ Asthma
- ○ Shortness of Breath
- ○ COPD
- ○ HIV/AIDS

Other:_____

Other:
- ○ Anxiety
- ○ Depression
- ○ Cancer

Chief Complaint: *Left knee pain*

Goals for Therapy: *To return to normal activity without pain or the sense of "giving way."*

In the last week, how many days have you had pain? *7*

Pain worst: *When attempting to fully straighten or fully flex the knee or twisting while weight bearing. General activity throughout the day increases discomfort and swelling.*

Numerical Pain Rating Scale (NPRS)[1]
The patient noted a constant 1/10 pain, which worsened to a 7/10 when he attempted to twist in a weight-bearing position. Pain is generally a 5/10 by the end of an active day.

SANE Functional Rating
Please rate your **ability** to use your injured area on a 0 to 100% scale with **0%** being unable to use the injured area and **100%** being normal use of injured area in your daily activity: *90%*

Also, if you exercise or have a sport activity or a job that requires special demands please rate your activity on the 0 to 100% scale: *70%*

Patient-Specific Functional Scale
Please list 3 activities that you find are difficult because of this problem and circle the number that corresponds with your ability to perform the activity.

	Unable								No limitations	
1. Running	1	2	③	4	5	6	7	8	9	10
2. Jumping	1	②	3	4	5	6	7	8	9	10
3. Climbing stairs	1	2	3	4	⑤	6	7	8	9	10

Unique Outcomes Measures
Lower extremity functional scale (LEFS)[2] = 47/80

Observation

The patient is 5 feet 8 inches and weighs 135 pounds (BMI = 20.5). His postural assessment showed apprehensiveness to weight bearing on the right lower extremity. Also, mild knee effusion was observed around the knee. He stands in a generally slouched position with sway-back and genu-recurvatum. When the patient steps up or down, a valgus movement with concomitant internal rotation is noted.

Patient History

The patient reports a traumatic mechanism to his injury sustained 8 days prior to the physical examination. When he jumped onto his bicycle, he says that he put his foot down at a "funny angle" and twisted his knee, causing the patella to dislocate and him to collapse to the ground. He was taken to the emergency department, where a physician reduced the dislocation, prescribed Vicodin for symptoms, and gave him crutches and a soft knee brace (immobilizer). The patient reports that there is always pain in the knee right now but that it comes and goes depending on position of the leg or activity level. He states that he has minimized some of his general activities and has been guarding his knee but still is allowing partial weight bearing with the crutches and has been doing isometric contractions of his quadriceps.

Mechanism: *Awkwardly getting on his bicycle*

Concordant Sign: *Weight bearing and end-range movements bother his knee the most.*

Nature of the Condition: *Currently this problem is disabling since the patient is unable to fully bear weight, needs crutches to feel safe to walk, and has pain with most physical activities.*

Behavior of the Symptoms: *The patient's symptoms are isolated to the left knee with some discomfort that extends up into the distal thigh and down into the proximal calf. The knee becomes quite stiff with prolonged positioning.*

Endnotes

1. Bolton JE. Accuracy of recall of usual pain intensity in back pain patients. Pain 1999;83:533–9.

2. Binkley JM, Stratford PW, Lott SA, Riddle DL. The lower extremity functional scale (LEFS): scale development, measurement properties, and clinical application. North American Orthopaedic Rehabilitation Research Network. Phys Ther. 1999;79:371–83.

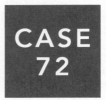

CASE 72

Setting: *Outpatient Orthopedics*

Date: *Present Day*

Medical Diagnosis: *Achilles Tendinitis*

Charted Data

Name:	*Alisha Samuelson*	New Injury:	*No*
Age:	*33 years*	General Health:	*Excellent*
MRN:	*75671*	Amount of Exercise:	*1–2 hours/day, 5 days/week*
Home Address:	*902 East Washington Way, Portland, OR*	Occupation:	*Accounts manager*
		Household:	*Single, lives alone with 2 dogs in single-story home*
Date of Injury:	*6 months ago*	Race:	*Caucasian*

Please fill in the location of your pain with a pencil.

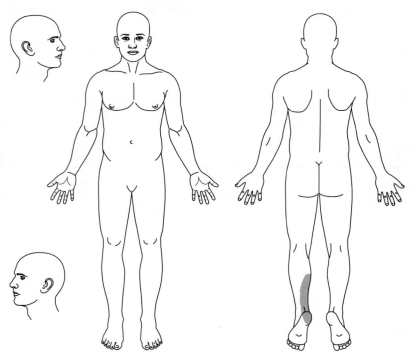

R Front L   L Back R

Pain Intensity Scale	
0	No Pain
1	Low-level pain, able to perform regular activities
2	
3	
4	Moderate-level pain, use of pain medication, activity limited but functional
(5)	
6	
7	High-level pain, use of pain medication, activity very limited—decreased function
8	
9	
10	Emergency Situation

Imaging Results
None performed.

Medications
Aleve (PRN), Albuterol (PRN)

Past Medical History (Please check any items that apply to you.)

Musculoskeletal:
- ○ Osteoarthritis
- ○ Rheumatoid Arthritis
- ○ Lupus/SLE
- ○ Fibromyalgia
- ○ Osteoporosis
- ○ Headaches
- ○ Bulging Disc
- ○ Leg Cramps
- ○ Restless Legs
- ○ Jaw Pain/TMJ
- ○ History of Falling
- ○ Use of Cane or Walker
- ○ Gout
- ○ Double Jointed

Other:

Neurological:
- ○ Stroke/TIA
- ○ Dementia

Neurological (continued)
- ○ Polio
- ○ Parkinson's Disease
- ○ Multiple Sclerosis
- ○ Epilepsy/Seizures
- ○ Concussion
- ○ Numbness
- ○ Tingling

Other:_____

Endocrine:
- ○ Diabetes
- ○ Kidney Dysfunction
- ○ Bladder Dysfunction
- ○ Liver Dysfunction
- ○ Thyroid Dysfunction

Other:_____

Cardiopulmonary:
- ○ Congestive Heart Failure
- ○ Heart Arrhythmia

Cardiopulmonary (continued)
- ○ Pacemaker
- ⊗ High Cholesterol
- ○ Blood Clots
- ○ Anemia
- ○ High Blood Pressure
- ⊗ Asthma
- ○ Shortness of Breath
- ○ COPD
- ○ HIV/AIDS

Other:_____

Other:
- ○ Anxiety
- ○ Depression
- ○ Cancer

Chief Complaint: *Comparable sign is pain between 1 and 2 inches proximal to the calcaneus that becomes worse with irritation and limits activity participation.*

Goals for Therapy: *To reduce the pain to allow full participation in recreational activities.*

In the last week, how many days have you had pain? **7**

Pain worst: *Most of the time, the pain is quite mild but when flared-up from running hills and jumping, it gets pretty severe.*

Numerical Pain Rating Scale[1] (NPRS)
The patient noted a constant sense of discomfort (not really pain) at 1/10 pain that worsens to a 5/10 when she attempts to run hills or jump, but the pain is usually is 3–4/10 with other activities.

SANE Functional Rating

Please rate your **ability** to use your injured area on a 0 to 100% scale with **0%** being unable to use the injured area and **100%** being normal use of injured area in your daily activity: 90%

Also, if you exercise or have a sport activity or a job that requires special demands please rate your activity on the 0 to 100% scale: 70%

Patient-Specific Functional Scale

Please list 3 activities that you find are difficult because of this problem and circle the number that corresponds with your ability to perform the activity.

	Unable									No limitations
1. Running hills	1	2	3	(4)	5	6	7	8	9	10
2. Jumping	1	2	3	(4)	5	6	7	8	9	10
3. Trail running	1	2	3	4	5	(6)	7	8	9	10

Unique Outcomes Measures

Victorian Institute of Sports Assessment-Achilles questionnaire (VISA-A)[2] = 45/100

The VISA-A is a 10-item visual analog questionnaire with each individual question having a range of score from 0–10 and a total of number of possible points from 0 to 100. Reliability (0.81 to 0.93) and validity (0.58 and −0.57) have been established and are acceptable for clinical practice.[2]

Observation

The patient is 5 feet 10 inches and weighs 162 pounds (BMI = 23.2). Her postural assessment showed generally good kinematics.

Patient History

The patient reports a progressive onset of symptoms over a period of months that began as mild soreness in her calf and Achilles tendon after activity. With time, this mild soreness became tightness and eventually pain after most activities. Certain recreational pursuits such as trail running, hill running, and jumping in her volleyball league are the worst and limit her activity the following day. She is now controlling her participation to manage the symptoms.

Mechanism: *Progressive problem with exercise and activity*

Concordant Sign: *End-range ankle dorsiflexion and repetitive motion and/or weight-bearing sport participation.*

Nature of the Condition: *The patient considers her condition somewhat disabling because she has had to reduce her hill running. She is still able to participate but not for as long and intensely as before and she usually has a fair amount of discomfort the following day, requiring longer recovery periods between training sessions.*

Behavior of the Symptoms: *The symptoms are a constant 1/10 pain that worsen throughout the day with activity, but the symptoms are maximized with hill running and especially just after getting out of bed the following morning.*

Endnotes

1. Bolton JE. Accuracy of recall of usual pain intensity in back pain patients. Pain. 1999;83:533–9.

2. Robinson JM, Cook JL, Purdam C, Visentini PJ, Ross J, Maffulli N, et al. The VISA-A questionnaire: a valid and reliable index of the clinical severity of Achilles tendinopathy. Br J Sports Med. 2001;35:335–41.

CASE 73

Setting: *Outpatient Orthopedics*

Date: *Present Day*

Medical Diagnosis: *Ankle Sprain*

Charted Data

Name:	*J. P. Smyth*	New Injury:	*Yes*
Age:	*16 years*	General Health:	*Excellent*
MRN:	*50546*	Amount of Exercise:	*1–2 hours/day, 6 days/week*
Home Address:	*1189 Livingston, Ann Arbor, Michigan*	Occupation:	*High school student*
		Household:	*Lives with family*
Date of Injury:	*Sprained ankle yesterday*	Hand Dominance:	*Right*
		Race:	*White*

Please fill in the location of your pain with a pencil.

R Front L   L Back R

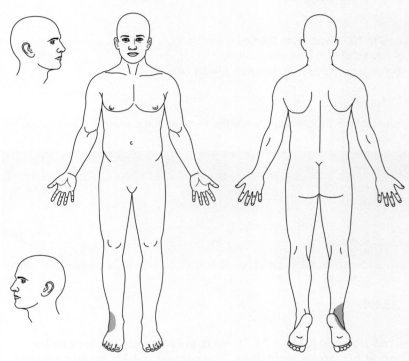

Pain Intensity Scale	
0	No Pain
1	Low-level pain, able to perform regular activities
2	
3	
4	Moderate-level pain, use of pain medication, activity limited but functional
⑤	
6	
7	High-level pain, use of pain medication, activity very limited—decreased function
8	
9	
10	Emergency Situation

Imaging Results
No imaging was performed.

Medications
None

Past Medical History (Please check any items that apply to you.)

Musculoskeletal:
- ○ Osteoarthritis
- ○ Rheumatoid Arthritis
- ○ Lupus/SLE
- ○ Fibromyalgia
- ○ Osteoporosis

Musculoskeletal (continued)
- ⊗ Headaches*
- ○ Bulging Disc
- ○ Leg Cramps
- ○ Restless Legs
- ○ Jaw Pain/TMJ

Musculoskeletal (continued)
- ○ History of Falling
- ○ Use of Cane or Walker
- ○ Gout
- ○ Double Jointed
- Other:_____

Neurological:

- o Stroke/TIA
- o Dementia
- o Polio
- o Parkinson's Disease
- o Multiple Sclerosis
- o Epilepsy/Seizures
- o Concussion
- o Numbness
- o Tingling

Other:_____

Endocrine:

- o Diabetes
- o Kidney Dysfunction

Endocrine (continued)

- o Bladder Dysfunction
- o Liver Dysfunction
- o Thyroid Dysfunction

Other:_____

Cardiopulmonary:

- o Congestive Heart Failure
- o Heart Arrhythmia
- o Pacemaker
- o High Cholesterol
- o Blood Clots
- o Anemia
- o High Blood Pressure
- o Asthma

Cardiopulmonary (continued)

- o Shortness of Breath
- o COPD
- o HIV/AIDS

Other:_____

Other:

- o Anxiety
- o Depression
- o Cancer

Suffers from Migraines

Chief Complaint: *Ankle pain during weight bearing*

Goals for Therapy: *To get back to playing soccer in 2 weeks.*

In the last week, how many days have you had pain? *1*

Pain worst: *All the time*

SANE Functional Rating

Please rate your **ability** to use your injured area on a 0 to 100% scale with **0%** being unable to use the injured area and **100%** being normal use of injured area in your daily activity: ____25%____

Also, if you exercise or have a sport activity or a job that requires special demands please rate your activity on the 0 to 100% scale: ____0%____

Patient-Specific Functional Scale

Please list 3 activities that you find are difficult because of this problem and circle the number that corresponds with your ability to perform the activity.

	Unable								No limitations	
1. Walking	1	2	(3)	4	5	6	7	8	9	10
2. Standing	1	2	3	(4)	5	6	7	8	9	10
3. Running	(1)	2	3	4	5	6	7	8	9	10

Unique Outcomes Measures

Lower extremity functional scale (LEFS) = 28/80

Observation

The patient is 5 feet 10 inches and weighs 165 pounds (BMI = 23.7). He is very fit and appears to be athletic. He exhibits ecchymosis and swelling at his lateral right foot. The patient avoids weight bearing, and walks (quite poorly) with a significant limp. He is in significant pain during weight bearing.

Patient History

He indicates that while jogging in the park he stepped in a hole and rolled his ankle into inversion. He immediately could not weight bear and had to receive assistance from his friends to get him back to his car. He still struggles with weight bearing (it is painful) but also notes significant swelling and the onset of stiffness at his ankle.

Mechanism: *The patient reports an inversion sprain that occurred 1 day ago.*

Concordant Sign: *The patient's worst pain occurs during weight bearing and during active dorsiflexion.*

Nature of the Condition: *The condition has only been present for 1 day. Still, the pain is fairly substantial and the patient reports a lot of discomfort when he tries to walk. When he stays off the foot, the pain is decreased.*

Behavior of the Symptoms: *There is no change in his condition since yesterday other than increased stiffness.*

CASE 74

Setting: *Home Health*
Date: *Present Day*
Medical Diagnosis: *Fifth Metatarsal Fracture*

Charted Data

Name:	*Berta McGuff*	New Injury:	*Yes*
Age:	*88 years*	General Health:	*Poor*
MRN:	*51536*	Amount of Exercise:	*None*
Home Address:	*456 Turtle Dove Drive, Stream, Colorado*	Occupation:	*Retired*
		Household:	*Lives with daughter in one-story home*
Date of Injury:	*Fractured foot 2 months ago. Was in walking boot*	Hand Dominance:	*Right*
		Race:	*Black*

Please fill in the location of your pain with a pencil.

R Front L

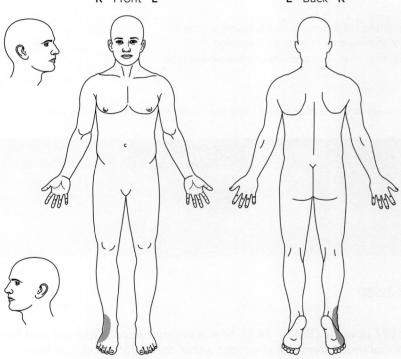

L Back R

Pain Intensity Scale

0	No Pain
1 2	Low-level pain, able to perform regular activities
③	
4 5 6	Moderate-level pain, use of pain medication, activity limited but functional
7 8 9	High-level pain, use of pain medication, activity very limited—decreased function
10	Emergency Situation

Imaging Results
Recent radiograph has indicated the fracture has healed well.

Medications
Rheumatrex oral, Precose, Lasix, Aspirin

Past Medical History (Please check any items that apply to you.)

Musculoskeletal:
- ○ Osteoarthritis
- ⊗ Rheumatoid Arthritis
- ○ Lupus/SLE
- ○ Fibromyalgia
- ○ Osteoporosis

Musculoskeletal (continued)
- ⊗ Headaches
- ○ Bulging Disc
- ○ Leg Cramps
- ○ Restless Legs
- ○ Jaw Pain/TMJ

Musculoskeletal (continued)
- ○ History of Falling
- ○ Use of Cane or Walker
- ○ Gout
- ○ Double Jointed
- Other:_____

201

Neurological:
- o Stroke/TIA
- o Dementia
- o Polio
- o Parkinson's Disease
- o Multiple Sclerosis
- o Epilepsy/Seizures
- o Concussion
- o Numbness
- o Tingling

Other:_____

Endocrine:
- ⊗ Diabetes
- o Kidney Dysfunction

Endocrine (continued)
- o Bladder Dysfunction
- o Liver Dysfunction
- o Thyroid Dysfunction

Other:_____

Cardiopulmonary:
- ⊗ Congestive Heart Failure
- o Heart Arrhythmia
- o Pacemaker
- o High Cholesterol
- o Blood Clots
- o Anemia
- o High Blood Pressure
- o Asthma

Cardiopulmonary (continued)
- o Shortness of Breath
- o COPD
- o HIV/AIDS

Other:_____

Other:
- o Anxiety
- o Depression
- o Cancer

*Suffers from migraines

Chief Complaint: *Stiffness and difficulty with weight bearing for long periods*

Goals for Therapy: *To walk around the house with a cane.*

In the last week, how many days have you had pain? *7*

Pain worst: *All the time*

SANE Functional Rating

Please rate your **ability** to use your injured area on a 0 to 100% scale with **0%** being unable to use the injured area and **100%** being normal use of injured area in your daily activity: ____*35%*____

Also, if you exercise or have a sport activity or a job that requires special demands please rate your activity on the 0 to 100% scale: ____*N/A*____

Patient-Specific Functional Scale

Please list 3 activities that you find are difficult because of this problem and circle the number that corresponds with your ability to perform the activity.

	Unable								No limitations	
1. Walking	1	2	(3)	4	5	6	7	8	9	10
2. Standing	1	2	3	(4)	5	6	7	8	9	10
3. Sitting to standing from toilet	1	2	3	(4)	5	6	7	8	9	10

Unique Outcomes Measures

Lower extremity functional scale (LEFS) = 22/80

Observation

The patient is 5 feet 3 inches and weighs 197 pounds (BMI = 34.9). She is visually deconditioned and has labored breathing. She demonstrates minimal movements of the right ankle and is fatigued just from sitting and talking during the interview.

Patient History

The patient indicates that she tripped on her dog (who is no longer living in the home) and fractured "a bone" in her foot. She was casted for 6 weeks, then given a walking boot to facilitate use. Because her ankle and foot have been stiff, she has avoided weight bearing. She is also scared that using the foot may lead to further fractures.

Mechanism: *More than 2 months ago, the patient tripped on her dog and fractured her foot.*

Concordant Sign: *Weight bearing and pushing off during walking (toe off)*

Nature of the Condition: *The nature of the condition is stiffness and her condition is relatively stable. She exhibits concomitant problems that contribute to her condition.*

Behavior of the Symptoms: *There is no true pattern other than the disuse of the ankle.*

CASE 75

Setting: *Outpatient Orthopedics*

Date: *Present Day*

Medical Diagnosis: *Achilles Tendon Rupture*

Name:	*William A. Jones*	New Injury:	*Yes*
Age:	*52*	General Health:	*Good*
MRN:	*076598887*	Amount of Exercise:	*High*
Home Address:	*352 West Blvd. Mount Pleasant, Michigan*	Occupation:	*College professor*
		Household:	*Single, lives with roommate*
Date of Injury:	*6 weeks prior*	Hand Dominance:	*Right*

Please fill in the location of your pain with a pencil.

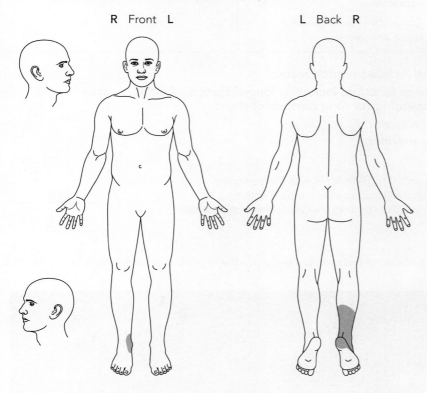

R Front L   L Back R

Pain Intensity Scale	
0	No Pain
1	Low-level pain, able to perform regular activities
2	
③	
4	Moderate-level pain, use of pain medication, activity limited but functional
5	
6	
7	High-level pain, use of pain medication, activity very limited—decreased function
8	
9	
10	Emergency Situation

Imaging Results

A radiograph of the right distal insertion of the Achilles tendon reveals the surgical repair has been completed with full reattachment just proximal to the calcaneal tuberosity.

Medications

Ibuprofen (PRN), Simvastatin, Lisinopril

Past Medical History (Please check any items that apply to you.)

Musculoskeletal:
- ○ Osteoarthritis
- ○ Rheumatoid Arthritis
- ○ Lupus/SLE
- ○ Fibromyalgia
- ○ Osteoporosis
- ○ Headaches
- ⊛ Bulging Disc
- ○ Leg Cramps
- ○ Restless Legs
- ○ Jaw Pain/TMJ
- ○ History of Falling
- ○ Use of Cane or Walker
- ⊛ Gout
- ○ Double Jointed
- Other:_____

Neurological:
- ○ Stroke/TIA
- ○ Dementia

Neurological (continued)
- ○ Polio
- ○ Parkinson's Disease
- ○ Multiple Sclerosis
- ○ Epilepsy/Seizures
- ○ Concussion
- ○ Numbness
- ○ Tingling
- Other:_____

Endocrine:
- ○ Diabetes
- ○ Kidney Dysfunction
- ○ Bladder Dysfunction
- ○ Liver Dysfunction
- ○ Thyroid Dysfunction
- Other:_____

Cardiopulmonary:
- ○ Congestive Heart Failure
- ○ Heart Arrhythmia

Cardiopulmonary (continued)
- ○ Pacemaker
- ⊛ High Cholesterol
- ○ Blood Clots
- ○ Anemia
- ⊛ High Blood Pressure
- ○ Asthma
- ○ Shortness of Breath
- ○ COPD
- ○ HIV/AIDS
- Other:_____

Other:
- ○ Anxiety
- ○ Depression
- ○ Cancer

Chief Complaint: *Ankle stiffness following Achilles tendon repair*

Goals for Therapy: *To return to prior level of function, including long-distance ambulation, stair negotiation, sprinting for softball, and standing for long periods of the day.*

In the last week, how many days have you had pain? *7*

Pain worst: *When standing initially in the morning*

SANE Functional Rating

Please rate your **ability** to use your injured area on a 0 to 100% scale with **0%** being unable to use the injured area and **100%** being normal use of injured area in your daily activity: ___25%___

Also, if you exercise or have a sport activity or a job that requires special demands please rate your activity on the 0 to 100% scale: ___25%___

Patient-Specific Functional Scale

Please list 3 activities that you find are difficult because of this problem and circle the number that corresponds with your ability to perform the activity.

	Unable								No limitations	
1. Standing	1	2	3	(4)	5	6	7	8	9	10
2. Walking	1	2	3	(4)	5	6	7	8	9	10
3. Up/Down stairs	1	2	3	(4)	5	6	7	8	9	10

Unique Outcomes Measures

Lower extremity functional scale (LEFS) = 35/80

Observation

The patient is 5 feet 8 inches tall and weighs 208 pounds (BMI = 31.6). He has a large forward protruding abdomen that causes increased lumbar lordosis when he stands. His right posterior lower leg reveals a well-healed surgical incision with minimal redness; skin is flaky and dry around the incision. His right calf is visibly smaller than his left. The patient wears a walking boot for ambulation at this time.

Patient History

The patient reports the initial tear occurred 6 weeks ago while playing softball. He began to sprint between bases when he tripped, heard an audible "snap," and fell immediately. He was immediately unable to bear weight through his right lower extremity when he attempted to stand. The patient was taken to and treated by a local emergency department with referral to orthopedic surgeon 2 days following the incident.

The patient underwent surgical repair 5 weeks ago. The physician has ordered partial weight bearing on the right lower extremity and instructions that all weight-bearing activities must be completed with his walking cast on and set for 20° plantarflexion. He has been performing light ROM activities as tolerated that were prescribed by his inpatient physical therapist. He was discharged post-op day 2 secondary to DVT concerns following surgery.

The patient states that he works as a college professor and ambulates from home to his classroom in a walking cast (~1 mile each way) and negotiates stairs to the 4th floor classroom. His major concern is that he cannot tolerate standing to teach for more than 10 minutes throughout the day. He is highly motivated and active, and anxious to return to his prior level of function.

Mechanism: *Suspected sudden push off with right lower extremity from baseball base with weight shifted anteriorly over forefoot and knee extended.*

Concordant Sign: *All active and passive ROM of the ankle.*

Nature of the Condition: *Typical Achilles rupture and repair; surgical precautions in place. The patient is not limited by pain and reports only mild discomfort with stretching exercises.*

Behavior of the Symptoms: *Symptoms slightly worsened after a long day of walking, stairs, and standing; patient is minimally irritable.*

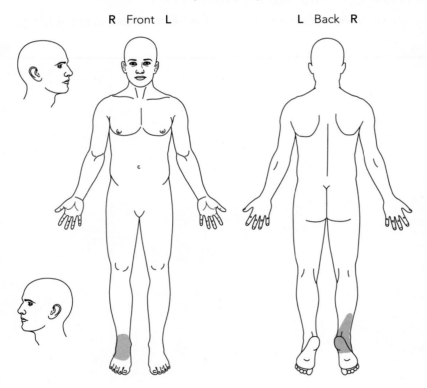

CASE 76

Setting: *Outpatient Orthopedics*

Date: *Present Day*

Medical Diagnosis: *Ankle Sprain*

Charted Data

Name:	*Garret Miser*	General Health:	*Good*
Age:	*20 years*	Amount of Exercise:	*2 hours/day, 6 days/week*
MRN:	*28766*	Occupation:	*College Linebacker*
Home Address:	*546 Martin Road, Pittsburgh, Pennsylvania*	Household:	*Lives in dorm room with roommate*
Date of Injury:	*3 days ago*	Hand Dominance:	*Right*
New Injury:	*Yes*	Race:	*White*

Please fill in the location of your pain with a pencil.

R Front L   L Back R

Pain Intensity Scale

0	No Pain
1	Low-level pain, able to perform regular activities
2	
3	
4	Moderate-level pain, use of pain medication, activity limited but functional
5	
6	
⑦	High-level pain, use of pain medication, activity very limited—decreased function
8	
9	
10	Emergency Situation

Imaging Results

A radiograph of the right ankle yields no fractures.

Medications

Ibuprofen (PRN)

Past Medical History (Please check any items that apply to you.)

Musculoskeletal:

- o Osteoarthritis
- o Rheumatoid Arthritis
- o Lupus/SLE
- o Fibromyalgia
- o Osteoporosis
- o Headaches
- o Bulging Disc
- o Leg Cramps
- o Restless Legs
- o Jaw Pain/TMJ
- o History of Falling
- o Use of Cane or Walker
- o Gout
- o Double Jointed

Other:_____

Neurological:

- o Stroke/TIA
- o Dementia
- o Polio

Neurological (continued)

- o Parkinson's Disease
- o Multiple Sclerosis
- o Epilepsy/Seizures
- ⊗ Concussion
- o Numbness
- o Tingling

Other:_____

Endocrine:

- o Diabetes
- o Kidney Dysfunction
- o Bladder Dysfunction
- o Liver Dysfunction
- o Thyroid Dysfunction

Other:_____

Cardiopulmonary:

- o Congestive Heart Failure
- o Heart Arrhythmia
- o Pacemaker

- o High Cholesterol
- o Blood Clots
- o Anemia
- o High Blood Pressure
- o Asthma
- o Shortness of Breath
- o COPD
- o HIV/AIDS

Other:_____

Other:

- o Anxiety
- o Depression
- o Cancer

Chief Complaint: *The patient has right foot pain and requires the use of crutches for ambulation and is unable to play football*

Goals for Therapy: *To decrease pain in order to discontinue use of crutches and to return to football.*

In the last week, how many days have you had pain? *3*

Pain worst: *With weight bearing*

SANE Functional Rating

Please rate your **ability** to use your injured area on a 0 to 100% scale with **0%** being unable to use the injured area and **100%** being normal use of injured area in your daily activity: *75%*

Also, if you exercise or have a sport activity or a job that requires special demands please rate your activity on the 0 to 100% scale: *50%*

Patient Specific Functional Scale

Please list 3 activities that you find are difficult because of this problem and circle the number that corresponds with your ability to perform the activity.

	Unable									No limitations
1. Walking	1	2	③	4	5	6	7	8	9	10
2. Running	①	2	3	4	5	6	7	8	9	10
3. Stairs	1	2	③	4	5	6	7	8	9	10

Unique Outcomes Measures

Lower extremity functional scale (LEFS) = 25/80

Observation

The patient is 6 feet 1 inch, weighs 220 pounds (BMI = 29.0), and appears in good overall health, muscular and fit. Edema and ecchymosis are noted in the region of the distal tibiofibular syndesmosis and extending up the anterior tibia. There is acute tenderness to palpation over the syndesmosis. The patient avoids right lower extremity weight bearing with use of crutches.

Patient History

This patient is a 20-year-old linebacker for his college football team. His medical history includes a mild concussion during high school football with no previous ankle pathology. He states that during his football game when attempting to tackle his opponent he pivoted on his right foot and fell to the ground in pain.

Mechanism: *The patient reports injuring his ankle 3 days ago during a football game.*

Concordant Sign: *He indicates that he has 7/10 pain that increases with weight bearing over his anterior ankle/lower leg.*

Nature of the Condition: *The patient's condition has been present for 3 days. He avoids right lower extremity weight bearing due to increases in pain.*

Behavior of the Symptoms: *Pain increasing with weight bearing is tender to palpation. The patient reports use of ice and rest for pain relief.*

CASE 77

Setting: *Outpatient Orthopedics*

Date: *Present Day*

Medical Diagnosis: *Left Ankle Injury*

Charted Data

Name:	*Jason Carper*	General Health:	*Good*
Age:	*17 years*	Amount of Exercise:	*2–3 hours/day, 5 days/week*
MRN:	*50490*	Occupation:	*High school student, soccer player*
Home Address:	*4012 State Street, Chicago, Illinois*	Household:	*Lives with parents and sister*
Date of Injury:	*2 weeks ago*	Hand Dominance:	*Right*
New Injury:	*Yes*	Race:	*White*

Please fill in the location of your pain with a pencil.

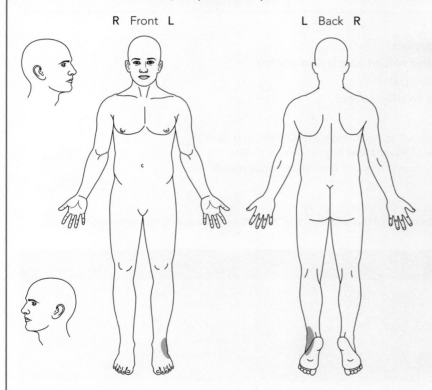

R Front L   L Back R

Pain Intensity Scale	
0	No Pain
1	Low-level pain, able to perform regular activities
2	
3	
4	Moderate-level pain, use of pain medication, activity limited but functional
5	
⑥	
7	High-level pain, use of pain medication, activity very limited—decreased function
8	
9	
10	Emergency Situation

Imaging Results

No imaging was performed.

Medications

Naproxen (PRN)

Past Medical History (Please check any items that apply to you.)

Musculoskeletal:
- ○ Osteoarthritis
- ○ Rheumatoid Arthritis
- ○ Lupus/SLE
- ○ Fibromyalgia
- ○ Osteoporosis
- ○ Headaches
- ○ Bulging Disc
- ○ Leg Cramps
- ○ Restless Legs
- ○ Jaw Pain/TMJ
- ○ History of Falling
- ○ Use of Cane or Walker
- ○ Gout
- ⊗ Double Jointed

Other: *Previous left ankle injury at the age of 12*

Neurological:
- ○ Stroke/TIA
- ○ Dementia

Neurological (continued)
- ○ Polio
- ○ Parkinson's Disease
- ○ Multiple Sclerosis
- ○ Epilepsy/Seizures
- ○ Concussion
- ○ Numbness
- ○ Tingling

Other:_____

Endocrine:
- ○ Diabetes
- ○ Kidney Dysfunction
- ○ Bladder Dysfunction
- ○ Liver Dysfunction
- ○ Thyroid Dysfunction

Other:_____

Cardiopulmonary:
- ○ Congestive Heart Failure
- ○ Heart Arrhythmia

Cardiopulmonary (continued)
- ○ Pacemaker
- ○ High Cholesterol
- ○ Blood Clots
- ○ Anemia
- ○ High Blood Pressure
- ○ Asthma
- ○ Shortness of Breath
- ○ COPD
- ○ HIV/AIDS

Other:_____

Other:
- ○ Anxiety
- ○ Depression
- ○ Cancer

Chief Complaint: *Left ankle pain, lateral aspect*

Goals for Therapy: *To reduce ankle pain and return to playing soccer.*

In the last week, how many days have you had pain? *7*

Pain worst: *After walking and attempting to play soccer*

SANE Functional Rating

Please rate your **ability** to use your injured area on a 0 to 100% scale with **0%** being unable to use the injured area and **100%** being normal use of injured area in your daily activity: *50%*

Also, if you exercise or have a sport activity or a job that requires special demands please rate your activity on the 0 to 100% scale: *25%*

Patient-Specific Functional Scale

Please list **3 activities** that you find are difficult because of this problem and circle the number that corresponds with your ability to perform the activity.

	Unable								No limitations	
1. Walking at school	1	2	3	4	(5)	6	7	8	9	10
2. Playing soccer	1	2	(3)	4	5	6	7	8	9	10
3. Getting in/out of car (driver's side)	1	2	3	4	(5)	6	7	8	9	10

Unique Outcomes Measures

Lower extremity functional scale (LEFS) = 50/80 (37% moderate disability)

Observation

The patient is 5 feet 10 inches and weighs 155 pounds (BMI = 22.2). He is fit and healthy. Currently the patient is weight bearing as tolerated (WBAT) and using bilateral axillary crutches to assist pain reduction in his left ankle. His left ankle appears to have moderate bruising and edema.

Patient History

The patient reports left lateral ankle pain; onset was 2 weeks ago when he injured his ankle during soccer practice. He reports "rolling" his ankle inward as he was about to kick the ball. It was immediately sore and began to swell. Per his coach's advice, he applied ice to his ankle periodically to assist with swelling and pain. The patient decided to use an old pair of crutches that he had at his house to decrease his weight on his ankle and decrease his pain. One week post-injury, the school athletic trainer saw him as he was having increased difficulty walking and could not participate in soccer. The trainer applied an ace wrap to the athlete's ankle; educated him on rest, ice, compression, and elevation of ankle; and encouraged him to seek medical treatment if the pain persisted.

Mechanism: The patient states that his ankle injury occurred at soccer practice after he prepared to kick a ball with his right foot. As he transferred weight to his left lower extremity, his left ankle rolled inward (patient demonstrated the injury as ankle inversion and slight plantarflexion).

Concordant Sign: He reports that his pain is initiated with weight bearing and putting on socks and shoes.

Nature of the Condition: The patient reports intermittent pain of 4/10 in the left lateral ankle at rest. After any weight bearing or attempting soccer activities, pain becomes 8/10, where he is unable to maintain standing on his ankle or participate in soccer activities.

Behavior of the Symptoms: His symptoms worsen during standing, ambulation, and soccer activities. His pain decreases with ice, Naproxen (PRN), and rest with elevation of left lower extremity in seated or supine position.

CASE 78

Setting: *Outpatient Orthopedics*

Date: *Present Day*

Medical Diagnosis: *Right Foot Pain*

Charted Data

Name:	*Cindy Reed*	General Health:	*Good*
Age:	*49 years*	Amount of Exercise:	*1 hour/day, 5 days/week*
MRN:	*86734*	Occupation:	*Chef*
Home Address:	*446 East Market Street, Nashville, Tennessee*	Household:	*Lives in a multi-level home with husband and three children*
Date of Injury:	*Insidious onset about 2 months ago*	Hand Dominance:	*Right*
New Injury:	*Yes*	Race:	*Black*

Please fill in the location of your pain with a pencil.

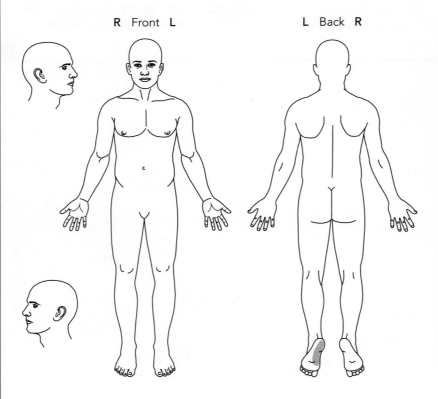

Pain Intensity Scale	
0	No Pain
1	Low-level pain, able to perform regular activities
2	
3	
4	Moderate-level pain, use of pain medication, activity limited but functional
5	
6	
⑦	High-level pain, use of pain medication, activity very limited—decreased function
8	
9	
10	Emergency Situation

Imaging Results

No imaging has been completed.

Medications

Prozac, Ibuprofen (PRN)

Past Medical History (Please check any items that apply to you.)

Musculoskeletal:

- ⊛ Osteoarthritis
- ○ Rheumatoid Arthritis
- ○ Lupus/SLE
- ○ Fibromyalgia
- ○ Osteoporosis
- ○ Headaches
- ○ Bulging Disc
- ○ Leg Cramps
- ○ Restless Legs
- ○ Jaw Pain/TMJ
- ○ History of Falling
- ○ Use of Cane or Walker
- ○ Gout
- ⊛ Double Jointed

Other:_____

Neurological:

- ○ Stroke/TIA
- ○ Dementia
- ○ Polio

Neurological (continued)

- ○ Parkinson's Disease
- ○ Multiple Sclerosis
- ○ Epilepsy/Seizures
- ○ Concussion
- ○ Numbness
- ○ Tingling

Other:_____

Endocrine:

- ○ Diabetes
- ○ Kidney Dysfunction
- ○ Bladder Dysfunction
- ○ Liver Dysfunction
- ○ Thyroid Dysfunction

Other:_____

Cardiopulmonary:

- ○ Congestive Heart Failure
- ○ Heart Arrhythmia
- ○ Pacemaker

Cardiopulmonary (continued)

- ○ High Cholesterol
- ○ Blood Clots
- ○ Anemia
- ⊛ High Blood Pressure
- ○ Asthma
- ○ Shortness of Breath
- ○ COPD
- ○ HIV/AIDS

Other:

Other:

- ○ Anxiety
- ○ Depression
- ○ Cancer

Chief Complaint: *The patient complains of inferior medial left foot pain described as throbbing and piercing with weight bearing*

Goals for Therapy: *To decrease pain in the left foot in order to return to 8-hour workdays and pain-free running.*

In the last week, how many days have you had pain? *7*

Pain worst: *In the morning and following periods of inactivity*

SANE Functional Rating

Please rate your **ability** to use your injured area on a 0 to 100% scale with **0%** being unable to use the injured area and **100%** being normal use of injured area in your daily activity:

_75%_

Also, if you exercise or have a sport activity or a job that requires special demands please rate your activity on the 0 to 100% scale:

_60%_

Patient-Specific Functional Scale

Please list 3 activities that you find are difficult because of this problem and circle the number that corresponds with your ability to perform the activity.

	Unable									No limitations
1. Work 8 hours	1	(2)	3	4	5	6	7	8	9	10
2. Run	(1)	2	3	4	5	6	7	8	9	10
3. Stairs	1	2	(3)	4	5	6	7	8	9	10

Unique Outcomes Measures

Lower extremity functional scale (LEFS) = 30/80

Observation

The patient is 5 feet 6 inches and weighs 145 pounds (BMI = 23.4). In weight bearing, the patient demonstrates genu valgus and foot pronation bilaterally. Her gait reveals minimal toe extension with a pre-swing, decreased heel strike, and excessive pronation during stance on the right.

Patient History

The patient is a 49-year old female with a 2-month history of left inferior-medial foot pain; she denies any history of numbness or tingling. She is required to stand for 8 hours a day as a chef in a local restaurant but has been forced to modify her schedule to accommodate her left foot pain and discomfort. She has also been forced to discontinue running. The patient has not tried orthotics.

Mechanism: *No specific incident triggered the onset. The patient reports gradual onset of pain about 2 months ago.*

Concordant Sign: *The patient states that the pain is the worst in the morning or after periods of inactivity during weight bearing. It is also exacerbated with increased activity such as stairs, running, and standing for extended periods of time.*

Nature of the Condition: *The 7/10 pain she reports occurs in the morning and while at work.*

Behavior of the Symptoms: *Symptoms are the worst in the morning or after periods of prolonged inactivity but lessen with further ambulation. Throughout the day her symptoms occur with activities requiring weight bearing, but the pain lessens with rest (sitting or lying down).*

CASE 79

Setting: *Outpatient Orthopedic Clinic*

Date: *Present Day*

Medical Diagnosis: *Turf Toe*

Charted Data

Name:	*Scott Liverpool*	General Health:	*Excellent*
Age:	*19 years*	Amount of Exercise:	*2 hours/day, 6 days/week*
MRN:	*50578*	Occupation:	*University student and taekwondo player*
Home Address:	*134 East Street, Hamilton, Georgia*	Household:	*Resident in college dormitory*
Date of Injury:	*30 days*	Hand Dominance:	*Right*
New Injury:	*Yes*	Race:	*Caucasian*

Please fill in the location of your pain with a pencil.

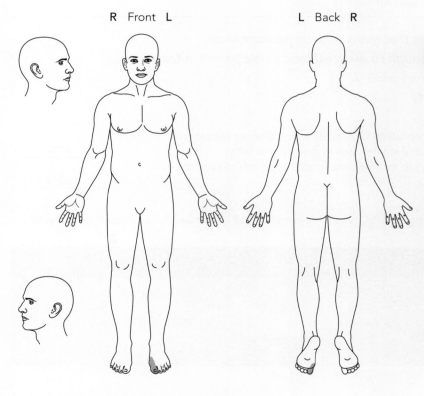

R Front L   L Back R

Pain Intensity Scale	
0	No Pain
1	Low-level pain, able to perform regular activities
2	
3	
4	Moderate-level pain, use of pain medication, activity limited but functional
5	
6	
(7)	High-level pain, use of pain medication, activity very limited— decreased function
8	
9	
10	Emergency Situation

Imaging Results

Radiographs of the left foot were taken, non-weight bearing and with weight bearing. Radiological findings suggest metatarsal-phalangeal (MTP) instability of the first phalange in weight bearing. The MRI shows edema surrounding the medial collateral ligament (MCL) of the MTP joint of the first phalange. The MRI also concluded that there was no fracture, dislocation, or contusion to the surrounding bony structures.

Medications

Ibuprofen PM

Past Medical History (Please check any items that apply to you.)

Unremarkable

Musculoskeletal:
- ○ Osteoarthritis
- ○ Rheumatoid Arthritis
- ○ Lupus/SLE
- ○ Fibromyalgia
- ○ Osteoporosis
- ○ Headaches
- ○ Bulging Disc
- ○ Leg Cramps
- ○ Restless Legs
- ○ Jaw Pain/TMJ
- ○ History of Falling
- ○ Use of Cane or Walker
- ○ Gout
- ○ Double Jointed

Other:_____

Neurological:
- ○ Stroke/TIA
- ○ Dementia

Neurological (continued)
- ○ Polio
- ○ Parkinson's Disease
- ○ Multiple Sclerosis
- ○ Epilepsy/Seizures
- ○ Concussion
- ○ Numbness
- ○ Tingling

Other:_____

Endocrine:
- ○ Diabetes
- ○ Kidney Dysfunction
- ○ Bladder Dysfunction
- ○ Liver Dysfunction
- ○ Thyroid Dysfunction

Other:_____

Cardiopulmonary:
- ○ Congestive Heart Failure
- ○ Heart Arrhythmia

Cardiopulmonary (continued)
- ○ Pacemaker
- ○ High Cholesterol
- ○ Blood Clots
- ○ Anemia
- ○ High Blood Pressure
- ○ Asthma
- ○ Shortness of Breath
- ○ COPD
- ○ HIV/AIDS

Other:_____

Other:
- ○ Anxiety
- ○ Depression
- ○ Cancer

Chief Complaint: *Pain in the left great toe that limits athletic performance*

Goals for Therapy: *To reduce the pain enough to allow athletic participation in taekwondo.*

In the last week, how many days have you had pain? *7*

Pain worst: *During weight-bearing activity*

SANE Functional Rating

Please rate your **ability** to use your injured area on a 0 to 100% scale with **0%** being unable to use the injured area and **100%** being normal use of injured area in your daily activity: _____ *65%* _____

Also, if you exercise or have a sport activity or a job that requires special demands please rate your activity on the 0 to 100% scale: _____ *25%* _____

Patient-Specific Functional Scale

Please list **3 activities** that you find are difficult because of this problem and circle the number that corresponds with your ability to perform the activity

	Unable								No limitations	
1. Running	1	2	③	4	5	6	7	8	9	10
2. Kicking with right foot	1	②	3	4	5	6	7	8	9	10
3. Jumping	1	2	③	4	5	6	7	8	9	10

Unique Outcomes Measures

Lower extremity functional scale (LEFS)[1] = 48/80

Foot and ankle disability index (FADI)[2] = 25/50

Observation

The patient is 6 feet 3 inches and weighs 185 pounds (BMI = 23.1). He presents with an antalgic gait, favoring his left lower extremity. His posture is normal. The left hallux valgus has visible edema at the MTP joint.

Patient History

The patient indicates onset within the last 30 days. The pain was initiated after he attempted to perform a round kick with his right lower extremity (RLE). He immediately had discomfort and experienced difficulty continuing taekwondo. The pain continuously increased over the past 30 days, making it difficult to return to sport.

Mechanism: *Discomfort and worsening pain following a round kick with his RLE.*

Concordant Sign: *Weight-bearing extension of his left great toe produces stabbing pain, whereas a non–weight-bearing position causes a dull ache.*

Nature of the Condition: *The patient's condition moderately limits his walking, steps, and daily activities, but severely limits running, jumping, and other athletic activity.*

Behavior of the Symptoms: *The pain worsens during weight bearing, walking on uneven surfaces, jumping, and sport-related activity.*

Endnotes

1. Binkley JM, Stratford PW, Lott SA, Riddle DL. The lower extremity functional scale (LEFS): scale development, measurement, properties, and clinical application. Phys Ther. 1999;79(4):371–83.

2. Hale SA, Hertel J. Reliability and sensitivity of the foot and ankle disability index in subjects with chronic ankle instability. J Athl Train. 2004;40:35–40.

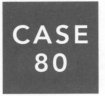

CASE 80

Setting: *Outpatient Clinic*

Date: *Present Day*

Medical Diagnosis: *Grade I Left Syndesmotic Ankle Sprain*

Charted Data

Name:	*Michael Scramm*	Amount of Exercise:	*3–4 hours/day, 6 days/week*
Age:	*27 years*	Occupation:	*Professional football running back*
MRN:	*50774*		
Home Address:	*234 Great Lakes Drive, Salt Lake City, Utah*	Household:	*Travels more than he is home, permanent address is with wife and 2 children*
Date of Injury:	*4 days*		
New Injury:	*Yes*	Hand Dominance:	*Right*
General Health:	*Excellent*	Race:	*Caucasian*

Please fill in the location of your pain with a pencil.

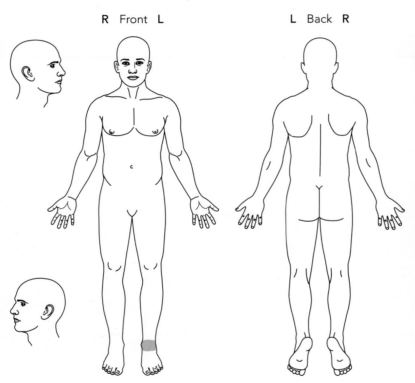

R Front L   L Back R

Pain Intensity Scale	
0	No Pain
1	Low-level pain, able to perform regular activities
2	
3	
4	Moderate-level pain, use of pain medication, activity limited but functional
5	
6	
⑦	High-level pain, use of pain medication, activity very limited—decreased function
8	
9	
10	Emergency Situation

Imaging Results

Anterior-posterior with external rotation and lateral left ankle radiographs rule out presence of fracture.

Medications

None

Past Medical History (Please check any items that apply to you.)

Musculoskeletal:

- ○ Osteoarthritis
- ○ Rheumatoid Arthritis
- ○ Lupus/SLE
- ○ Fibromyalgia
- ○ Osteoporosis
- ○ Headaches
- ○ Bulging Disc
- ○ Leg Cramps
- ○ Restless Legs
- ○ Jaw Pain/TMJ
- ○ History of Falling
- ○ Use of Cane or Walker
- ○ Gout
- ○ Double Jointed

Other: *Recurrent (L) Ankle Sprains*

Neurological:

- ○ Stroke/TIA
- ○ Dementia

Neurological (continued)

- ○ Polio
- ○ Parkinson's Disease
- ○ Multiple Sclerosis
- ○ Epilepsy/Seizures
- ○ Concussion
- ○ Numbness
- ○ Tingling

Other:_____

Endocrine:

- ○ Diabetes
- ○ Kidney Dysfunction
- ○ Bladder Dysfunction
- ○ Liver Dysfunction
- ○ Thyroid Dysfunction

Other:_____

Cardiopulmonary:

- ○ Congestive Heart Failure
- ○ Heart Arrhythmia

Cardiopulmonary (continued)

- ○ Pacemaker
- ○ High Cholesterol
- ○ Blood Clots
- ○ Anemia
- ○ High Blood Pressure
- ○ Asthma
- ○ Shortness of Breath
- ○ COPD
- ○ HIV/AIDS

Other:_____

Other:

- ○ Anxiety
- ○ Depression
- ○ Cancer

Chief Complaint: *Sharp 7/10 pain that is localized right about at the height of the dome of the talus on the dorsal side of the left foot*

Goals for Therapy: *To return to playing football.*

In the last week, how many days have you had pain? *4*

Pain worst: *Weight bearing*

SANE Functional Rating

Please rate your **ability** to use your injured area on a 0 to 100% scale with **0%** being unable to use the injured area and **100%** being normal use of injured area in your daily activity: *60%*

Also, if you exercise or have a sport activity or a job that requires special demands please rate your activity on the 0 to 100% scale: *10%*

Patient-Specific Functional Scale

Please list 3 activities that you find are difficult because of this problem and circle the number that corresponds with your ability to perform the activity.

	Unable									No limitations
1. Walking	1	2	(3)	4	5	6	7	8	9	10
2. Running	(1)	2	3	4	5	6	7	8	9	10
3. 3-point football stance	1	(2)	3	4	5	6	7	8	9	10

Unique Outcome Measures

Lower extremity functional scale (LEFS)[1] = 22/80

Foot and ankle disability index (FADI)[2] = 31/50

Observation

The patient is 6 feet 5 inches and weighs 240 pounds (BMI = 28.5). His gait is altered by a shorter stance phase on his left lower extremity. Heel-strike is absent; instead, stance phase on the left is initiated by metatarsal heads. Minimal edema is noted. Sensory screen reveals that sensation in the area is intact. Dorsal pedal pulse is palpable. Active and passive ROM does not increase pain, with the exception of passive dorsiflexion, which causes an increase in pain over the anterior tibiofibular ligament. Palpation of malleoli and tarsals is not provocative. Palpation of anterior talofibular and calcaneofibular ligaments is nonprovocative.

Patient History

The patient's overall general health is excellent. He is a young, professional football player who is highly active. Review of symptoms and past medical history are negative, with the exception of frequent left ankle sprains.

Mechanism: *In an attempt to elude a tackle during practice, the patient pivoted on his left lower extremity (LE). He does not recall hearing any noises such as a "pop."*

Concordant Sign: *Concordant pain over the dorsal talar dome of the left ankle is reproduced with dorsiflexion, whether passive or active in weight bearing.*

Nature of the Condition: *Acute injury*

Behavior of the Symptoms: *The patient reports that the 3-point football stance, which he must assume multiple times during practices and games, increases his pain. Any kind of weight-bearing activity as well as passive dorsiflexion also increase his symptoms. Pain is relieved by complete rest and immobilization of the left ankle.*

Endnotes

1. Binkley JM, Stratford PW, Lott SA, Riddle DL. The lower extremity functional scale (LEFS): scale development, measurement, properties, and clinical application. Phys Ther. 1999;79(4):371–83.

2. Hale SA, Hertel J. Reliability and sensitivity of the foot and ankle disability index in subjects with chronic ankle instability. J Athl Train. 2004;40:35–40.

CASE 81

Setting: *Outpatient Orthopedics*

Date: *Present Day*

Medical Diagnosis: *Hypomobile Talocrural Postrecurrent Ankle Sprains*

Charted Data

Name:	*Brady Li*	General Health:	*Excellent*
Age:	*20 years*	Amount of Exercise:	*30 minutes to 1 hour/day, 4 days/week*
MRN:	*50501*		
Home Address:	*643 Miller Drive, Herndon, VA*	Occupation:	*College student*
		Household:	*Single, lives alone*
Date of Injury:	*2 months ago*	Hand Dominance:	*Right*
New Injury:	*No*	Race:	*Asian*

Please fill in the location of your pain with a pencil.

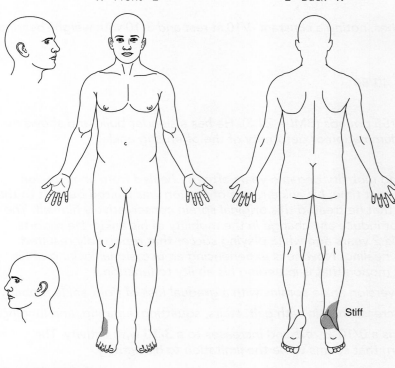

Stiff

Pain Intensity Scale	
0	No Pain
1	Low-level pain, able to perform regular activities
2	
3	
4	Moderate-level pain, use of pain medication, activity limited but functional
5	
6	
(7)	High-level pain, use of pain medication, activity very limited—decreased function
8	
9	
10	Emergency Situation

Imaging Results
Radiographs revealed slight narrowing of the joint space of the talocrural joint space.

Medications
None

Past Medical History (Please check any items that apply to you.)

Musculoskeletal:
- ○ Osteoarthritis
- ○ Rheumatoid Arthritis
- ○ Lupus/SLE
- ○ Fibromyalgia
- ○ Osteoporosis

Musculoskeletal (continued)
- ○ Headaches
- ○ Bulging Disc
- ○ Leg Cramps
- ○ Restless Legs
- ○ Jaw Pain/TMJ

Musculoskeletal (continued)
- ○ History of Falling
- ○ Use of Cane or Walker
- ○ Gout
- ○ Double Jointed
- Other: *Lateral Ankle Sprain x2*

Neurological:

- o Stroke/TIA
- o Dementia
- o Polio
- o Parkinson's Disease
- o Multiple Sclerosis
- o Epilepsy/Seizures
- o Concussion
- o Numbness
- o Tingling

Other:_____

Endocrine:

- o Diabetes
- o Kidney Dysfunction

Endocrine (continued)

- o Bladder Dysfunction
- o Liver Dysfunction
- o Thyroid Dysfunction

Other:_____

Cardiopulmonary:

- o Congestive Heart Failure
- o Heart Arrhythmia
- o Pacemaker
- o High Cholesterol
- o Blood Clots
- o Anemia
- o High Blood Pressure
- o Asthma

Cardiopulmonary (continued)

- o Shortness of Breath
- o COPD
- o HIV/AIDS

Other:_____

Other:

- o Anxiety
- o Depression
- o Cancer

Chief Complaint: *Limited right ankle mobility and pain anteriorly*

Goals for Therapy: *To improve mobility and the ability to ambulate, do stairs, and participate in sport-related activities.*

In the last week, how many days have you had pain? *4*

Pain worst: *During stair climbing, squatting, and lunging*

Numerical Pain Rating Scale (NPRS)[1]

The patient related this scale to his headaches, noting a constant 0/10 at rest and 3/10 with weight-bearing activity.

Unique Outcomes Measures

Lower extremity functional scale (LEFS)[2] = 40/80

Observation

The patient is 5 feet 7 inches and weighs 155 pounds (BMI = 24.3). He has a slender build and shows no signs of discomfort. There is no sign of inflammation or deformity of the offending ankle.

Patient History

The patient reports that his pain and limited mobility began 6 years after he healed from an inversion ankle sprain he acquired while running. At that time, his ankle range of motion was limited but not to the degree it is presently. The patient reports that he treated this original sprain conservatively himself. The treatment resulted in pain relief but did not induce any change in the mobility of his ankle. He reports a second inversion sprain of the same ankle 2 years ago while playing soccer that reportedly resulted in further reduction of ankle mobility after healing. Now he is experiencing an occasional locking of his ankle and a significantly noticeable loss of motion that is impeding his ability to function.

Mechanism: *There are repeated chronic inversion ankle sprains with a gradual loss of right ankle mobility.*

Concordant Sign: *The patient reports an increase in pain with gait, stairs, squatting, jumping, and lunging.*

Nature of the Condition: *The pain intensity is a 0/10 at rest and increases to a 3/10 with activity. The sensation of stiffness is the primary concern that seems to be the limitation to his activity.*

Behavior of the Symptoms: *The patient's symptoms worsen with activity and are not present at rest.*

Endnotes

1. Bolton JE. Accuracy of recall of usual pain intensity in back pain patients. Pain 1999;83:533–9.

2. Binkley, J. The lower extremity functional scale (LEFS): scale development, measurement properties, and clinical application. Phys Ther. 79.4 (1999):371–83.

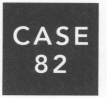

CASE 82

Setting: *Outpatient Orthopedics*

Date: *Present Day*

Medical Diagnosis: *Lower Leg Pain*

Charted Data

Name:	*Daryl Jacobs*	General Health:	*Good*
Age:	*42 years*	Amount of Exercise:	*30–35 minutes of walking/ day, 5 days/week*
MRN:	*50501*	Occupation:	*Desk work*
Home Address:	*317 Eden Court, Trenton, New Jersey*	Household:	*Married, lives with wife and 2 children*
Date of Injury:	*6 months ago*	Hand Dominance:	*Right*
New Injury:	*Yes*	Race:	*Caucasian*

Please fill in the location of your pain with a pencil.

R Front L   L Back R

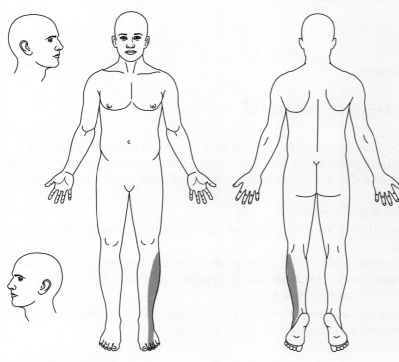

Pain Intensity Scale	
0	No Pain
1 2 3	Low-level pain, able to perform regular activities
4 5 6	Moderate-level pain, use of pain medication, activity limited but functional
⑦ 8 9	High-level pain, use of pain medication, activity very limited—decreased function
10	Emergency Situation

Imaging Results

Radiographs of the knee/ankle-foot complex were obtained and the impression was normal.

Medications

Ibuprofen (PRN)

Past Medical History (Please check any items that apply to you.)

Musculoskeletal:
- o Osteoarthritis
- o Rheumatoid Arthritis
- o Lupus/SLE
- o Fibromyalgia
- o Osteoporosis

Musculoskeletal (continued)
- ⊗ Headaches
- o Bulging Disc
- o Leg Cramps
- o Restless Legs
- o Jaw Pain/TMJ

Musculoskeletal (continued)
- o History of Falling
- o Use of Cane or Walker
- o Gout
- o Double Jointed
- Other:_____

Neurological:

- o Stroke/TIA
- o Dementia
- o Polio
- o Parkinson's Disease
- o Multiple Sclerosis
- o Epilepsy/Seizures
- o Concussion
- o Numbness
- o Tingling

Other:_____

Endocrine:

- o Diabetes
- o Kidney Dysfunction

Endocrine (continued)

- o Bladder Dysfunction
- o Liver Dysfunction
- o Thyroid Dysfunction

Other:_____

Cardiopulmonary:

- o Congestive Heart Failure
- o Heart Arrhythmia
- o Pacemaker
- o High Cholesterol
- o Blood Clots
- o Anemia
- o High Blood Pressure
- o Asthma

Cardiopulmonary (continued)

- o Shortness of Breath
- o COPD
- o HIV/AIDS

Other:_____

Other:

- ⊗ Anxiety
- o Depression
- o Cancer

Chief Complaint: *Pain in the lower third of the left lower extremity, lateral aspect of the fibula extending to the second and third toes*

Goals for Therapy: *To be able to push down on the gas pedal and brake while driving and be able to sit or walk for more than 1 hour.*

In the last week, how many days have you had pain? *7*

Pain worst: *After sitting or walking for more than 1 hour*

Outcome Measures

Visual analog scale (VAS)[1] = 6.3 cm

Unique Outcomes Measures

Lower extremity functional scale (LEFS)[2] = 59/80

Observation

The patient is 6 feet 2 inches and weighs 214 pounds (BMI = 27.5).

Patient History

The patient reports that his symptoms have been present for a total of 6 months. During the initial 3 months, his symptoms worsened each day until plateauing. His symptoms gradually progressed and are located on his left lower leg, approximately the distal third to the second and third toes. Rest relieves his pain within 50 seconds.

Mechanism: *The patient could not recall any specific incident.*

Concordant Sign: *Walking or sitting for more than 1 hour. The patient has difficulty pushing down on the break and accelerator pedals while driving.*

Nature of the Condition: *The patient's symptoms rated as a 6.3 cm on the VAS are intermittent and are provoked by sitting or walking for more than 1 hour. Upon assuming a resting position, the symptoms are relieved in 50 seconds. The LEFS score for disability was a 59/80.*

Behavior of the Symptoms: *The 24-hour behavior pattern varies day to day depending on the activity. The symptoms, though, are consistently aggravated by prolong sitting or walking.*

Endnotes

1. Bijur PE, Silver W, Gallagher EJ. Reliability of the visual analog scale for measurement of acute pain. Acad Emerg Med. 2002;8:1153–7.

2. Binkley, J. The lower extremity functional scale (LEFS): scale development, measurement properties, and clinical application." Phys Ther. 79.4 (1999):371–83.

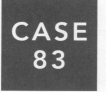

CASE 83

Setting: *Acute Rehab Facility*

Date: *Present Day*

Medical Diagnosis: *Stage IIB Osteosarcoma of Left Femur Following Total Femur Replacement*

Charted Data

Name:	*Douglas Wright*
Age:	*62 years*
MRN:	*226518*
Home Address:	*1879 Copley Street, Des Moines, Iowa*
Date of Injury:	*8 days post-op*
New Injury:	*Progressive cancer requiring surgical intervention*
General Health:	*Poor*
Amount of Exercise:	*0 hours/day, 0 days/week*
Occupation:	*Fast-food restaurant manager*

Household: *Married with 4 adult children living in state. 40 pack-year smoking history, quit when diagnosed with osteosarcoma. He lives in a 2-story house with 7 steps to enter/exit his home. Patient was functionally independent prior to surgery at home and in the community using a straight cane.*

Hand Dominance: *Right*

Race: *White*

Please fill in the location of your pain with a pencil.

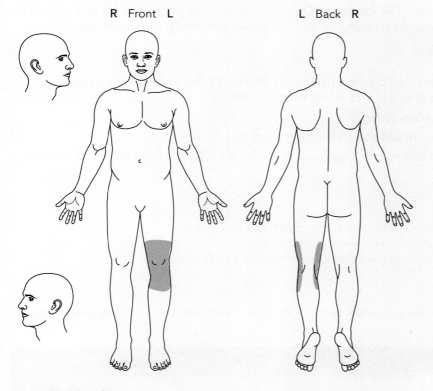

R Front L   L Back R

Pain Intensity Scale

0	No Pain
1	Low-level pain, able to perform regular activities
2	
3	
4	Moderate-level pain, use of pain medication, activity limited but functional
5	
6	
⑦	High-level pain, use of pain medication, activity very limited—decreased function
8	
9	
10	Emergency Situation

Imaging Results
No imaging was performed.

Medical Testing Results
Hemoglobin = 16 (reference 14–17 g/100 ml)[1]
Hematocrit = 48 (reference 41%–51%)[1]

Medications

Extra Strength Tylenol, Lopressor, Lovenox, Singulair, Micronase. Scheduled for future radiation therapy when stable.

Past Medical History (Please check any items that apply to you.)

Musculoskeletal:

- o Osteoarthritis
- o Rheumatoid Arthritis
- o Lupus/SLE
- o Fibromyalgia
- o Osteoporosis
- o Headaches
- o Bulging Disc
- o Leg Cramps
- o Restless Legs
- o Jaw Pain/TMJ
- o History of Falling
- o Use of Cane or Walker
- o Gout
- o Double Jointed

Other:_____

Neurological:

- o Stroke/TIA
- o Dementia
- o Polio

Neurological (continued)

- o Parkinson's Disease
- o Multiple Sclerosis
- o Epilepsy/Seizures
- o Concussion
- o Numbness
- o Tingling

Other:_____

Endocrine:

- ⊗ Diabetes
- o Kidney Dysfunction
- o Bladder Dysfunction
- o Liver Dysfunction
- o Thyroid Dysfunction

Other:_____

Cardiopulmonary:

- ⊗ Hypertension
- o Coronary Artery Disease
- o Congestive Heart Failure

Cardiopulmonary (continued)

- o Heart Arrhythmia
- o Pacemaker
- ⊗ High Cholesterol
- o Blood Clots
- o Anemia
- o High Blood Pressure
- ⊗ Asthma
- o Shortness of Breath
- o COPD
- o HIV/AIDS

Other:_____

Other:

- o Anxiety
- o Depression
- ⊗ Cancer

Patient Presentation

The patient is currently on a surgical ward. The current MD orders are for the patient to be out of bed as tolerated. He may try touching down weight bearing on the left lower extremity. No active straight leg raises or hip abduction against gravity.

Observation

The patient is 6 feet 2 inches and weighs 165 pounds (BMI = 21.2). He is lying in bed with a Foley catheter in place. Surgical incisions are dressed and intact over his left hip.

Chief Complaint: *"Feels weird to have a bionic leg."*

Goals for Therapy: *"To walk my daughter down the aisle at her wedding."*

In the last week, how many days have you had pain? *"I've been weak for so long it's hard to tell how many days it's been."*

Pain worst: *When medication wears off*

SANE Functional Rating

Please rate your **ability** to use your injured area on a 0 to 100% scale with **0%** being unable to use the injured area and **100%** being normal use of injured area in your daily activity: *20%*

Also, if you exercise or have a sport activity or a job that requires special demands please rate your activity on the 0 to 100% scale: *N/A*

Patient-Specific Functional Scale

Please list **3 activities** that you find are difficult because of this problem and circle the number that corresponds with your ability to perform the activity.

	Unable									No limitations
1. Walking	1	(2)	3	4	5	6	7	8	9	10
2. Standing	1	2	3	(4)	5	6	7	8	9	10
3. Moving in bed	1	(2)	3	4	5	6	7	8	9	10

Standardized Tests

Musculoskeletal Tumour Society (MTS) rating scale[2] = 19 / 30

Endnotes

1. Acute Care Section Lab Values Resource Update 2012, American Physical Therapy Association.

2. Enneking WF. Staging musculoskeletal tumors. In: Enneking WF (ed.) Musculoskeletal Tumor Surgery. New York; Churchill Livingstone, 1983:69–88.

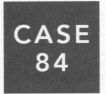

CASE 84

Setting: *Skilled Nursing Facility*

Date: *Present Day*

Medical Diagnosis: *Right Femur Fracture with ORIF*

Charted Data

Name:	*Bob Brown*	Occupation:	*Retired attorney*
Age:	*77 years*	Household:	*Married with 4 adult children living both in and out of state. Lives in a 2-story home and prior to surgery was functionally independent at home and in the community without any assistive devices.*
MRN:	*2568903*		
Home Address:	*1200 Quincy Avenue, Rockville, Maryland*		
Date of Injury:	*5 days ago*		
New Injury:	*Yes*		
General Health:	*Good*	Hand Dominance:	*Right*
Amount of Exercise:	*1 hour/day, 5 days/week "Mall walker"*	Race:	*White*

Please fill in the location of your pain with a pencil.

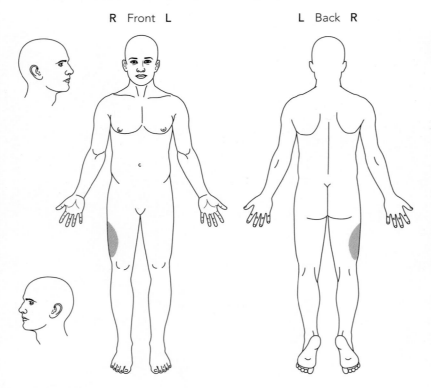

R Front L   L Back R

Pain Intensity Scale

0	No Pain
1	Low-level pain, able to perform regular activities
②	
3	
4	Moderate-level pain, use of pain medication, activity limited but functional
5	
6	
7	High-level pain, use of pain medication, activity very limited—decreased function
8	
9	
10	Emergency Situation

Imaging Results
No imaging was performed.

Medical Testing Results
- *Hemoglobin = 16 (reference 14–17 g/100 ml)[1]*
- *Hematocrit = 50 (reference 41%–51%)[1]*

Medications
Lopressor, Metformin, ASA

Past Medical History (Please check any items that apply to you.)

Musculoskeletal:
- ○ Osteoarthritis
- ○ Rheumatoid Arthritis
- ○ Lupus/SLE
- ○ Fibromyalgia
- ○ Osteoporosis
- ○ Headaches
- ○ Bulging Disc
- ○ Leg Cramps
- ○ Restless Legs
- ○ Jaw Pain/TMJ
- ○ History of Falling
- ○ Use of Cane or Walker
- ○ Gout
- ○ Double Jointed

Neurological:
- ○ Stroke/TIA
- ○ Dementia
- ○ Polio

Neurological (continued)
- ○ Parkinson's Disease
- ○ Multiple Sclerosis
- ○ Epilepsy/Seizures
- ○ Concussion
- ○ Numbness
- ○ Tingling

Other:_____

Endocrine:
- ⊗ Diabetes
- ○ Kidney Dysfunction
- ○ Bladder Dysfunction
- ○ Liver Dysfunction
- ○ Thyroid Dysfunction

Other:_____

Cardiopulmonary:
- ⊗ Hypertension
- ⊗ Coronary Artery Disease

Cardiopulmonary (continued)
- ○ Congestive Heart Failure
- ○ Heart Arrhythmia
- ○ Pacemaker
- ○ High Cholesterol
- ○ Blood Clots
- ○ Anemia
- ○ High Blood Pressure
- ○ Asthma
- ○ Shortness of Breath
- ○ COPD
- ○ HIV/AIDS

Other:_____

Other:
- ○ Anxiety
- ○ Depression
- ○ Cancer

Patient Presentation

Current MD orders are for patient to be out of bed as tolerated with progressive activity. Patient can be partial weight bearing (PWB) on right lower extremity (RLE).

The patient is 6 feet 2 inches and weighs 205 pounds (BMI = 26.3). He is sitting up in the chair watching TV. His surgical incisions are dressed and intact over his right femur.

Chief Complaint: *"I'm limping."*

Goals for Therapy: *To "walk like I used to."*

In the last week, how many days have you had pain? *"My leg has been sore since I fell and broke it."*

Pain worst: *"When I go to get out of bed, after lying down for a while."*

SANE Functional Rating

Please rate your **ability** to use your injured area on a 0 to 100% scale with **0%** being unable to use the injured area and **100%** being normal use of injured area in your daily activity: _65%_

Also, if you exercise or have a sport activity or a job that requires special demands please rate your activity on the 0 to 100% scale: _N/A_

Patient-Specific Functional Scale

Please list 3 activities that you find are difficult because of this problem and circle the number that corresponds with your ability to perform the activity.

	Unable								No limitations	
1. Walking	1	2	3	4	5	6	(7)	8	9	10
2. Standing	1	2	3	4	5	6	7	8	(9)	10
3. Moving in bed	1	2	3	(4)	5	6	7	8	9	10

Standardized Tests

Functional Independence Measure (FIM) mobility subscale = 68 points/91 points

Endnotes

1. Acute Care Section Lab Values Resource Update 2012, American Physical Therapy Association.

CASE 85

Setting: *Acute Care Facility*

Date: *Present Day*

Medical Diagnosis: *Multi-trauma*

Charted Data

Name: *Bobby Jones*

Age: *62 years*

MRN: *11032*

Home Address: *75 North Street, Springfield, Illinois*

Date of Injury: *1 day(s)*

New Injury: *Yes*

General Health: *Poor*

Amount of Exercise: *1 hour/day, 3 days /week*

Occupation: *Real estate agent*

Household: *Married with 4 adult children living in the region. Family is very supportive. 30 pack-year smoking history, but quit 5 years ago after his myocardial infarction (MI). He lives in a 2-story house with a full bathroom on both floors. There are 5 steps to enter/ exit his home.*

Hand Dominance: *Right*

Race *African American*

Please fill in the location of your pain with a pencil.

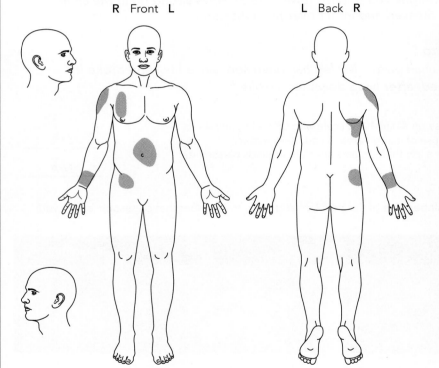

R Front L   L Back R

Pain Intensity Scale	
0	No Pain
1	Low-level pain, able to perform regular activities
2	
3	
4	Moderate-level pain, use of pain medication, activity limited but functional
5	
(6)	
7	High-level pain, use of pain medication, activity very limited—decreased function
8	
9	
10	Emergency Situation

Imaging Results

No imaging was performed.

History of Present Illness

The patient is a 62-year-old male admitted to the emergency room for status post-multi-trauma resulting from motorcycle accident. He was helmeted and had a brief loss of consciousness (LOC) at the scene. The emergency room (ER) assessment revealed the following:

- Diffuse ecchymosis throughout
- Rib fractures on the right with hemopneumothorax
- Displaced right proximal humeral head fracture
- Right Colles' fracture
- Right lateral compression fracture of pelvis with oblique pubic ramus fracture
- Acute abdomen

Management in the ER included stabilization of bleeding, chest tube insertion, IV fluids, and pain management. Upper extremity fractures were immobilized until further surgical consult. After stabilization, the patient was brought to the operating room (OR) for exploratory laparotomy and possible management of orthopedic injuries. The exploratory laparotomy revealed a splenic laceration and resulted in a splenectomy. An open reduction external fixation (OREF) of the Colles' fracture was also performed.

Surgical repair of the right humeral fracture was deferred until patient was more hemodynamically stable—approximately 2 days later when the open reduction internal fixation (ORIF) was performed on the humeral head fracture.

Current MD orders are for patient to be out of bed as tolerated with progressive activity in preparation for discharge. Patient can be weight bearing as tolerated (WBAT) on RLE. Right UE to remain in sling immobilization at all times, except for therapy, dressing, and bathing.

Medical Testing Results

- Radiographs: resolving hemopneumothorax, hardware in place right radioulnar joint and proximal humerus
- PT/INR = 2.2 (reference 0.9–1.1)[1]
- Hemoglobin = 17 (reference 14–17 g/100 ml)[1]
- Hematocrit = 44 (reference 41%–51%)[1]

Medications

NTG PRN, Ventolin, Beclovent nebulizers, Dilaudid, periodic blood transfusions, Lovenox

Past Medical History (Please check any items that apply to you.)

Musculoskeletal:

- ○ Osteoarthritis
- ⊗ Rheumatoid Arthritis
- ○ Lupus/SLE
- ○ Fibromyalgia
- ○ Osteoporosis
- ○ Headaches
- ○ Bulging Disc
- ○ Leg Cramps
- ○ Restless Legs
- ○ Jaw Pain/TMJ
- ○ History of Falling
- ○ Use of Cane or Walker
- ○ Gout
- ○ Double Jointed

Other:_____

Neurological:

- ○ Stroke/TIA
- ○ Dementia
- ○ Polio

Neurological (continued)

- ○ Parkinson's Disease
- ○ Multiple Sclerosis
- ○ Epilepsy/Seizures
- ○ Concussion
- ○ Numbness
- ○ Tingling

Other:_____

Endocrine:

- ⊗ Diabetes
- ○ Kidney Dysfunction
- ○ Bladder Dysfunction
- ○ Liver Dysfunction
- ○ Thyroid Dysfunction

Other:_____

Cardiopulmonary:

- ⊗ Hypertension
- ⊗ Coronary Artery Disease
- ○ Congestive Heart Failure

Cardiopulmonary (continued)

- ○ Heart Arrhythmia
- ○ Pacemaker
- ⊗ High Cholesterol
- ○ Blood Clots
- ○ Anemia
- ○ High Blood Pressure
- ⊗ Asthma
- ○ Shortness of Breath
- ⊗ COPD
- ○ HIV/AIDS

Other: 1 Heart attack, just quit smoking 1 pack/day for 35 years

Other:

- ○ Anxiety
- ○ Depression
- ○ Cancer

Patient Presentation in Surgical Ward

The patient is 5 feet 10 inches and weighs 185 pounds (BMI = 26.5). He is lying in bed with the following equipment in place:

Lines and Tubes: peripheral IV in left wrist, chest tube on right side (water seal), Foley catheter, JP drain abdomen, RUQ

EKG: fluctuates between NSR, atrial fibrillation, and occasional runs of unsustained couplets.

O_2 *saturation on 2 liters of oxygen via nasal prongs = 96%*
His surgical incisions are dressed and intact over his abdomen, right humerus, and right wrist. His right upper extremity is in a sling for immobilization and his right wrist is in a splint.

Chief Complaint: *Really sore and feels weak*

Goals for Therapy: *To get walking and out of the hospital.*

In the last week, how many days have you had pain? *"I think 5."*

Pain worst: *When medication wears off*

SANE Functional Rating

Please rate your **ability** to use your injured area on a 0 to 100% scale with **0%** being unable to use the injured area and **100%** being normal use of injured area in your daily activity: *N/A*

Also, if you exercise or have a sport activity or a job that requires special demands please rate your activity on the 0 to 100% scale: *N/A*

Patient-Specific Functional Scale

Please list **3 activities** that you find are difficult because of this problem and circle the number that corresponds with your ability to perform the activity.

	Unable								No limitations	
1. Walking	1	(2)	3	4	5	6	7	8	9	10
2. Standing	1	(2)	3	4	5	6	7	8	9	10
3. Moving in bed	1	2	(3)	4	5	6	7	8	9	10

Standardized Tests (performed 1 day apart)

Timed up and go test (TUG) = 55 seconds (requires rolling walker and contact guard x1)
Berg balance scale (BBS) = 7/56 high risk for falls

Endnotes

1. Acute Care Section Lab Values Resource Update 2012, American Physical Therapy Association.

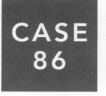

CASE 86

Setting: *Acute Rehabilitation Facility*

Date: *Present Day*

Medical Diagnosis: *Multi-trauma*

Charted Data

Name: *Juan Ramirez*

Age: *22 years*

MRN: *1760528*

Home Address: *13 South Street, Springfield, California*

Date of Injury: *44 days ago*

New Injury: *Yes*

General Health: *Good*

Amount of Exercise: *Several hours/day, 7 days/ week*

Occupation: *U.S. Army Soldier*

Household: *Single male, previously living in barracks before going overseas for combat in Iraq*

Hand Dominance: *Right*

Race: *Hispanic*

Please fill in the location of your pain with a pencil.

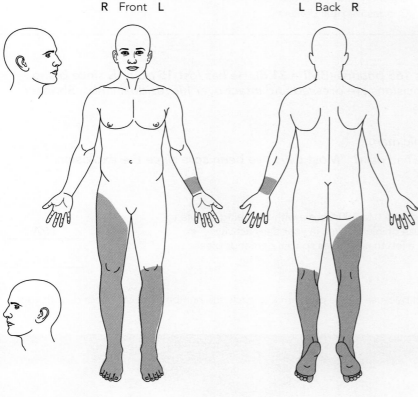

R   Front   L   L   Back   R

Pain Intensity Scale	
0	No Pain
1	Low-level pain, able to perform regular activities
2	
3	
4	Moderate-level pain, use of pain medication, activity limited but functional
5	
⑥	
7	High-level pain, use of pain medication, activity very limited—decreased function
8	
9	
10	Emergency Situation

History of Present Illness

The patient is a 22-year-old[1] male soldier transferred to acute rehabilitation 22 days after sustaining blast injuries during overseas combat. He was initially stabilized in the field then transferred to Germany for further management. After stabilization at the medical facility in Germany, he was transferred to the United States for the remainder of his medical care and rehabilitation. Injuries sustained resulted in (1) left transradial amputation, (2) right hip disarticulation, and (3) left knee disarticulation.

Current MD orders are for patient to be out of bed as tolerated with progressive activity. Patient can be weight bearing as tolerated (WBAT) on all affected extremities. Dressing changes to be made to affected extremities and residual limbs.

Medications
Gabapentin

Past Medical History (Please check any items that apply to you.)

Musculoskeletal:
- ○ Osteoarthritis
- ○ Rheumatoid Arthritis
- ○ Lupus/SLE
- ○ Fibromyalgia
- ○ Osteoporosis
- ○ Headaches
- ○ Bulging Disc
- ○ Leg Cramps
- ○ Restless Legs
- ○ Jaw Pain/TMJ
- ○ History of Falling
- ○ Use of Cane or Walker
- ○ Gout
- ○ Double Jointed

Other:_____

Neurological:
- ○ Stroke/TIA
- ○ Dementia
- ○ Polio

Neurological (continued)
- ○ Parkinson's Disease
- ○ Multiple Sclerosis
- ○ Epilepsy/Seizures
- ○ Concussion
- ○ Numbness
- ○ Tingling

Other:_____

Endocrine:
- ○ Diabetes
- ○ Kidney Dysfunction
- ○ Bladder Dysfunction
- ○ Liver Dysfunction
- ○ Thyroid Dysfunction

Other:_____

Cardiopulmonary:
- ○ Hypertension
- ○ Coronary Artery Disease
- ○ Congestive Heart Failure

Cardiopulmonary (continued)
- ○ Heart Arrhythmia
- ○ Pacemaker
- ○ High Cholesterol
- ○ Blood Clots
- ○ Anemia
- ○ High Blood Pressure
- ○ Asthma
- ○ Shortness of Breath
- ○ COPD
- ○ HIV/AIDS

Other:_____

Other:
- ○ Anxiety
- ○ Depression
- ○ Cancer

Observation

The patient is 6 feet 1 inch and weighs 165 pounds (BMI = 21.8). He has lost 15 pounds since being injured and hospitalized. His surgical incisions are dressed and intact over his residual limbs. Shrinker socks are also applied to residual limbs.

Chief Complaint: *"Kind of out of it"*

Goals for Therapy: *"To be the next bionic man."*

In the last week, how many days have you had pain? *"Most days I've been sore since the explosion."*

Pain worst: *When medication wears off*

SANE Functional Rating

Please rate your **ability** to use your injured area on a 0 to 100% scale with **0%** being unable to use the injured area and **100%** being normal use of injured area in your daily activity: _____ *N/A*

Also, if you exercise or have a sport activity or a job that requires special demands please rate your activity on the 0 to 100% scale: _____ *N/A*

Patient-Specific Functional Scale

Please list 3 activities that you find are difficult because of this problem and circle the number that corresponds with your ability to perform the activity.

	Unable								No limitations	
1. Walking	(1)	2	3	4	5	6	7	8	9	10
2. Standing	(1)	2	3	4	5	6	7	8	9	10
3. Moving in bed	1	(2)	3	4	5	6	7	8	9	10

Standardized Tests

Orthotic and prosthetic user's survey (OPUS)[2]

Lower extremity functional measure = 94 (Scores 20–100)

Health-related quality of life measure = 97 (Scores 23–115)

Endnotes

1. Goff BJ, Bergeron A, Ganz O, Gambel JM. Rehabilitation of a US Army soldier with traumatic triple major limb amputations: a case report. J Prosthetics Orthotics. 2008;20(4):142–9.

2. Heinemann AW, Bode RK, O'Reilly C. Development and measurement properties of the orthotics and prosthetics users' survey (OPUS): a comprehensive set of clinical outcome instruments. Prosthetics Orthotics Internat. 2003; 27:191–206

CASE 87

Setting: *Outpatient Orthopedics*

Date: *Present Day*

Medical Diagnosis: *Fibromyalgia*

Charted Data

Name:	*Amber Gray*	New Injury:	*No*
Age:	*32 years*	General Health:	*Good*
MRN:	*68203*	Amount of Exercise:	*0 days/week*
Home Address:	*4563 Smith Drive, Lima, Ohio*	Occupation:	*Cleans houses*
		Household:	*Lives with husband and 2 children*
Date of Injury:	*No specific date of onset, ongoing since car accident 6 months ago*	Hand Dominance:	*Right*
		Race:	*White*

Please fill in the location of your pain with a pencil.

R Front L   L Back R

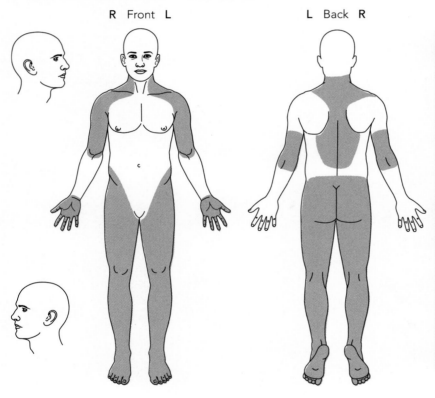

Pain Intensity Scale

0	No Pain
1	Low-level pain, able to perform regular activities
2	
3	
4	Moderate-level pain, use of pain medication, activity limited but functional
5	
6	
7	High-level pain, use of pain medication, activity very limited—decreased function
(8)	
9	
10	Emergency Situation

Imaging Results
No imaging was performed.

Medications
Citalopram, Lopressor

Past Medical History (Please check any items that apply to you.)

Musculoskeletal:
- ○ Osteoarthritis
- ○ Rheumatoid Arthritis
- ○ Lupus/SLE
- ⊗ Fibromyalgia
- ○ Osteoporosis
- ⊗ Headaches
- ○ Bulging Disc
- ○ Leg Cramps
- ⊗ Restless Legs
- ○ Jaw Pain/TMJ
- ○ History of Falling
- ○ Use of Cane or Walker
- ○ Gout
- ○ Double Jointed

Other:_____

Neurological:
- ○ Stroke/TIA
- ○ Dementia
- ○ Polio

Neurological (continued)
- ○ Parkinson's Disease
- ○ Multiple Sclerosis
- ○ Epilepsy/Seizures
- ○ Concussion
- ○ Numbness
- ○ Tingling

Other:_____

Endocrine:
- ○ Diabetes
- ○ Kidney Dysfunction
- ○ Bladder Dysfunction
- ○ Liver Dysfunction
- ○ Thyroid Dysfunction

Other:_____

Cardiopulmonary:
- ○ Congestive Heart Failure
- ○ Heart Arrhythmia
- ○ Pacemaker

Neurological (continued)
- ○ High Cholesterol
- ○ Blood Clots
- ○ Anemia
- ○ High Blood Pressure
- ○ Asthma
- ○ Shortness of Breath
- ○ COPD
- ○ HIV/AIDS

Other: *Irregular heartbeat*

Other:
- ⊗ Anxiety
- ⊗ Depression
- ○ Cancer

Chief Complaint: *Widespread pain*

Goals for Therapy: *To reduce the pain in my body so I can sleep at night, clean houses, and take care of my family/my own house.*

In the last week, how many days have you had pain? *7*

Pain worst: *Mornings and evenings*

SANE Functional Rating

Please rate your **ability** to use your injured area on a 0 to 100% scale with **0%** being unable to use the injured area and **100%** being normal use of injured area in your daily activity: *65%*

Also, if you exercise or have a sport activity or a job that requires special demands please rate your activity on the 0 to 100% scale: *55%*

Patient-Specific Functional Scale

Please list 3 activities that you find are difficult because of this problem and circle the number that corresponds with your ability to perform the activity.

	Unable									No limitations
1. Sleeping	1	(2)	3	4	5	6	7	8	9	10
2. Cleaning houses	1	2	3	4	5	(6)	7	8	9	10
3. Sitting	1	2	3	4	(5)	6	7	8	9	10

Unique Outcomes Measures

Fibromyalgia impact questionnaire = 50/80 (moderate effect on functioning)

McGill pain questionnaire = 56/78

Observation

The patient is 5 feet 3 inches and weighs 130 pounds (BMI = 23). She appears stressed and anxious over her condition. She is unable to sit still and has a flat affect.

Patient History

The patient reports widespread pain that seemed to appear about 6 months ago after a recent car accident. She states that she "walks the floors" at night because she is in so much pain and cannot sleep. She describes her pain as "achy" and a feeling of muscle stiffness throughout. When she awakes in the morning she feels stiff, but it seems to get better throughout the day. By the end of the day she is very fatigued. Her physician prescribed an anti-depressant to help calm her symptoms and recommended physical therapy.

Mechanism: *Although there was no specific incident, this patient indicates that she did not have this pain until after she was in a bad car accident 6 months ago.*

Concordant Sign: *She indicates that her pain is initiated after a stressful day of cleaning houses, doing laundry, cooking, and taking care of her two children.*

Nature of the Condition: *The 8/10 pain she reports occurs as deep muscle aching and is at specific areas on her body that seem to be very tender to the touch.*

Behavior of the Symptoms: *The patient's symptoms worsen in times of stress or toward the end of the day after she has done physically demanding activities. The symptoms seem to lessen mid-day. She is unable to sleep through the night or sit still because of the pain. Cold weather also increases her symptoms.*

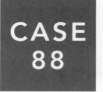

CASE 88

Setting: *Inpatient Rehabilitation*

Date: *Present Day*

Medical Diagnosis: *Right Transfemoral Amputation and Mild Traumatic Brain Injury*

Charted Data

Name:	*Carter Burke*	General Health:	*Good*
Age:	*25 years*	Amount of Exercise:	*1–2 hours/day, 7 days/ week prior to accident*
MRN:	*56841*	Occupation:	*Army, Combat—active duty*
Home Address:	*305 High Street, Columbus, Kansas*	Household:	*Single*
Date of Injury:	*2 1/2 weeks ago*	Hand Dominance:	*Right*
New Injury:	*Yes*	Race:	*White*

Please fill in the location of your pain with a pencil.

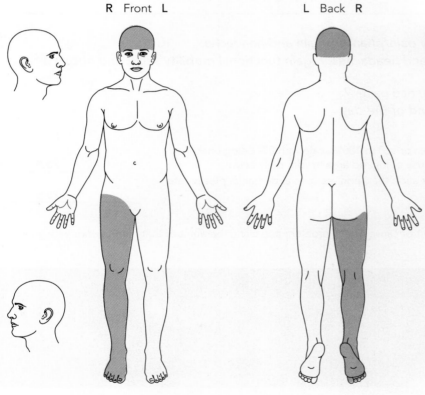

R Front L   L Back R

Pain Intensity Scale	
0	No Pain
1	Low-level pain, able to perform regular activities
2	
3	
4	Moderate-level pain, use of pain medication, activity limited but functional
5	
6	
7	High-level pain, use of pain medication, activity very limited—decreased function
(8)	
9	
10	Emergency Situation

Imaging Results

Radiographs, CT scan, and MRI completed acutely and confirmed the absence of a skull fracture, cervical instability, intracranial hemorrhage, and significant edema. A minor contusion in the frontal lobe was found on imaging.

Medications

Neurontin, Percocet PRN, Tylenol

Past Medical History (Please check any items that apply to you.)

Musculoskeletal:
- ○ Osteoarthritis
- ○ Rheumatoid Arthritis
- ○ Lupus/SLE
- ○ Fibromyalgia
- ○ Osteoporosis
- ○ Headaches
- ○ Bulging Disc
- ○ Leg Cramps
- ○ Restless Legs
- ○ Jaw Pain/TMJ
- ○ History of Falling
- ○ Use of Cane or Walker
- ○ Gout
- ○ Double Jointed

Other:_____

Neurological:
- ○ Stroke/TIA
- ○ Dementia
- ○ Polio

Neurological (continued)
- ○ Parkinson's Disease
- ○ Multiple Sclerosis
- ○ Epilepsy/Seizures
- ○ Concussion
- ○ Numbness
- ○ Tingling

Other: _Concussions x1_

Endocrine:
- ○ Diabetes
- ○ Kidney Dysfunction
- ○ Bladder Dysfunction
- ○ Liver Dysfunction
- ○ Thyroid Dysfunction

Other:_____

Cardiopulmonary:
- ○ Congestive Heart Failure
- ○ Heart Arrhythmia
- ○ Pacemaker

Cardiopulmonary (continued)
- ○ High Cholesterol
- ○ Blood Clots
- ○ Anemia
- ○ High Blood Pressure
- ○ Asthma
- ○ Shortness of Breath
- ○ COPD
- ○ HIV/AIDS

Other:_____

Other:
- ○ Anxiety
- ○ Depression
- ○ Cancer

Chief Complaint: _Right lower extremity pain/phantom pain and headaches_

Goals for Therapy: _To reduce the pain and headaches, regain functional mobility skills, and obtain a prosthetic device._

In the last week, how many days have you had pain? _7_

Pain worst: _Early morning and at the end of the day_

SANE Functional Rating

Please rate your **ability** to use your injured area on a 0 to 100% scale with **0%** being unable to use the injured area and **100%** being normal use of injured area in your daily activity: _25%_

Also, if you exercise or have a sport activity or a job that requires special demands please rate your activity on the 0 to 100% scale: _25%_

Patient-Specific Functional Scale

Please list 3 activities that you find are difficult because of this problem and circle the number that corresponds with your ability to perform the activity.

	Unable									No limitations
1. Walking	1	(2)	3	4	5	6	7	8	9	10
2. Using the computer	1	2	3	(4)	5	6	7	8	9	10
3. Stairs	(1)	2	3	4	5	6	7	8	9	10

Unique Outcomes Measures

Amputee mobility predictor (AMPnoPRO) = 27/43 without prosthesis (K2 level = has the potential to ambulate curbs, stairs, and uneven surfaces)

Glasgow coma scale = 14 (mild traumatic brain injury [TBI])

Observation

The patient is 5 feet 11 inches and weighs 175 pounds (BMI = 24.4). He has a muscular build with no apparent postural abnormalities. He presents with a recent right transfemoral amputation that is covered with a shrinker. The patient presents to therapy in a wheelchair but he has crutches with him.

Patient History

The patient reports being stationed in Afghanistan and sustaining his injuries from an attack on his unit. He states that he remembers being thrown from his vehicle after a "blast" and when he woke up he was in the hospital. He reports sustaining a concussion from this event and also reports a previous concussion that was sustained when he was a football player in high school. He believes that his memory is not as "sharp" as it was prior to his accident and he forgets his daily routine. Currently, the patient reports that he has been able to use crutches to ambulate minimally due to the pain in his right leg as well as the occasional dizziness he experiences. He also reports that he feels like his right calf is cramping and itching even though he knows it is no longer present. He takes Neurontin 1–2 times a day, which helps with pain management but makes him drowsy. The patient also reports his headaches are still present but the intensity is beginning to decrease, and his tolerance to bright lights and noises is increasing.

Mechanism: *The patient was involved in a combat attack on his unit while stationed in Afghanistan in which he was thrown from his vehicle.*

Concordant Sign: *He indicates that the pain in his right leg is constant. His headaches are initiated after using the computer and after watching television for prolonged periods of time.*

Nature of the Condition: *The 8/10 pain the patient reports occurs after increased activity with his lower extremities as well as with his headaches. His headaches become severe enough that he must stop watching television or using the computer. When his lower extremity pain is severe, he takes his pain medication.*

Behavior of the Symptoms: *Symptoms in the patient's right leg worsen after ambulation and improve with rest and pain medications. His headaches initiate and worsen with prolonged television or computer use and improve if he rests in a quiet and dimly lit room.*

CASE 89

Setting: *Outpatient Orthopedic Clinic*

Date: *Present Day*

Medical Diagnosis: *Polyarthrodial Juvenile Rheumatoid Arthritis (JRA)*

Charted Data

Name:	*Annie Cortina*	New Injury:	*No*
Age:	*12 years*	General Health:	*Good*
MRN:	*52578*	Amount of Exercise:	*2 hours/day, 5 days/week*
Home Address:	*123 St. Charles Street, Anacortes, Washington*	Occupation:	*Sixth-grade student*
		Household:	*Lives with parents*
		Hand Dominance:	*Right*
Date of Injury:	*9 months*	Race:	*Hispanic*

Please fill in the location of your pain with a pencil.

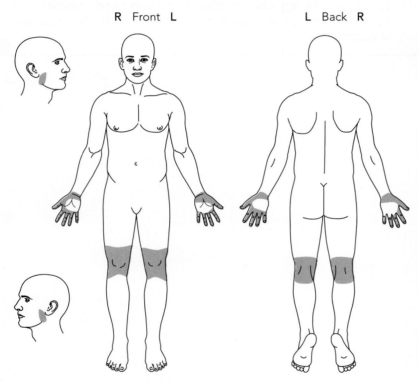

Pain Intensity Scale	
0	No Pain
1	Low-level pain, able to perform regular activities
2	
3	
(4)	Moderate-level pain, use of pain medication, activity limited but functional
5	
6	
7	High-level pain, use of pain medication, activity very limited—decreased function
8	
9	
10	Emergency Situation

Imaging Results

No imaging. A pediatric ophthalmologist has ruled out iridocyclitis at this time. Lab results have been positive for IgM rheumatoid factor RF for the past 6 months.

Medications

Ibuprofen (PRN), Etanercept (15mg subcutaneous, biweekly)[1]

Past Medical History (Please check any items that apply to you.)

Musculoskeletal:
- o Osteoarthritis
- ⊗ Rheumatoid Arthritis
- o Lupus/SLE
- o Fibromyalgia
- o Osteoporosis
- o Headaches
- o Bulging Disc
- o Leg Cramps
- o Restless Legs
- ⊗ Jaw Pain/TMJ
- o History of Falling
- o Use of Cane or Walker
- o Gout
- o Double Jointed

Other:_____

Neurological:
- o Stroke/TIA
- o Dementia

Neurological (continued)
- o Polio
- o Parkinson's Disease
- o Multiple Sclerosis
- o Epilepsy/Seizures
- o Concussion
- o Numbness
- o Tingling

Other:_____

Endocrine:
- o Diabetes
- o Kidney Dysfunction
- o Bladder Dysfunction
- o Liver Dysfunction
- o Thyroid Dysfunction

Other:_____

Cardiopulmonary:
- o Congestive Heart Failure
- o Heart Arrhythmia

Cardiopulmonary (continued)
- o Pacemaker
- o High Cholesterol
- o Blood Clots
- o Anemia
- o High Blood Pressure
- o Asthma
- o Shortness of Breath
- o COPD
- o HIV/AIDS

Other:_____

Other:
- ⊗ Anxiety
- ⊗ Depression
- o Cancer
- ⊗ Recurrent Fever

Chief Complaint: *Pain and stiffness in the morning and worsening joint pain throughout her day at school*

Goals for Therapy: *To reduce stiffness and reduce pain with functional activities.*

In the last week, how many days have you had pain? **7**

Pain worst: *In morning and during prolonged weight-bearing activity.*

SANE Functional Rating

Please rate your **ability** to use your injured area on a 0 to 100% scale with **0%** being unable to use the injured area and **100%** being normal use of injured area in your daily activity: *85%*

Also, if you exercise or have a sport activity or a job that requires special demands please rate your activity on the 0 to 100% scale: *60%*

Patient-Specific Functional Scale

Please list 3 activities that you find are difficult because of this problem and circle the number that corresponds with your ability to perform the activity.

	Unable									No limitations
1. Going up and down stairs, especially in the morning	1	2	3	(4)	5	6	7	8	9	10
2. Running in gym class	1	2	3	(4)	5	6	7	8	9	10
3. Tying shoes and writing (dexterous hand activities)	1	2	(3)	4	5	6	7	8	9	10

Unique Outcomes Measures
Functional disability inventory = 45/60 68²

Observation

The patient is 4 feet 7 inches and weighs 85 pounds (BMI = 23.1). She presents with an antalgic gait. Forward head posture is noted but it is not severe. The patient exhibits bilateral (B) genu valgus, elbow flexion contractures, and interphalangeal (IP) flexion contractures. Visible edema is present at IP joints in both hands as well as at both radiocarpal joints. The patient is also exhibiting edema in both tibiofemoral joints. Edema is symmetrical (B). Joints do not appear red and are not painful to light touch.

Patient History

The patient had experienced mild joint pain on and off for several years. Nine months ago a pediatric rheumatologist diagnosed her as having RF-positive, polyarthritis. Her pain has since been controlled with NSAIDS and the juvenile rheumatoid arthritis (JRA) (sometimes called juvenile idiopathic arthritis [JIA]) is being treated with etanercept injections but is yet to go into remission. The patient and her family are currently working with a child and family psychologist due to anxiety and depression issues that have resulted from years of uncontrolled pain.

Mechanism: *The patient's stiffness is worst in the morning and worsens with inactivity. Her joint pain throughout the day limits her ability to participate in physical education activities and to complete hand functions that require dexterity. This causes the child to ambulate slower than the other children at school.*

Concordant Sign: *The constant, dull ache is mostly in her knees and hands. She also mentions occasional bilateral jaw pain that feels like an annoying ache.*

Nature of the Condition: *The condition moderately limits ambulation on even surfaces and severely limits ambulation up and down stairs. The patient is independent with all ADLs, but functional movements of the Upper Extremity (UE) are limited by flexor contractures and edema in the hands.*

Behavior of the Symptoms: *Stiffness in the morning takes 1 to 2 hours to dissipate but it never fully goes away. Her pain never fully goes away but it is worse with prolonged standing, ambulation, writing, and so on. The child's pain is made better with ibuprofen and frequent rest breaks.*

Endnotes

1. Lovell DJ, Giannini EH, Reiff A, Cawkwell GD, Silverman ED, Nocton JJ, Stein LD, Gedalia A, Llowite NT, Wallace CA, Whitmore J, Finck BK. Etanercept in children with polyarticular juvenile rheumatoid arthritis. N Engl J Med. 2000;342:763–9.

2. Feinstein AB, Forman EM, Masuda A, Cohen LL, Herbert JD, Moorthy LN, Goldsmith DP. Pain intensity, psychological inflexibility, and acceptance of pain as predictors of functioning in adolescents with juvenile idiopathic arthritis: a preliminary investigation. J Clin Psychol Med Settings 2011;18:291–8.

CASE 90

Setting: *Outpatient Orthopedic Office*

Date: *Present Day*

Medical Diagnosis: *Nonspecific Low Back Pain*

Charted Data

Name:	*Millie Thompson*	General Health:	*Poor*
Age:	*53 years*	Amount of Exercise:	*0 hours/day, 0 days/week*
MRN:	*96375*	Occupation:	*Disabled (depression and chronic pain)*
Home Address:	*2165 West Allegheny Drive, Smithtown, Pennsylvania*	Household:	*Lives alone in low-income apartment*
Date of Injury:	*15 years ago*	Hand Dominance:	*Right*
New Injury:	*Pain increased 1 month ago*	Race	*Black*

Please fill in the location of your pain with a pencil.

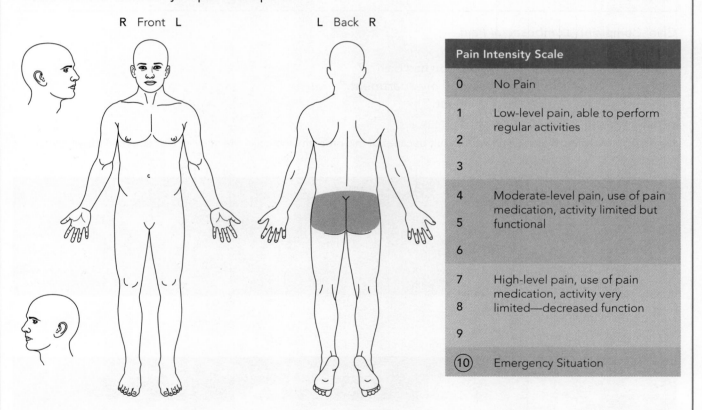

R   Front   L   L   Back   R

Pain Intensity Scale

0	No Pain
1	Low-level pain, able to perform regular activities
2	
3	
4	Moderate-level pain, use of pain medication, activity limited but functional
5	
6	
7	High-level pain, use of pain medication, activity very limited—decreased function
8	
9	
(10)	Emergency Situation

Imaging Results

Radiographs were negative for pathology but the patient was told she has some degenerative changes of her spine. She had an MRI several years ago but reports she is frustrated because it was also negative and "they couldn't find her pain."

Medications

Celexa, Lithium, Trazodone

Past Medical History (Please check any items that apply to you.)

Musculoskeletal:
- ⊗ Osteoarthritis
- ○ Rheumatoid Arthritis
- ○ Lupus/SLE
- ⊗ Fibromyalgia
- ○ Osteoporosis
- ○ Headaches
- ○ Bulging Disc
- ○ Leg Cramps
- ⊗ Restless Legs
- ○ Jaw Pain/TMJ
- ○ History of Falling
- ○ Use of Cane or Walker
- ○ Gout
- ○ Double Jointed

Other:_____

Neurological:
- ○ Stroke/TIA
- ○ Dementia
- ○ Polio

Neurological (continued)
- ○ Parkinson's Disease
- ○ Multiple Sclerosis
- ○ Epilepsy/Seizures
- ○ Concussion
- ⊗ Numbness
- ⊗ Tingling

Other:_____

Endocrine:
- ○ Diabetes
- ○ Kidney Dysfunction
- ○ Bladder Dysfunction
- ○ Liver Dysfunction
- ○ Thyroid Dysfunction

Other:_____

Cardiopulmonary:
- ○ Congestive Heart Failure
- ○ Heart Arrhythmia
- ○ Pacemaker

Cardiopulmonary (continued)
- ○ High Cholesterol
- ○ Blood Clots
- ⊗ Anemia
- ○ High Blood Pressure
- ○ Asthma
- ○ Shortness of Breath
- ○ COPD
- ○ HIV/AIDS

Other:_____

Other:
- ⊗ Anxiety
- ⊗ Depression
- ○ Cancer
- ⊗ Bipolar Disorder

Chief Complaint: *Lumbosacral Pain*

Goals for Therapy: **To reduce the pain.**

In the last week, how many days have you had pain? *7*

Pain worst: *"When walking outside of my apartment."*

Pain best: *"When inside my apartment."*

Patient-Specific Functional Scale

Please list 3 activities that you find are difficult because of this problem and circle the number that corresponds with your ability to perform the activity

	Unable								No limitations	
1. Walking	(1)	2	3	4	5	6	7	8	9	10
2. Standing	(1)	2	3	4	5	6	7	8	9	10
3. Lying supine	1	2	(3)	4	5	6	7	8	9	10

Unique Outcomes Measures

Pain Catastrophizing Scale

	Not at all	To a slight degree	To a moderate degree	To a great degree	All the time
I worry all the time about whether the pain will end.	0	1	2	3	(4)
I feel I can't go on.	0	1	(2)	3	4
It's terrible and I think it's never going to get any better.	0	1	(2)	3	4
It's awful and I feel that it overwhelms me.	0	1	(2)	3	4

	Not at all	To a slight degree	To a moderate degree	To a great degree	All the time
I feel I can't stand it anymore.	0	1	(2)	3	4
I become afraid that the pain will get worse.	0	1	(2)	3	4
I keep thinking of other painful events.	0	(1)	2	3	4
I anxiously want the pain to go away.	0	1	(2)	3	4
I can't seem to keep it out of my mind.	0	1	2	(3)	4
I keep thinking about how much it hurts.	0	1	2	(3)	4
I keep thinking about how badly I want the pain to stop.	0	1	2	(3)	4
There's nothing I can do to reduce the intensity of the pain.	0	1	2	(3)	4
I wonder whether something serious may happen.	0	1	(2)	3	4

Observation

The patient is 5 feet 2 inches and weighs 100 pounds (BMI = 18.3). She is seated on the table in a "slump" position with mildly rounded shoulders. She appears very nervous and fidgety. She does not make eye contact during the history taking.

Patient History

The patient indicates she has a long history of low back pain. She states that 15 years ago, she was in a domestic altercation with her spouse, who beat her severely. Following this incident, she suffered from low back pain that eventually became unmanageable (she was not diagnosed with any significant pathology of her spine but did suffer broken bones in her face and multiple ribs) and she qualified for disability (which was also supported by her comorbidity of bipolar disorder). The patient states that the pain has become insidiously more severe over the past month and says that her ex-spouse was released from prison one month ago. When asked the question, "Do you feel the two are related?" she shrugs her shoulders and says, "Maybe. But I know I'm not crazy."

Mechanism: *The pain is long-standing and the only physical mechanism of injury appears to be potential soft tissue damage following the domestic assault. Note that she has identified a potential correlation between increased symptoms and her ex-spouse being released from prison. Also note that she reported in her pain scale that her pain is worse when "walking outside."*

Concordant Sign: *The patient's symptoms are reproduced when hands are placed on her low back to perform mobility testing. She is very irritable with light touch in wide regions throughout the entire lumbar spine. She begins to cry as pressure is applied, so the manual assessment should be discontinued. She tells the therapist, "That is it. That is the pain I feel."*

Nature of the Condition: *This condition is very debilitating for this patient. She is avoiding leaving her apartment due to increased symptoms. She indicates that standing, walking, and lying are all painful.*

Behavior of the Symptoms: *The patient has a high amount of irritability and symptoms do not appear to be simply movement specific. The context of being "outside" appears to be a variable that she perceives as influencing her symptoms.*

Setting: *Outpatient Orthopedic Office*

Date: *Present Day*

Medical Diagnosis: *Complex Regional Pain Syndrome-Type 1*

Charted Data

Name:	Robert Williams	New Injury:	*Developed complex regional pain syndrome –type 1(CRPS-1) since surgery*
Age:	*34 years*		
MRN:	*96223*		
Home Address:	*615 E. Main Street, Cold Spring, Alabama*	General Health:	*Poor*
		Amount of Exercise:	*0 hours/days, 0 days/week*
Date of Injury:	*Lateral release of patella 1 year ago following work-related accident (patellar dislocation)*	Occupation:	*Disabled since accident*
		Household:	*Married, no children*
		Hand Dominance:	*Right*
		Race	*Caucasian*

Please fill in the location of your pain with a pencil.

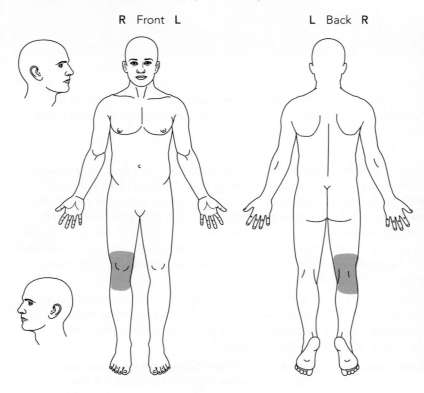

R Front L   L Back R

Pain Intensity Scale

0	No Pain
1	Low-level pain, able to perform regular activities
2	
3	
4	Moderate-level pain, use of pain medication, activity limited but functional
5	
6	
7	High-level pain, use of pain medication, activity very limited— decreased function
8	
9	
10	Emergency Situation

Imaging Results
MRI indicates generalized joint effusion, but ligaments and meniscus are within normal limits.

Medications
Methadone, Hydromorphone

Past Medical History (Please check any items that apply to you.)

Musculoskeletal:
- o Osteoarthritis
- o Rheumatoid Arthritis
- o Lupus/SLE
- o Fibromyalgia
- o Osteoporosis
- o Headaches
- o Bulging Disc
- o Leg Cramps
- ⊗ Restless Legs
- o Jaw Pain/TMJ
- o History of Falling
- o Use of Cane or Walker
- o Gout
- o Double Jointed

Other:_____

Neurological:
- o Stroke/TIA
- o Dementia

Neurological (continued)
- o Polio
- o Parkinson's Disease
- o Multiple Sclerosis
- o Epilepsy/Seizures
- o Concussion
- o Numbness
- ⊗ Tingling

Other:_____

Endocrine:
- o Diabetes
- o Kidney Dysfunction
- o Bladder Dysfunction
- o Liver Dysfunction
- o Thyroid Dysfunction

Other:_____

Cardiopulmonary:
- o Congestive Heart Failure
- o Heart Arrhythmia

Cardiopulmonary (continued)
- o Pacemaker
- o High Cholesterol
- o Blood Clots
- o Anemia
- o High Blood Pressure
- o Asthma
- o Shortness of Breath
- o COPD
- o HIV/AIDS

Other:_____

Other:
- ⊗ Anxiety
- ⊗ Depression
- o Cancer
- ⊗ CRPS-1

Chief Complaint: *Severe left leg pain*

Goals for Therapy: *To reduce left leg pain and return to work.*

In the last week, how many days have you had pain? *7*

Pain worst: *"Always"*

Pain best: *"It never goes away."*

Patient-Specific Functional Scale

Please list 3 activities that you find are difficult because of this problem and circle the number that corresponds with your ability to perform the activity.

	Unable									No limitations
1. Standing	(1)	2	3	4	5	6	7	8	9	10
2. Lifting left leg	(1)	2	3	4	5	6	7	8	9	10
3. Walking	(1)	2	3	4	5	6	7	8	9	10

Unique Outcomes Measures

Pain Catastrophizing Scale

	Not at all	To a slight degree	To a moderate degree	To a great degree	All the time
I worry all the time about whether the pain will end.	0	1	2	3	(4)
I feel I can't go on.	0	1	2	3	(4)
It's terrible and I think it's never going to get any better.	0	1	2	3	(4)
It's awful and I feel that it overwhelms me.	0	1	2	3	(4)

	Not at all	To a slight degree	To a moderate degree	To a great degree	All the time
I feel I can't stand it anymore.	0	1	2	3	(4)
I become afraid that the pain will get worse.	0	1	2	3	(4)
I keep thinking of other painful events.	0	1	2	3	(4)
I anxiously want the pain to go away.	0	1	2	3	(4)
I can't seem to keep it out of my mind.	0	1	2	3	(4)
I keep thinking about how much it hurts.	0	1	2	3	(4)
I keep thinking about how badly I want the pain to stop.	0	1	2	3	(4)
There's nothing I can do to reduce the intensity of the pain.	0	1	2	3	(4)
I wonder whether something serious may happen.	0	1	2	3	(4)

Observation

The patient is a large Caucasian male who is 6 feet tall and weighs 240 pounds. He walks from the waiting room to his room, utilizing a cane in his right hand. He literally "drags" his left lower extremity through the swing phase of his gait cycle. He sits onto the plinth and uses both hands to position his left lower extremity flat onto the table. His left knee has two small port site scars that have healed but his knee appears to be very swollen and has a purplish hue. This discoloration extends from his suprapatellar border into the mid-shin/calf region.

Patient History

The patient reports he injured his left knee in a work-related accident last year. He describes the accident as a fall directly onto his knee, while attempting to move a piece of furniture. He states he heard a "pop" and noticed that his patella dislocated to the side of his knee. He reported that he "froze," not knowing what to do, and asked a coworker to call an ambulance. He was taken by ambulance to a local emergency room, where his patella was relocated and it was recommend that he have an arthroscopic procedure to loosen structures on the lateral aspect of his knee. He reports he was released from the hospital with a narcotic pain medication, and was scheduled to have the procedure performed a few days later. Following the surgery, the patient reports he began to develop severe pain in his patella, which the surgeon said was normal. He says this pain became disabling and within a month he was unable to weight-bear through that lower extremity. On a subsequent office visit, the surgeon told the patient that the surgery was successful and that he should not have pain, because everything had healed. He did offer a referral to pain management, which the patient accepted.

After his first visit to pain management, the patient was diagnosed with complex regional pain syndrome and began a cocktail of narcotic pain medications. He reports these barely work and he believes he is going to have to live with this pain for the rest of his life. He states he has considered cutting his leg off. When questioned further, he states he is serious and believes this is his only option.

Mechanism: *Development of CRPS following an arthroscopic knee procedure for a patellar dislocation.*

Concordant Sign: *The patient's symptoms are constant and he is extremely irritable to any form of light touch.*

Nature of the Condition: *This condition has resulted in the patient being unable to work, and the pain has led to catastrophic thoughts such as "The only way to get rid of this pain is to remove the limb."*

Behavior of the Symptoms: *The patient's symptoms, primarily pain, are very irritable.*

CASE 92

Setting: *Outpatient Orthopedic Office*

Date: *Present Day*

Medical Diagnosis: *Left Saturday Night Palsy (Radial Neuropathy)*

Charted Data

Name:	*Walter Booth*	General Health:	*Poor*
Age:	*48 years*	Amount of Exercise:	*0 hours/day, 0 days/week*
MRN:	*86443*	Occupation:	*Archeologist*
Home Address:	*1726 E. Main Street, Batavia, New York*	Household:	*Single; currently has a non–live-in girlfriend*
Date of Injury:	*2 months ago*	Hand Dominance:	*Right*
New Injury:	*Pain got worse over past month and patient developed CRPS-2*	Race	*Caucasian*

Please fill in the location of your pain with a pencil.

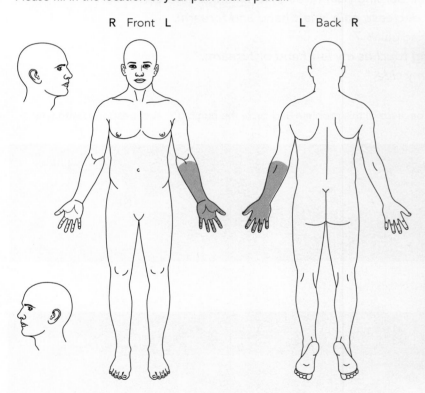

R Front L   L Back R

Pain Intensity Scale	
0	No Pain
1	Low-level pain, able to perform regular activities
2	
3	
4	Moderate-level pain, use of pain medication, activity limited but functional
5	
6	
7	High-level pain, use of pain medication, activity very limited—decreased function
8	
9	
10	Emergency Situation

Imaging Results

The patient had a CT scan on his brain following the accident that was negative for pathology. He also had negative radiographs on his left shoulder for fracture or dislocation, a negative MRI for rotator cuff or labral pathology, and a positive EMG for significant radial nerve damage.

Medications

Lithium

Past Medical History (Please check any items that apply to you)

Musculoskeletal:

- ○ Osteoarthritis
- ○ Rheumatoid Arthritis
- ○ Lupus/SLE
- ○ Fibromyalgia
- ○ Osteoporosis
- ○ Headaches
- ○ Bulging Disc
- ○ Leg Cramps
- ○ Restless Legs
- ○ Jaw Pain/TMJ
- ○ History of Falling
- ○ Use of Cane or Walker
- ○ Gout
- ○ Double Jointed

Other:_____

Neurological:

- ○ Stroke/TIA
- ○ Dementia

Neurological (continued)

- ○ Polio
- ○ Parkinson's Disease
- ○ Multiple Sclerosis
- ○ Epilepsy/Seizures
- ○ Concussion
- ⊗ Numbness
- ○ Tingling

Other: _Inability to move (L) arm_

Endocrine:

- ○ Diabetes
- ○ Kidney Dysfunction
- ○ Bladder Dysfunction
- ○ Liver Dysfunction
- ○ Thyroid Dysfunction

Other:_____

Cardiopulmonary:

- ○ Congestive Heart Failure
- ○ Heart Arrhythmia

Cardiopulmonary (continued)

- ○ Pacemaker
- ○ High Cholesterol
- ○ Blood Clots
- ○ Anemia
- ○ High Blood Pressure
- ○ Asthma
- ○ Shortness of Breath
- ○ COPD
- ○ HIV/AIDS

Other:_____

Other:

- ⊗ Anxiety
- ⊗ Depression
- ○ Cancer
- ⊗ Bipolar Disorder

Chief Complaint: _Unable to move left arm. Burning pain through left hand and forearm_

Goals for Therapy: _To move left arm and decrease pain in left hand and forearm._

In the last week, how many days have you had pain? _7_

Pain worst: _"Constant pain when anything touches my left hand or forearm."_

Pain best: _"When arm hangs loosely by my side."_

Patient-Specific Functional Scale

Please list 3 activities that you find are difficult because of this problem and circle the number that corresponds with your ability to perform the activity.

	Unable								No limitations	
1. Putting on a shirt	①	2	3	4	5	6	7	8	9	10
2. Lifting objects off the ground	①	2	3	4	5	6	7	8	9	10
3. Carrying things	①	2	3	4	5	6	7	8	9	10

Unique Outcomes Measures

Pain Catastrophizing Scale

	Not at all	To a slight degree	To a moderate degree	To a great degree	All the time
I worry all the time about whether the pain will end.	0	1	2	3	④
I feel I can't go on.	0	1	2	3	④
It's terrible and I think it's never going to get any better.	0	1	2	3	④
It's awful and I feel that it overwhelms me.	0	1	2	3	④

	Not at all	To a slight degree	To a moderate degree	To a great degree	All the time
I feel I can't stand it anymore.	0	1	2	3	(4)
I become afraid that the pain will get worse.	0	1	2	3	(4)
I keep thinking of other painful events.	0	1	2	3	(4)
I anxiously want the pain to go away.	0	1	2	3	(4)
I can't seem to keep it out of my mind.	0	1	2	3	(4)
I keep thinking about how much it hurts.	0	1	2	3	(4)
I keep thinking about how badly I want the pain to stop.	0	1	2	3	(4)
There's nothing I can do to reduce the intensity of the pain.	0	1	2	3	(4)
I wonder whether something serious may happen.	0	1	2	3	(4)

Observation

The patient is an ectomorphic male. He appears to be very anxious at rest and appears to have difficulty paying attention to questions asked by the therapist. He is seated in a chair and his left arm is hanging flaccidly by his side. His left hand and wrist look very red and swollen. The patient appears to have changes in his nails on the left (they are more yellow and worn as compared to his nails on the right). He nervously shakes his right foot at rest.

Patient History

The patient reports that he had a long night of binge drinking and does not remember much of what happened after that. He states that his girlfriend found him in an empty bathtub, with his left arm draped over the side. He suspects he may have been in this position for 6–8 hours. He reports when he was attempting to get out of the bathtub, his left arm "would not wake up." He states that this was very concerning, so his girlfriend took him to the emergency room. When the patient arrived, the attending physician was concerned about a CVA; thus, a CT scan was performed on his brain. The patient reports that nothing was found, so radiographs were performed on his left arm, which were negative for fracture or dislocation. The physician ordered an MRI, which was also negative for pathology. The patient was discharged home and referred to an orthopedic surgeon.

When following up with the surgeon, he ordered an EMG, which indicated significant radial nerve damage. The patient was sent to physical therapy, which he attended for a couple of weeks, but reports that his left hand began to swell and hurt. He reports the therapist was applying moist heat to his left arm, neuromuscular electrical stimulation (NMES) on his left shoulder and aggressive active-assisted range of motion activities. He reports he followed up with his physician, who then recommended he be evaluated by another physical therapist and was referred to the current facility.

Mechanism: *It is likely that direct compression of the radial nerve led to this patient's damage. It is suspected that he developed CRPS-2 secondary to this and that it may or may not be a result of aggressive physical therapy.*

Concordant Sign: *The patient complains of reproduction of severe pain with any light touch of the left hand or wrist.*

Nature of the Condition: *This condition is currently very disabling. The patient is having difficulty with the performance of ADLs such as dressing and cooking. He is currently very depressed and reports this is secondary to this arm.*

Behavior of the Symptoms: *The patient's condition is irritable. Because his left arm is currently flaccid, an assessment of the activity of symptoms with active movement is not possible.*

CASE 93

Setting: *Outpatient Orthopedic Office*

Date: *Present Day*

Medical Diagnosis: *Motor Weakness of Right Arm*

Charted Data

Name:	*Donald Mazur*	General Health:	*Poor*
Age:	*78 years*	Amount of Exercise:	*0 hours/day, 0 days/week*
MRN:	*36227*	Occupation:	*Retired*
Home Address:	*599 Willow Run Drive, Lancaster, Ohio*	Household:	*Lives alone. Recently widowed*
Date of Injury:	*2 months ago*	Hand Dominance:	*Right*
New Injury:	*Yes*	Race:	*Caucasian*

Please fill in the location of your pain with a pencil.

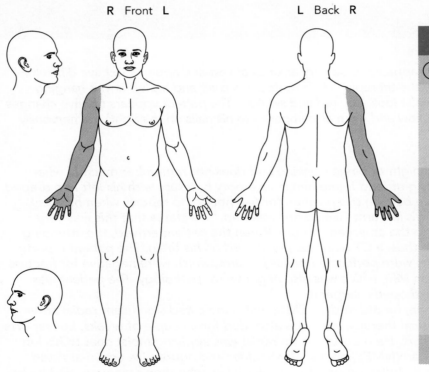

R Front L   L Back R

Pain Intensity Scale	
⓪	No Pain
1 2	Low-level pain, able to perform regular activities
3	
4 5	Moderate-level pain, use of pain medication, activity limited but functional
6	
7 8	High-level pain, use of pain medication, activity very limited— decreased function
9	
10	Emergency Situation

Imaging Results

Radiographs of the right shoulder and cervical spine indicated normal degenerative changes. MRI of the right shoulder, cervical spine, and brain indicate no abnormal pathology.

Medications

Atenolol, baby aspirin

Past Medical History (Please check any items that apply to you.)

Musculoskeletal:

- ⊗ Osteoarthritis
- ○ Rheumatoid Arthritis
- ○ Lupus/SLE
- ○ Fibromyalgia
- ○ Osteoporosis
- ○ Headaches
- ○ Bulging Disc
- ○ Leg Cramps
- ○ Restless Legs
- ○ Jaw Pain/TMJ
- ○ History of Falling
- ○ Use of Cane or Walker
- ○ Gout
- ○ Double Jointed

Other:_____

Neurological:

- ○ Stroke/TIA
- ○ Dementia

Neurological (continued)

- ○ Polio
- ○ Parkinson's Disease
- ○ Multiple Sclerosis
- ○ Epilepsy/Seizures
- ○ Concussion
- ⊗ Numbness
- ○ Tingling

Other:_____

Endocrine:

- ○ Diabetes
- ○ Kidney Dysfunction
- ○ Bladder Dysfunction
- ○ Liver Dysfunction
- ○ Thyroid Dysfunction

Other:_____

Cardiopulmonary:

- ○ Congestive Heart Failure
- ○ Heart Arrhythmia

Cardiopulmonary (continued)

- ○ Pacemaker
- ⊗ High Cholesterol
- ○ Blood Clots
- ○ Anemia
- ⊗ High Blood Pressure
- ○ Asthma
- ○ Shortness of Breath
- ○ COPD
- ○ HIV/AIDS

Other:_____

Other:

- ○ Anxiety
- ○ Depression
- ○ Cancer
- ○ Bipolar Disorder

Chief Complaint: *Inability to lift right arm*

Goals for Therapy: *To improve use of right arm.*

In the last week, how many days have you had pain? *0*

Pain worst: *N/A*

Pain best: *N/A*

PHQ-2 (Depression Screen)

Over the past 2 weeks, how often have you been bothered by any of the following problems?

	Not at All	Several Days	More than Half the Days	Nearly Every Day
1. Little interest or pleasure in doing things	0	1	2	③
2. Feeling down, depressed, or hopeless	0	1	2	③

Scoring of PHQ-2[1]

Major Depressive Episode				Any Depressive Disorder			
PHQ-2 Score	Sens.	Spec.	+ Pred. Value	PHQ-2 Score	Sens.	Spec.	+ Pred. Value
1	97.6	59.2	15.4	1	90.6	65.4	36.9
2	92.7	73.7	21.1	2	82.1	80.4	48.3
3	82.9	90	38.4	3	62.3	95.4	75.0
4	73.2	93.3	45.5	4	50.9	97.9	81.2
5	53.7	96.8	56.4	5	31.1	98.7	84.6
6	26.8	99.4	78.6	6	12.3	99.8	92.9

Patient-Specific Functional Scale

Please list **3 activities** that you find are difficult because of this problem and circle the number that corresponds with your ability to perform the activity.

	Unable									No limitations
1. Dressing	1	(2)	3	4	5	6	7	8	9	10
2. Driving	1	2	3	4	(5)	6	7	8	9	10
3. Cooking	1	2	(3)	4	5	6	7	8	9	10

Observation

The patient is 5 feet 10 inches and weighs 130 pounds (BMI = 18.7). He appears to be frail and nervous for the examination. He is very soft spoken and doesn't make much eye contact when talking.

Patient History

The patient reports that a couple of months ago his right upper extremity lost the ability to move. It all began when he walked into his bedroom to wake up his long-time girlfriend but she did not respond. He reports he got very nervous and called 911. While waiting for the paramedics, he attempted to pick her up into his arms. At this time, she was still unresponsive but he did not know what to do. Once the paramedics arrived, he was instructed that she did not have a pulse and was rushed to a local hospital. Upon arriving to the hospital, she was pronounced dead. A family friend drove him home and when he arrived home, he noticed difficulty moving his right arm. He suspected he injured it while lifting his girlfriend but "ignored" the deficit until after her funeral.

Following the burial, he went to his physician's office but reports that his MD was unsure of the reason for paralysis. He ordered images (radiographs and MRIs) to assess for a plethora of conditions, such as a CVA, rotator cuff tear, and so on, but all the images were negative for pathology. He and his physician were perplexed. The patient was referred to another physician, who also put him through additional testing but in the end was also unable to come to a pathoanatomical diagnosis. After ruling out major pathology, the physician suggested that this was possibly a conversion disorder.

Mechanism: *The patient suspected his symptoms were related to lifting his girlfriend out of bed. The physical therapist suspected the same, but did not believe it was simply due to mechanical damage. It is possible that a psychosocial influence may potentially be resulting in motor changes.*

Concordant Sign: *The patient is unable to actively lift his arm and it lays flaccid by his side.*

Nature of the Condition: *This condition is disabling and has limited the patient's ability to perform simple ADLs without difficulty.*

Behavior of the Symptoms: *These symptoms do not appear to be mechanical. The flaccidity likely indicates some form of neurological deficit between the central and peripheral nervous system.*

Endnotes

1. Kroenke K, Spitzer RL, Williams JB. The patient health questionnaire-2: validity of a two-item depression screener. Medical Care. 2003;41:1284–94.

CASE 94

Setting: *Outpatient Orthopedic Office*

Date: *Present Day*

Medical Diagnosis: *Multiple Myeloma Resulting in Thoracic Spine Cord Compression*

Charted Data

Name:	*Lucy Offerdahl*	General Health:	*Average*
Age:	*64 years*	Amount of Exercise:	*1 hour/day, 3 days/week*
MRN:	*83967*	Occupation:	*Retired; was going to school abroad in Mexico*
Home Address:	*515 West Andover Drive, Bainbridge, Ohio*	Household:	*Married and lives with husband*
Date of Injury:	*3 weeks ago*	Hand Dominance:	*Right*
New Injury:	*Acute onset of diffuse, thoracic spine pain*	Race	*Caucasian*

Please fill in the location of your pain with a pencil.

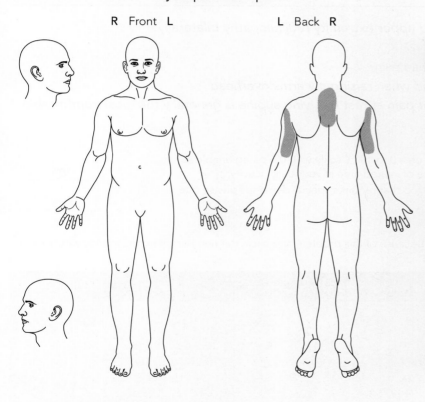

R Front L   L Back R

Pain Intensity Scale	
0	No Pain
1	Low-level pain, able to perform regular activities
2	
3	
4	Moderate-level pain, use of pain medication, activity limited but functional
(5)	
6	
7	High-level pain, use of pain medication, activity very limited—decreased function
8	
9	
10	Emergency Situation

Imaging Results

Radiographs were taken by a chiropractor in Mexico, where the patient was attending school. The chiropractor reported to her that she had a subluxation in the mid-thoracic spine. Radiographs were also taken in the emergency room when the patient returned to the United States—they, too, were negative.

Medications

Synthroid

Past Medical History (Please check any items that apply to you.)

Musculoskeletal:
- ○ Osteoarthritis
- ○ Rheumatoid Arthritis
- ○ Lupus/SLE
- ○ Fibromyalgia
- ○ Osteoporosis
- ○ Headaches
- ○ Bulging Disc
- ○ Leg Cramps
- ○ Restless Legs
- ○ Jaw Pain/TMJ
- ○ History of Falling
- ○ Use of Cane or Walker
- ○ Gout
- ○ Double Jointed

Other:_____

Neurological:
- ○ Stroke/TIA
- ○ Dementia

Neurological (continued)
- ○ Polio
- ○ Parkinson's Disease
- ○ Multiple Sclerosis
- ○ Epilepsy/Seizures
- ○ Concussion
- ○ Numbness
- ○ Tingling

Other:_____

Endocrine:
- ○ Diabetes
- ○ Kidney Dysfunction
- ○ Bladder Dysfunction
- ○ Liver Dysfunction
- ○ Thyroid Dysfunction

Other:_____

Cardiopulmonary:
- ○ Congestive Heart Failure
- ○ Heart Arrhythmia

Cardiopulmonary (continued)
- ○ Pacemaker
- ○ High Cholesterol
- ○ Blood Clots
- ○ Anemia
- ○ High Blood Pressure
- ⊗ Asthma
- ○ Shortness of Breath
- ○ COPD
- ○ HIV/AIDS

Other:_____

Other:
- ○ Anxiety
- ○ Depression
- ○ Cancer
- ○ Bipolar Disorder
- ⊗ Thyroid Disorder

Chief Complaint: *Thoracic spine pain and upper extremity radiculopathy bilaterally*

Goals for Therapy: *To reduce pain.*

In the last week, how many days have you had pain? *7*

Pain worst: *"When pushing myself up and when raising my arms overhead."*

Pain best: *"It varies. I'll have intermittent pain at rest but lying supine is generally the most comfortable position."*

SANE Functional Rating

Please rate your **ability** to use your injured area on a 0 to 100% scale with **0%** being unable to use the injured area and **100%** being normal use of injured area in your daily activity: ___*30%*___

Also, if you exercise or have a sport activity or a job that requires special demands please rate your activity on the 0 to 100% scale: ___*40%*___

Patient-Specific Functional Scale

Please list **3 activities** that you find are difficult because of this problem and circle the number that corresponds with your ability to perform the activity.

	Unable								No limitations	
1. Walking	1	2	3	4	5	6	7	8	(9)	10
2. Raising arms above shoulders to don/doff shirt	1	2	(3)	4	5	6	7	8	9	10
3. Pushing self up	(1)	2	3	4	5	6	7	8	9	10

Unique Outcomes Measures
Pain Catastrophizing Scale

	Not at all	To a slight degree	To a moderate degree	To a great degree	All the time
I worry all the time about whether the pain will end.	0	(1)	2	3	4
I feel I can't go on.	0	(1)	2	3	4
It's terrible and I think it's never going to get any better.	0	(1)	2	3	4
It's awful and I feel that it overwhelms me.	0	1	(2)	3	4
I feel I can't stand it anymore.	(0)	1	2	3	4
I become afraid that the pain will get worse.	0	(1)	2	3	4
I keep thinking of other painful events.	(0)	1	2	3	4
I anxiously want the pain to go away.	0	(1)	2	3	4
I can't seem to keep it out of my mind.	(0)	1	2	3	4
I keep thinking about how much it hurts.	(0)	1	2	3	4
I keep thinking about how badly I want the pain to stop.	(0)	1	2	3	4
There's nothing I can do to reduce the intensity of the pain.	(0)	1	2	3	4
I wonder whether something serious may happen.	(0)	1	2	3	4

Observation

The patient is 5 feet 3 inches and weighs 130 pounds (BMI = 23.0). She is seated in an unsupported position on the edge of a plinth and appears to be very guarded. She keeps her neck very stiff when the therapist walks into the room and does not appear to turn her head as the subjective history is conducted. When her gait is assessed, she appears to have a significant degree of difficulty going from sit to stand and once she reaches a standing position, she reaches to prevent a fall. When she begins to walk, her gait is very clumsy and ataxic, requiring guarding. The patient was adamant that she will not use an assistive device and that this gait pattern is due to "just being tired."

Patient History

The patient reports that she noticed an onset of thoracic spine pain while studying abroad in Mexico. She attributes the pain to sitting over a desk for prolonged periods of time and "ignoring her posture." She reports that she was leaving school one day and was crossing the street and was nearly hit by a car. She is unsure of how she reacted, but reports this event made her symptoms much more severe. She went to an emergency room but was discharged with a diagnosis of a thoracic sprain and given a prescription of Meloxicam.

The patient followed up with a chiropractor who took a radiograph of her spine and told her that she had a subluxed vertebrae in the thoracic spine. She reports that her cervical, thoracic, and lumbar spines were adjusted and that the chiropractor placed an electrical stimulation over her thoracic region. She states this felt good temporarily, but once removed, her symptoms got even worse. Her husband became very concerned for her health, so he booked a flight back to the United States. Upon returning, she went to an emergency room, where radiographs were taken of the thoracic spine, but she states the attending physician was much more concerned about a cardiovascular condition. The patient states that she underwent electromyography (EMG) analysis as well as a stress test, both of which were normal. She was released with a prescription for physical therapy. She now reports that she has experienced night sweats recently and attributes this to increased stress. She denies all other red-flag questions on intake forms as well as during the interview. She states that she is concerned that she has had a difficult time concentrating recently but attributes this to stress.

Mechanism: *Insidious, acute onset of thoracic pain after prolonged sitting over a desk.*

Concordant Sign: *The symptoms through this patient's thoracic spine appear to be in widespread distributions. She experiences an "electric-like" pain when asked to move her neck into flexion. Slight knee extension sensitizes this. She reports she occasionally feels this but keeps her neck stiff to avoid this sensation. The patient also reports that when her knee is passively bent, this is the worse pain she has experienced to date.*

Nature of the Condition: *The nature of this condition appears to be neurological.*

Behavior of the Symptoms: *This patient has a high amount of irritability following the assessment of her cervical spine.*

CASE 95

Setting: *Outpatient Orthopedic Office*

Date: *Present Day*

Medical Diagnosis: *Nonspecific Hip Pain of Mechanical Origin*

Charted Data

Name:	*Clarice Jones*	General Health:	*Excellent*
Age:	*23 years*	Amount of Exercise:	*1.5–2 hours/day, 7 days/week*
MRN:	*76399*		
Home Address:	*2609 Kenmore Avenue, Buffalo, New York*	Occupation:	*Student*
		Household:	*Dormitory, lives with a roommate*
Date of Injury:	*7 months ago*		
New Injury:	*Pain increased 1 month ago*	Hand Dominance:	*Right*
		Race:	*Caucasian*

Please fill in the location of your pain with a pencil.

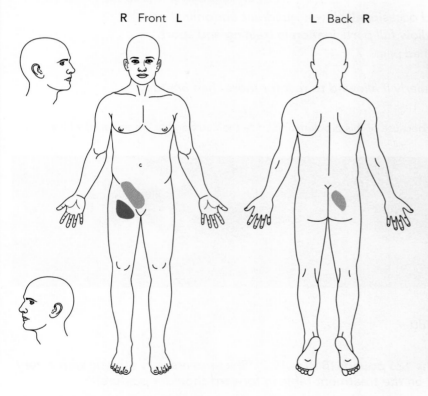

R Front L   L Back R

Pain Intensity Scale	
0	No Pain
1	Low-level pain, able to perform regular activities
2	
3	
4	Moderate-level pain, use of pain medication, activity limited but functional
5	
6	
⑦	High-level pain, use of pain medication, activity very limited—decreased function
8	
9	
10	Emergency Situation

Imaging Results

Radiographs were negative for significant pathology but MRI revealed an area of increased signal over the right superolateral edge of the pubis.

Medications

Aleve PRN

Past Medical History (Please check any items that apply to you.)

Musculoskeletal:

- o Osteoarthritis
- o Rheumatoid Arthritis
- o Lupus/SLE
- o Fibromyalgia
- o Osteoporosis
- o Headaches
- o Bulging Disc
- o Leg Cramps
- o Restless Legs
- o Jaw Pain/TMJ
- o History of Falling
- o Use of Cane or Walker
- o Gout
- o Double Jointed

Other: _LBP, ACL tear with reconstruction, repeated ankle sprains_

Neurological:

- o Stroke/TIA
- o Dementia

Neurological (continued)

- o Polio
- o Parkinson's Disease
- o Multiple Sclerosis
- o Epilepsy/Seizures
- o Concussion
- o Numbness
- o Tingling

Other:_____

Endocrine:

- o Diabetes
- o Kidney Dysfunction
- o Bladder Dysfunction
- o Liver Dysfunction
- o Thyroid Dysfunction

Other:_____

Cardiopulmonary:

- o Congestive Heart Failure
- o Heart Arrhythmia

Cardiopulmonary (continued)

- o Pacemaker
- o High Cholesterol
- o Blood Clots
- o Anemia
- o High Blood Pressure
- o Asthma
- o Shortness of Breath
- o COPD
- o HIV/AIDS

Other:_____

Other:

- o Anxiety
- o Depression
- o Cancer
- o Bipolar Disorder

Chief Complaint: *Anterior hip, groin, and occasionally lower quadrant abdominal pain*

Goals for Therapy: *To eliminate pain to allow full participation in training and sport.*

In the last week, how many days have you had pain? *7*

Pain worst: *During training*

Pain best: *During periods of rest, particularly if allowed to rest for more than one day.*

Patient-Specific Functional Scale[1]

Please list 3 activities that you find are difficult because of this problem and circle the number that corresponds with your ability to perform the activity.

	Unable								No limitations	
1. Sprinting	1	2	3	4	(5)	6	7	8	9	10
2. Jumping	1	2	3	4	(5)	6	7	8	9	10
3. Quick change of direction (cutting)	1	2	3	(4)	5	6	7	8	9	10

Unique Outcomes Measures

Lower extremity functional scale[2] = 57/80

Observation

The patient is 5 feet 8 inches and weighs 126 pounds (BMI = 19.2). She appears very athletic with a very low body fat percentage. She is seated on the treatment table in forward shoulder posture.

Patient History

The patient indicates she has a history of multiple episodes of low back pain and lower extremity injuries but this has not been a problem recently nor has it limited her daily activity or participation in sport. She states that 5 years ago, she experienced a noncontact ACL tear while playing soccer in high school that was repaired with a patella tendon graft. She missed 9 months of competition but returned to play as soon as she was allowed. She also has experienced several inversion sprains in both ankles over the past 8 years. On occasion, she experiences low back pain that has not been associated with a particular injury but comes and goes with higher-intensity competition. To date, this back pain hasn't limited her activity but it has been a nuisance. In college, she has focused on track and field and is currently a middle distance runner with the 1,500 and 5,000 being her primary events.

During the last 7 months, the patient has experienced a gradual increase in groin and hip pain that occasionally refers to the right lower quadrant of the abdomen. It began insidiously following a minor tweak of her hip when she slipped running on icy trails this past winter. The pain has progressively worsened to the point, during the last month, where participation in longer training runs has been hard to handle.

Mechanism: The pain is long-standing and the only physical mechanism of injury appears to be potential soft tissue damage possibly associated with overuse in sport and training. The patient has identified activities that make her pain worse, including some running and jumping, and squatting being the worst activity.

Concordant Sign: Squatting, running and jumping increase pain in the low back, thigh or groin region.

Nature of the Condition: This condition is very limiting for higher-level function, but for everyday activity, it has only been a nuisance. Running for distance, jumping, squatting, and lifting weights are all painful, but walking and general self-care are essentially normal.

Behavior of the Symptoms: The patient has a mild to moderate amount of irritability, and symptoms appear to be specific to movement and activity specific.

Endnotes

1. Chatman AB, Hyams SP, Neel JM, Binkley JM, Stratford PW, Schomberg A, et al. The patient-specific functional scale: measurement properties in patients with knee dysfunction. Phys Ther. 1997;77:820–9.

2. Binkley JM, Stratford PW, Lott SA, Riddle DL. The lower extremity functional scale (LEFS): scale development, measurement properties, and clinical application. North American Orthopaedic Rehabilitation Research Network. Phys Ther. 1999;79:371–83.

CASE 96

Setting: *Acute Care Facility*

Date: *Present Day*

Medical Diagnosis: *Kyphoplasty for Vertebral Compression Fracture*

Charted Data

Name:	*Patty Brown*
Age:	*67 years*
MRN:	*3578213*
Home Address:	*12 Stowe Avenue, Ardmore, Oklahoma*
Date of Injury:	*Yesterday*
New Injury:	*Yes, elective surgery*
General Health:	*Good*
Amount of Exercise:	*1 hour/day, 6 days/week; "Mall walker"*

Occupation:	*Retired nurse*
Household:	*Married with 2 adult children living both in and out of state; lives in a single-level home and prior to surgery she was functionally independent at home and in the community without any assistive devices*
Hand Dominance:	*Right*
Race	*Caucasian*

Current MD orders are for patient to be out of bed as tolerated with progressive activity. No lifting greater than 10 pounds.

Please fill in the location of your pain with a pencil.

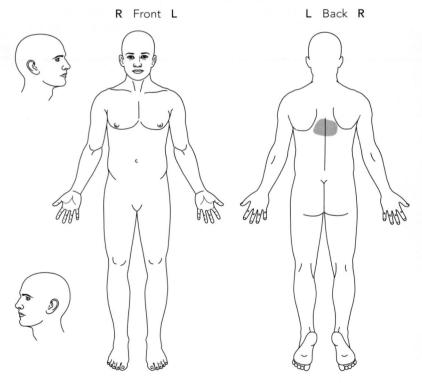

R Front L   L Back R

Pain Intensity Scale	
0	No Pain
1	Low-level pain, able to perform regular activities
②	
3	
4	Moderate-level pain, use of pain medication, activity limited but functional
5	
6	
7	High-level pain, use of pain medication, activity very limited— decreased function
8	
9	
10	Emergency Situation

Medical Testing Results

Hemoglobin = 14 (reference 12–16 g/100 ml)[1]

Hematocrit = 44% (reference 36%–47%)[1]

Medications

Lopressor, ASA, Risedronate

Past Medical History (Please check any items that apply to you.)

Musculoskeletal:
- ○ Osteoarthritis
- ○ Rheumatoid Arthritis
- ○ Lupus/SLE
- ○ Fibromyalgia
- ⊗ Osteoporosis
- ○ Headaches
- ○ Bulging Disc
- ○ Leg Cramps
- ○ Restless Legs
- ○ Jaw Pain/TMJ
- ○ History of Falling
- ○ Use of Cane or Walker
- ○ Gout
- ○ Double Jointed

Neurological:
- ○ Stroke/TIA
- ○ Dementia
- ○ Polio

Neurological (continued)
- ○ Parkinson's Disease
- ○ Multiple Sclerosis
- ○ Epilepsy/Seizures
- ○ Concussion
- ○ Numbness
- ○ Tingling

Other:_____

Endocrine:
- ○ Diabetes
- ○ Kidney Dysfunction
- ○ Bladder Dysfunction
- ○ Liver Dysfunction
- ○ Thyroid Dysfunction

Other:_____

Cardiopulmonary:
- ⊗ Hypertension
- ○ Coronary Artery Disease
- ○ Congestive Heart Failure

Cardiopulmonary (continued)
- ○ Heart Arrhythmia
- ○ Pacemaker
- ○ High Cholesterol
- ○ Blood Clots
- ○ Anemia
- ○ High Blood Pressure
- ○ Asthma
- ○ Shortness of Breath
- ○ COPD
- ○ HIV/AIDS

Other:_____

Other:
- ○ Anxiety
- ○ Depression
- ○ Cancer

Chief Complaint: *"I'm a bit sore but not too bad."*

Goals for Therapy: *"To move around without back pain."*

In the last week, how many days have you had pain? *"I've had this nagging back pain for a while and that's why I had the surgery. Hopefully, in a few weeks I'll feel better."*

Pain worst: *"When I roll in bed and when I take a deep breath."*

SANE Functional Rating

Please rate your **ability** to use your injured area on a 0 to 100% scale with **0%** being unable to use the injured area and **100%** being normal use of injured area in your daily activity: _75%_

Also, if you exercise or have a sport activity or a job that requires special demands please rate your activity on the 0 to 100% scale: _N/A_

Patient-Specific Functional Scale

Please list 3 activities that you find are difficult because of this problem and circle the number that corresponds with your ability to perform the activity.

	Unable									No limitations
1. Walking	1	2	3	4	5	6	7	(8)	9	10
2. Standing	1	2	3	4	5	6	7	8	(9)	10
3. Moving in Bed	1	2	3	4	5	6	(7)	8	9	10

Outcomes Measures
FIM mobility subscale = 70 points/91 points

Observations
The patient is 5 feet 2 inches and weighs 135 pounds (BMI = 26.3). She is lying in bed reading a book. Her surgical incisions are dressed and intact over her thoracic spine.

Endnotes

1. Acute Care Section Lab Values Resource Update 2012, American Physical Therapy Association.

CASE 97

Setting: *Outpatient Orthopedic Office*

Date: *Present Day*

Medical Diagnosis: *Scapular Weakness*

Charted Data

Name:	*Frederick Pfannenschmidt*		
Age:	*58 years*	Amount of Exercise:	*Currently unable to exercise; used to be very active*
MRN:	*79322*		
Home Address:	*1964 Gossamer Court, Boulder, Colorado*	Occupation:	*Currently not working*
Date of Injury:	*Insidious onset 2 years ago*	Household:	*Lives with wife in 2-story home*
New Injury:	*Pain returned 2 months ago*		
General Health:	*Good except for neurological abnormalities*	Hand Dominance:	*Right*
		Race:	*Caucasian*

Please fill in the location of your pain with a pencil.

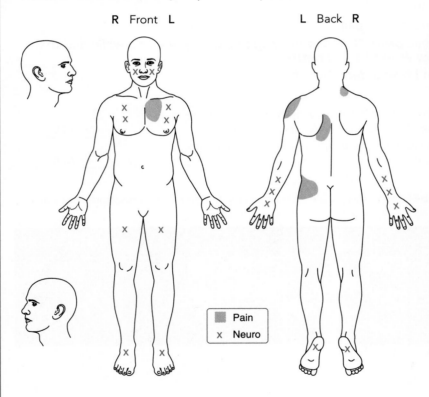

R Front L   L Back R

Pain
x Neuro

Pain Intensity Scale	
0	No Pain
1	Low-level pain, able to perform regular activities
②	
3	
4	Moderate-level pain, use of pain medication, activity limited but functional
5	
6	
7	High-level pain, use of pain medication, activity very limited— decreased function
8	
9	
10	Emergency Situation

Imaging Results

MRI of the cervical spine revealed minor degenerative processes with mild stenosis and mild to moderate left foraminal stenosis at C3–C4; mild to moderate stenosis and moderately severe left foraminal stenosis at C5–C6; and minimal left foraminal stenosis at C6–C7. MRI suggested disc bulge at T2–T3 that did not encroach on the spinal cord.

Medications

Intravenous immunoglobulin (IVIG), Ibuprofen PRN

Past Medical History (Please check any items that apply to you)

Musculoskeletal:
- o Osteoarthritis
- o Rheumatoid Arthritis
- o Lupus/SLE
- o Fibromyalgia
- o Osteoporosis
- o Headaches
- o Bulging Disc
- o Leg Cramps
- o Restless Legs
- o Jaw Pain/TMJ
- o History of Falling
- o Use of Cane or Walker
- o Gout
- o Double Jointed

Other: _____

Neurological:
- o Stroke/TIA
- o Dementia
- o Polio

Neurological (continued)
- o Parkinson's Disease
- o Multiple Sclerosis
- o Epilepsy/Seizures
- o Concussion
- o Numbness
- o Tingling

Other: *small fiber polyneuropathy*

Endocrine:
- o Diabetes
- o Kidney Dysfunction
- o Bladder Dysfunction
- o Liver Dysfunction
- o Thyroid Dysfunction

Other: _____

Cardiopulmonary:
- o Congestive Heart Failure
- o Heart Arrhythmia
- o Pacemaker

Cardiopulmonary (continued)
- o High Cholesterol
- o Blood Clots
- o Anemia
- o High Blood Pressure
- o Asthma
- o Shortness of Breath
- o COPD
- o HIV/AIDS

Other: _____

Other:
- o Anxiety
- o Depression
- o Cancer
- o Bipolar Disorder

Chief Complaint: *Sensation of discomfort in the thoracic spine between the shoulder blades on the left side and pain in the left-sided chest with weakness and loss of function in the left shoulder. Globally, a general sense that there is something very wrong through the left upper quadrant of the trunk. In addition, hypersensitivity is found in the hands and feet from the small fiber polyneuropathy.*

Goals for Therapy: *To reduce the loss of movement and strength in the left quadrant and return to a vigorous lifestyle, including exercise and golf.*

In the last week, how many days have you had pain? 7

Pain worst: *During any functional movement requiring the left arm and when rolling onto the left shoulder while sleeping.*

Pain best: *During periods of rest*

SANE Functional Rating

Please rate your **ability** to use your injured area on a 0 to 100% scale with **0%** being unable to use the injured area and **100%** being normal use of injured area in your daily activity: 65%

Also, if you exercise or have a sport activity or a job that requires special demands please rate your activity on the 0 to 100% scale: 40%

Patient-Specific Functional Scale[1]

Please list 3 activities that you find are difficult because of this problem and circle the number that corresponds with your ability to perform the activity.

	Unable									No limitations
1. Golfing	1	2	3	4	(5)	6	7	8	9	10
2. Lifting objects	1	2	(3)	4	5	6	7	8	9	10
3. Walking	1	2	3	(4)	5	6	7	8	9	10

Unique Outcomes Measures

Oswestry Disability Index (ODI) = 36%

Although the ODI was developed and validated for the lumbar spine, this patient has back pain related dysfunction consistent with the constructs contained in the ODI.

QuickDASH = 27.27

Observation

The patient is 5 feet 8 inches and weighs 164 pounds (BMI = 24.9). He appears healthy but there is mild atrophy visible in the left shoulder girdle. Posture is generally good with mild forward head and rounded shoulders. His skin looks good with no visible discoloration or trophic changes in the distal extremities

Patient History

The patient has a long and complicated medical history related to this problem. Approximately 4 years ago he took an antibiotic and began to lose feeling in both his hands and feet, which was subsequently diagnosed as small fiber polyneuropathy. Most of these symptoms resolved over the course of the following 6 months, and although he did not make a 100% recovery, a general return to all functional activities, including work, occurred. Approximately 2 years ago, he began to develop upper back and chest pain on the left side and a concomitant return of some of the neurological symptoms occurred. A full medical work-up found antibodies for myasthenia gravis. The treatment included physical therapy for the pain and IVIG for the neurological symptoms. About 18 months ago, while playing golf, the patient felt a popping sensation in the shoulder that would not allow him to continue playing. More recently, he experienced a popping sensation in the thoracic spine while reaching forward. Although it was extremely painful, it resolved in a couple of days.

Currently, the shoulder is very painful to sleep on, generally disturbs sleep, and is weak enough to limit function, and the intermittent back and chest pain limit participation, including work. It is difficult for him to determine how much of the limitation is due to pain and weakness and how much to attribute to the neurological diagnosis, which has not entirely subsided despite the continued IVIG therapy and autoimmune diet. The patient also reports a history of shingles approximately 3 years ago as well. The pain and rash from the shingles included the left side in the upper thoracic spine.

Mechanism: The pain is long-standing and associated with general shoulder weakness and potential overuse but may be tied to the diagnosis of small fiber polyneuropathy. It is apparent that all activities are limited by the neurological diagnosis, but this condition with back and chest pain and shoulder dysfunction are substantially worse.

Concordant Sign: Any shoulder activity but also trunk movements increase pain in the back and chest.

Nature of the Condition: Depending on activity level, this condition ranges from a nuisance to disabling—the greater the activity, the greater the limitation. It has prevented the patient from participating in normal recreational activity and from returning to work.

Behavior of the Symptoms: The condition has irritable features in that once the symptoms are exacerbated, it takes some time to settle them back down with rest. It also does not take a lot of activity to irritate the pain in the back and chest. Gentle palpation stimulated symptoms.

Endnotes

1. Chatman AB, Hyams SP, Neel JM, Binkley JM, Stratford PW, Schomberg A, et al. The patient-specific functional scale: measurement properties in patients with knee dysfunction. Phys Ther. 1997;77:820–9.

CASE 98

Setting: *Outpatient Orthopedic Office*

Date: *Present Day*

Medical Diagnosis: *Cervical Degenerative Joint Disease*

Charted Data

Name:	*Margaret Feldenstein*	General Health:	*Good*
Age:	*51 years*	Amount of Exercise:	*Currently avoiding but typically 30 minutes/day, 4 days/week*
MRN:	*73998*		
Home Address:	*218 Skyline Drive, Winchester, Virginia*	Occupation:	*Software engineer*
		Household:	*Lives with husband and 3 children in 2-story home*
Date of Injury:	*8 months ago*		
New Injury:	*Arm symptoms began 3 weeks ago*	Hand Dominance:	*Left*
		Race:	*Caucasian*

Please fill in the location of your pain with a pencil.

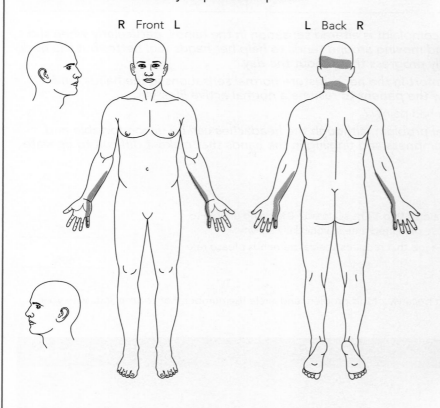

R Front L   L Back R

Pain Intensity Scale	
0	No Pain
1	Low-level pain, able to perform regular activities
2	
(3)	
4	Moderate-level pain, use of pain medication, activity limited but functional
5	
6	
7	High-level pain, use of pain medication, activity very limited—decreased function
8	
9	
10	Emergency Situation

Imaging Results

Radiographs of the cervical spine revealed mild degenerative changes with mild osteophyte formation on C5–C6. Nerve conduction velocity (NCV) revealed no changes in the upper extremities.

Medications

Ibuprofen PRN

Past Medical History (Please check any items that apply to you.)

Musculoskeletal:
- ○ Osteoarthritis
- ○ Rheumatoid Arthritis
- ○ Lupus/SLE
- ○ Fibromyalgia
- ○ Osteoporosis
- ⊗ Headaches
- ○ Bulging Disc
- ○ Leg Cramps
- ○ Restless Legs
- ⊗ Jaw Pain/TMJ
- ○ History of Falling
- ○ Use of Cane or Walker
- ○ Gout
- ○ Double Jointed

Other: _____

Neurological:
- ○ Stroke/TIA
- ○ Dementia
- ○ Polio

Neurological (continued)
- ○ Parkinson's Disease
- ○ Multiple Sclerosis
- ○ Epilepsy/Seizures
- ○ Concussion
- ○ Numbness
- ○ Tingling

Other: _____

Endocrine:
- ○ Diabetes
- ○ Kidney Dysfunction
- ○ Bladder Dysfunction
- ○ Liver Dysfunction
- ○ Thyroid Dysfunction

Other:_____

Cardiopulmonary:
- ○ Congestive Heart Failure
- ○ Heart Arrhythmia
- ○ Pacemaker

Cardiopulmonary (continued)
- ○ High Cholesterol
- ○ Blood Clots
- ○ Anemia
- ○ High Blood Pressure
- ○ Asthma
- ○ Shortness of Breath
- ○ COPD
- ○ HIV/AIDS

Other:_____

Other:
- ○ Anxiety
- ⊗ Depression
- ○ Cancer
- ○ Bipolar Disorder

Chief Complaint: *The patient's primary complaint is altered sensation in the hands, particularly when she first wakes in the morning. Being up and moving around tends to help her hands feel better but the neck discomfort and the headaches gradually progress throughout the day.*

Goals for Therapy: *To reduce the discomfort in the neck, restore normal sensations in the hands, and restore sleeping patterns that will allow the patient to resume a normal active lifestyle.*

In the last week, how many days have you had pain? *7*

Pain worst: *The discomfort isn't the real problem, although the headaches can be uncomfortable and distracting. The main problem is the numbness and tingling in the hands that make it difficult to operate the keyboard.*

Pain best: *Late morning*

SANE Functional Rating

Please rate your **ability** to use your injured area on a 0 to 100% scale with **0%** being unable to use the injured area and **100%** being normal use of injured area in your daily activity: _____60%_____

Also, if you exercise or have a sport activity or a job that requires special demands please rate your activity on the 0 to 100% scale: _____60%_____

Patient-Specific Functional Scale[1]

Please list 3 activities that you find are difficult because of this problem and circle the number that corresponds with your ability to perform the activity.

	Unable								No limitations	
1. Sleeping	1	2	③	4	5	6	7	8	9	10
2. Lifting weights	1	2	3	4	⑤	6	7	8	9	10
3. Operating keyboard at work	1	2	3	④	5	6	7	8	9	10

Unique Outcomes Measures
NDI[2] = 20/50 (signifies moderate disability)
QuickDASH[3] = 27.27

Observation

The patient is 5 feet 5 inches and weighs 144 pounds (BMI = 24.0). She appears healthy and fit. Posture is generally good with a mild forward head and rounded shoulders, which is common with people who work on computers much of the day. Her skin looks good with no visible discoloration or trophic changes in the distal hands that would suggest a vascular problem.

Patient History

The patient reports that 8 months ago she was involved in a car accident. At the time, she was experiencing a fair amount of neck pain but imaging revealed normal degenerative changes that weren't "out of the ordinary for someone her age." The neck pain and headaches subsided for the most part and weren't particularly troubling after about 2 months. But then she began to experience numbness and tingling in her hands, particularly in the ring and little fingers that would wake her from a sound sleep. After a couple of months of gradual progression, she returned to her physician, who was concerned about the neurological changes. More testing was performed, including an NCV and an MRI—both were negative for major pathology. She has basically been dealing with ongoing symptoms since that time, and since no major problem has been noted, she was referred to physical therapy for conservative care

Mechanism: *A general posture disorder with degenerative changes in the cervical spine was aggravated as a result of a car accident, which started placing undo stress on the nervous tissues of the upper extremity. With time and continual aggravation from sleeping and work postures, the abnormal neural tension condition developed*

Concordant Sign: *The patient's sleeping posture, especially when her arms are raised out to her sides or above her head when she sleeps on her side or stomach.*

Nature of the Condition: *In general, this condition is a nuisance but if the patient spends too much time in front of the computer without adequate breaks, it can become disabling. Time and activity management are required to keep symptoms at a level that allows a relatively normal workday.*

Behavior of the Symptoms: *The condition is not irritable but can compromise normal function. The lack of proper sleep may be the most disturbing component of the condition. The patient finds herself very tired by mid-afternoon, making concentration at work difficult and slow.*

Endnotes

1. Chatman AB, Hyams SP, Neel JM, Binkley JM, Stratford PW, Schomberg A, et al. The patient-specific functional scale: measurement properties in patients with knee dysfunction. Phys Ther. 1997;77:820–9.

2. Vernon H, Mior S. The neck disability index: a study of reliability and validity. J Manipulative Physiol Ther. 1991;14:409–15.

3. Beaton DE, Wright JG, Katz JN, Upper Extremity Collaborative G. Development of the QuickDASH: comparison of three item-reduction approaches. J Bone Joint Surg. 2005;87:1038–46.

CASE 99

Setting: *Outpatient Orthopedics*

Date: *Present Day*

Medical Diagnosis: *Neck Strain*

Charted Data

Name:	*Janie Morckel*	General Health:	*Very good*
Age:	*24 years*	Amount of Exercise:	*30 minutes/day, 5 days/ week*
MRN:	*93017*		
Home Address:	*16 Glacier Road, Juneau, Alaska*	Occupation:	*Bush pilot*
		Household:	*Married with 3 kids*
Date of Injury:	*2-year history of problems*	Hand Dominance:	*Right*
New Injury:	*Yes, last week*	Race:	*White*

Please fill in the location of your pain with a pencil.

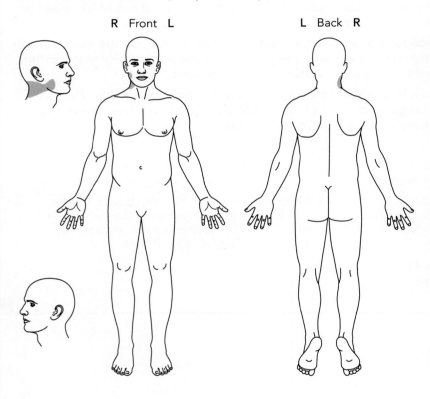

R Front L   L Back R

Pain Intensity Scale

0	No Pain
1	Low-level pain, able to perform regular activities
2	
3	
4	Moderate-level pain, use of pain medication, activity limited but functional
5	
(6)	
7	High-level pain, use of pain medication, activity very limited—decreased function
8	
9	
10	Emergency Situation

Imaging Results

Radiographs of the patient's temporomandibular joint (TMJ) were unremarkable.

Medications

Tylenol (PRN)

Past Medical History (Please check any items that apply to you.)

Musculoskeletal:
- ○ Osteoarthritis
- ○ Rheumatoid Arthritis
- ○ Lupus/SLE
- ○ Fibromyalgia
- ○ Osteoporosis
- ○ Headaches
- ○ Bulging Disc
- ○ Leg Cramps
- ○ Restless Legs
- ○ Jaw Pain/TMJ
- ○ History of Falling
- ○ Use of Cane or Walker
- ○ Gout
- ⊗ Double Jointed

Other:_____

Neurological:
- ○ Stroke/TIA
- ○ Dementia
- ○ Polio

Neurological (continued)
- ○ Parkinson's Disease
- ○ Multiple Sclerosis
- ○ Epilepsy/Seizures
- ○ Concussion
- ○ Numbness
- ○ Tingling

Other:_____

Endocrine:
- ○ Diabetes
- ○ Kidney Dysfunction
- ○ Bladder Dysfunction
- ○ Liver Dysfunction
- ○ Thyroid Dysfunction

Other:_____

Cardiopulmonary:
- ○ Congestive Heart Failure
- ○ Heart Arrhythmia
- ○ Pacemaker

Cardiopulmonary (continued)
- ○ High Cholesterol
- ○ Blood Clots
- ○ Anemia
- ○ High Blood Pressure
- ○ Asthma
- ○ Shortness of Breath
- ○ COPD
- ○ HIV/AIDS

Other:_____

Other:
- ⊗ Anxiety
- ○ Depression
- ○ Cancer

Chief Complaint: *Right-sided orofacial pain*

Goals for Therapy: *To reduce pain and decrease muscle tension and restrictions in the neck and facial muscles, allowing the patient to eat and speak without limitations.*

In the last week, how many days have you had pain? *7*

Pain worst: *Heightened stress levels, bruxism, and dietary choices that included eating hard foods and chewing gum contributed to the pain*

SANE Functional Rating

Please rate your **ability** to use your injured area on a 0 to 100% scale with **0%** being unable to use the injured area and **100%** being normal use of injured area in your daily activity: *85%*

Also, if you exercise or have a sport activity or a job that requires special demands please rate your activity on the 0 to 100% scale: *80%*

Numerical Pain Rating Scale (NPRS)[1]

This patient noted an intermittent pain that ranged from a 0–8/10 orofacial pain.

Patient-Specific Functional Scale

Please list **3 activities** that you find are difficult because of this problem and circle the number that corresponds with your ability to perform the activity.

	Unable									No limitations
1. Eating foods I want	1	2	③	4	5	6	7	8	9	10
2. Speaking for longer periods	1	2	3	④	5	6	7	8	9	10
3. Studying for school	1	2	3	4	5	⑥	7	8	9	10

PSFS initial score = 4.33

Observation

The patient is 5 feet 4 inches and weighs 135 pounds (BMI = 23.2). Her postural assessment showed excessive forward head position and a flexed lower cervical spine. Thoracic kyphosis also was noted. She presented very anxious and demonstrated constant fidgeting.

Patient History

The patient reports her symptoms began approximately 2 years ago for no apparent reason but believes her condition is strongly related to stress and grinding her teeth. Intermittent clicking was her initial symptom that progressed into pain over time. As the pain worsened, she noticed an inability chew her food while eating and was limited with prolonged speaking. She reports at times of stress that she grinds her teeth, which increases her symptoms as well. She relieves her stress by smoking cigarettes. A bruxism splint appliance was prescribed by her dentist but was not worn during the night because of added discomfort and loss of sleep.

Mechanism; *Insidious onset but stress and anxiety reported to be contributing.*

Concordant Sign: *Active mouth opening and mandibular left lateral deviation to the left.*

Nature of the Condition: *The patient's condition is irritable, as minimal provocative activity will elicit her symptoms. Once provoked, pain and mouth opening limitations will persist for several hours.*

Behavior of the Symptoms: *The symptoms are an intermittent 0–8/10 pain. Symptoms are always present in the morning but decrease by mid-morning dependent on the level of activity. The end of each day is similar to the morning hours.*

Endnotes

1. Bolton JE. Accuracy of recall of usual pain intensity in back pain patients. Pain. 1999;83:533–9.

CASE 100

Charted Data

Name:	*Rachael Davenport*		
Age:	*44 years*	General Health:	*Good*
MRN:	*16929*	Amount of Exercise:	*1 hour/day, 5 days/week*
Home Address:	*413 Cranberry Court, East Lansing, Michigan*	Occupation:	*Physical therapist*
		Household:	*Married, lives in one-story home*
Date of Injury:	*No specific injury*		
New Injury:	*Progressive pain over the past 10 years*	Hand Dominance:	*Right*
		Race:	*Caucasian*

Please fill in the location of your pain with a pencil.

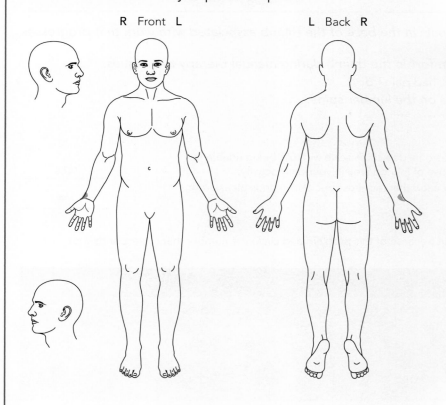

R Front L   L Back R

Pain Intensity Scale	
0	No Pain
1 2 3	Low-level pain, able to perform regular activities
④ 5 6	Moderate-level pain, use of pain medication, activity limited but functional
7 8 9	High-level pain, use of pain medication, activity very limited—ecreased function
10	Emergency Situation

Imaging Results
Radiographs of the wrist and hand revealed mild osteoarthritic changes in the CMC joint.

Medications
NSAIDS (PRN), aspirin daily

Past Medical History (Please check any items that apply to you.)

Musculoskeletal:
- ⊗ Osteoarthritis
- ○ Rheumatoid Arthritis
- ○ Lupus/SLE
- ○ Fibromyalgia
- ○ Osteoporosis
- ⊗ Headaches
- ○ Bulging Disc
- ○ Leg Cramps
- ○ Restless Legs
- ○ Jaw Pain/TMJ
- ○ History of Falling
- ○ Use of Cane or Walker
- ○ Gout
- ○ Double Jointed

Other: _____

Neurological:
- ○ Stroke/TIA
- ○ Dementia
- ○ Polio

Neurological (continued)
- ○ Parkinson's Disease
- ○ Multiple Sclerosis
- ○ Epilepsy/Seizures
- ○ Concussion
- ○ Numbness
- ○ Tingling

Other: _____

Endocrine:
- ○ Diabetes
- ○ Kidney Dysfunction
- ○ Bladder Dysfunction
- ○ Liver Dysfunction
- ○ Thyroid Dysfunction

Other:_____

Cardiopulmonary:
- ○ Congestive Heart Failure
- ⊗ Heart Arrhythmia
- ○ Pacemaker

Cardiopulmonary (continued)
- ⊗ High Cholesterol
- ○ Blood Clots
- ○ Anemia
- ○ High Blood Pressure
- ○ Asthma
- ○ Shortness of Breath
- ○ COPD
- ○ HIV/AIDS

Other:_____

Other:
- ○ Anxiety
- ○ Depression
- ○ Cancer
- ○ Bipolar Disorder

Chief Complaint: *Primary complaint is pain in the base of the thumb associated with work that progresses throughout the day.*

Goals for Therapy: *To reduce the discomfort in the thumb during manual therapy techniques.*

In the last week, how many days have you had pain? *5*

Pain worst: *When performing PA glides on the lumbar spine.*

Pain best: *With rest on days off*

SANE Functional Rating

Please rate your **ability** to use your injured area on a 0 to 100% scale with **0%** being unable to use the injured area and **100%** being normal use of injured area in your daily activity: _____ *90%* _____

Also, if you exercise or have a sport activity or a job that requires special demands please rate your activity on the 0 to 100% scale: _____ *70%* _____

Patient-Specific Functional Scale[1]

Please list 3 activities that you find are difficult because of this problem and circle the number that corresponds with your ability to perform the activity.

	Unable								No limitations	
1. PA glides	1	2	(3)	4	5	6	7	8	9	10
2. Gripping dumbbells when exercising	1	2	3	4	5	6	(7)	8	9	10
3. Operating keyboard at work	1	2	3	4	5	(6)	7	8	9	10

Unique Outcomes Measures

QuickDASH[2] = 11.36 and 37.5 work subscale

Observation

The patient is 5 feet 7 inches and weighs 170 pounds (BMI = 26.6). She appears slightly overweight but also athletic and fit. Posture is generally good with mild forward head and rounded shoulders.

Patient History

The patient reports that over the past 10 years of work she has experienced a gradual onset and progression of pain at the base of her right thumb with work-related manual therapy activities. She is an outpatient orthopedic therapist and routinely uses her thumbs to mobilize joints of her patients. Over the past 9 months, the pain has gotten substantially worse and her attempts to treat herself have generally failed, so she decided that she would seek help from another clinician, knowing that she would follow their treatment program and get superior results. She reports that there are no neurological symptoms.

Mechanism: *Overuse of the thumbs with occupational requirements*

Concordant Sign: *Compressive loading of the CMC of the right thumb*

Nature of the Condition: *The condition is a nuisance in the patient's personal life, resulting in mild difficulty with gripping heavier objects, but it is becoming more an impairment or mildly disabling for work-related activities.*

Behavior of the Symptoms: *Her pain is generally nonexistent in the morning and she is bothered only when her hand is used for heavier lifting tasks or during manual therapy tasks at work. As the day progresses, the pain becomes more severe.*

Endnotes

1. Chatman AB, Hyams SP, Neel JM, Binkley JM, Stratford PW, Schomberg A, et al. The patient-specific functional scale: measurement properties in patients with knee dysfunction. Phys Ther. 1997;77:820–9.

2. Beaton DE, Wright JG, Katz JN, Upper Extremity Collaborative G. Development of the QuickDASH: comparison of three item-reduction approaches. J Bone Joint Surg. 2005;87:1038–46.

LAB PRACTICAL CASES

CASE 1

(Please act out the following findings if working with a learning partner in a laboratory environment.)

Step One: Sinister Findings Assessment
Although not suspected, if the clinician performs a neurological test (such as cranial nerve testing) results should exhibit negative findings throughout. There should be no laxity or other structural problems if tested.

Active Physiological Findings
Active cervical flexion is restricted (0°–35°) and concordant for stiffness. Active side flexion is less restricted but also symptomatic (0°–18° left, 0°–17° right).

Manual Muscle Testing
3+/5: flexion, 4/5: extension, 4–/5: side flexion and rotation bilaterally

Passive Physiological Findings
Passive physiological findings are similar to those found during the active examination. Passive movements into flexion are restricted but "feel good" to the patient.

Passive Accessory Findings
There are no passive accessory test findings that are concordant to the patient.

Special Tests
The patient demonstrates a negative flexion/rotation test for cervicogenic headaches. Palpation of the trigger points does reproduce her concordant complaints of headache. Deep neck flexor endurance test of 9 seconds.

CASE 2

PATIENT'S PAPER

(Please act out the following findings if working with a learning partner in a laboratory environment.)

Step One: Sinister Findings Assessment
The patient has no unconcealed considerations that would warrant a red flag assessment. Because of his age one might consider a test for myelopathy such as Hoffmann's, the inverted supinator sign, or hyper-reflexia.

Active Physiological Findings
Active cervical side flexion and rotation to the right are restricted and concordant. Movements are limited to 37° right rotation and 13° right side bending. Flexion is 45° and extension is 28° with a slight left deviation.

Manual Muscle Testing
Flexion is 4/5; extension is 4/5; left rotation and side bending are 4/5; and right rotation and side bending are 3+/5.

Passive Physiological Findings

Passive physiological findings are similar to those found during the active examination. In particular, the restriction seems to manifest at C6–C7. Repeated movements actually improve overall range of motion.

Passive Accessory Findings

Concordant pain is reproduced with a right unilateral posterior-anterior mobilization at C6–C7. Repeated mobilizations decrease his pain and also improve the range of motion of side flexion by 6° and rotation by 13° when retested.

Special Tests

There is a positive Spurling's sign on the right. Traction is inconclusive. No other special tests yield positive results.

CASE 3

PATIENT'S PAPER

(Please act out the following findings if working with a learning partner in a laboratory environment.)

Step One: Sinister Findings Assessment

Any myelopathic tests should be negative. Also, any tests for stability or vertebrobasilar insufficiency should be negative.

Active Physiological Findings

Active cervical side flexion and rotation to the right are restricted and concordant. Movements to the right side are limited by one-half available range of motion at 35° rotation and 15° side flexion. Left rotation is 70° and side flexion is 24°.

Manual Muscle Testing

Flexion is 4/5, extension is 4–/5; and side flexion and rotation to the right are 3/5.

Passive Physiological Findings

Passive physiological findings are similar to those found during the active examination. In particular, the restriction seems to manifest at C5–C6 and C6–C7. Repeated movements actually improve overall range of motion.

Passive Accessory Findings

Concordant pain is reproduced with a right unilateral posterior-anterior mobilization at C5–C6 and C6–C7. Repeated mobilizations decrease the patient's pain and also improve the range of motion of side flexion and rotation (when retested).

Special Tests

There is a painful Spurling's test on the right at the neck but the pain does not go into the arm. Traction is also positive for reduction of neck pain. No other special tests yield positive results. The patient demonstrated a deep cervical flexor endurance test of 15 seconds.

CASE 4

PATIENT'S PAPER

(Please act out the following findings if working with a learning partner in a laboratory environment.)

Step One: Sinister Findings Assessment

With two motor vehicle accidents in the last two years, the clinician should consider assessing the ligamentous integrity of the cervical spine, since radiographs fail to assess this. Coronary artery dysfunction testing should also be done. All findings are negative.

Active Physiological Findings

Active cervical side flexion and rotation are restricted; the right side is worse than the left. During extension movements, her neck "fulcrums" (or bends) at the C5–C6 and C6–C7 levels, suggesting that the majority of movement occurs at these segments.

Passive Physiological Findings

Passive physiological findings are similar to those found during the active examination. The patient's neck pops and snaps during assessment of side flexion and extension.

Passive Accessory Findings

Concordant pain is reproduced at the C5–C6 and C6–C7 region. With vigorous pressures, the symptoms worsen. With light mobilizations, the patient reports a decrease in symptoms.

Special Tests

If tested, there is a negative flexion/rotation test for cervicogenic headaches. There is a negative Spurling's test, a positive cervical distraction test, and a positive upper limb tension sign for arm symptoms (that are not concordant). The patient is unable to hold a neck flexion endurance test.

CASE 5

PATIENT'S PAPER

(Please act out the following findings if working with a learning partner in a laboratory environment.)

Step One: Sinister Findings Assessment

The nebulous nature of the problem demands a neurological examination, including cranial nerve testing. Although the tests are negative, he does exhibit asymmetry of the face, which suggests further exploration and a temporomandibular joint examination. Tests for a recent monohemispheric lesion (arm roll, finger roll, etc.) are all negative.

Active Physiological Findings

Active cervical spine movements are all negative for concordant symptoms. The active temporomandibular joint examination is inconclusive.

Passive Physiological Findings

Passive physiological findings for the cervical spine are similar to those found during the active examination. The passive temporomandibular joint findings are not for movement but for the contact pressure on the jaw of the patient.

Passive Accessory Findings
All passive accessory findings for the cervical spine and temporomandibular joint are negative.

Special Tests
The only positive, concordant test involves palpation to the jaw (lateral mandible), which yields tenderness and a palpable hardened mass below the soft tissue.

CASE 6

PATIENT'S PAPER

(Please act out the following findings if working with a learning partner in a laboratory environment.)

Step One: Sinister Findings Assessment
Vertebral basilar insufficiency (cervical artery dysfunction) testing will yield negative results. Neurological testing reveals positive findings for inverted supinator sign, hyperreflexia, Babinski test, and left ankle clonus. Cranial nerve testing was negative.

Active Physiological Findings
All cervical and lumbar motions are globally restricted, specifically extension. No specific movements are concordant for low back pain.

Passive Physiological Findings
Passive physiological findings are similar to those found during the active examination.

Passive Accessory Findings
No passive accessory motions were completed secondary to positive neurological testing.

Special Tests
The patient demonstrates positive inverted supinator sign, Babinski test, and left ankle clonus.

CASE 7

PATIENT'S PAPER

(Please act out the following findings if working with a learning partner in a laboratory environment.)

Step One: Sinister Findings Assessment
Difficulty sleeping could indicate possible cancer origin. To rule out cancer, ask about recent weight loss/ gain within the last 6 months and positions of discomfort. To rule out cardiogenic causes, ask questions pertaining to exertion versus symptom provocation.

Active Physiological Findings
Active range of motion in all planes of shoulder movements are within normal limits. No shoulder movements produce concordant symptoms. Active cervical flexion is within normal limits, but increases symptom with repetitive motion. Active cervical extension is limited to 20°. Active cervical side bending to the right and left are limited to 30° and increase symptoms with repeated testing. With repetitive testing, active cervical rotation movements to the left increase symptoms. Active cervical rotation to the right does not provoke symptoms, but is limited to 65°. Active cervical retraction is limited by pain. Repeated retraction increased cervical pain.

Passive Physiological Findings

Passive physiological findings are similar to those found during the active examination.

Passive Accessory Findings

Hypomobility was noted in C4–C5 and C5–C6. Hypermobility was noted in C2–C3, C3–C4, C6–C7, and C7–T1. Posterior-anterior assessment of C6–C7 reproduced the patient's concordant symptoms.

Special Tests

The patient demonstrates a positive Spurling's compression sign, positive upper limb tension sign, positive cervical distraction test. Hawkins-Kennedy and Neer's test were negative.

CASE 8

PATIENT'S PAPER

(Please act out the following findings if working with a learning partner in a laboratory environment.)

Step One: Sinister Findings Assessment

Imaging of the patient's cervical spine exhibited two cervical disc herniations. A palpable mass was noted in the right cervical region, 3–4 cm in size, and the therapist's decision was to treat and refer back to the patient's physician for further testing. The patient was referred to a neurosurgeon, who ordered an MRI of the mass and found it to be only a benign tumor. Screening for signs and symptoms of ischemia was performed, including subjective questioning for facial parasthesiae, dysarthria, dysphagia, syncope, dysphonia, and drop attacks, which was negative. Neurocardiogenic testing was performed by measuring blood pressure in a seated/resting position and then again in a standing position, noting any drop in systolic pressure. No significant change in blood pressure was noted for this patient, thus ruling out the presence of orthostatic hypotension. Assessing the patient's ability to perform rapid alternating movements and other additional limb ataxia tests the integrity of the cerebellum. These tests were all negative. A cranial nerve screen was also performed without eliciting any positive findings. A positive finding was observed during the Romberg's test for testing postural control. With her eyes open, the patient was only able to maintain a normal upright position for 6 seconds and only 5 seconds subsequently with eyes closed. All positional testing for benign paroxysmal positional vertigo were negative. Vertebral basilar insufficiency tests were not performed due to the inconsistency between the patient's clinical presentation and potential vascular involvement.

Active Physiological Findings

Flexion is 40°, extension is 55°, and 40° degrees of side bending bilateral. Rotation right was 75°, and left was 90°. Repeated cervical neck retractions with extension decreased the right cervical spine pain.

Passive Physiological Findings

Decreased upper cervical flexion.

Passive Accessory Findings

Hypomobility of the patient's left CO–C1 side bending, right C1–C2 rotation, and right C4–C5 side bending

Special Tests

Muscle-length testing resulted in identified shortness of suboccipital, sternocleidomastoid, and pectoralis minor muscle. The patient demonstrated a positive deep flexor endurance test and cranio-cervical flexion test. It was identified as positive because the patient was unable to contract her deep cervical flexors independent of her sternocleidomastoid muscles. Testing for cervical radiculopathy via the Spurling's test was negative. This test has a low sensitivity for ruling out radiculopathy but a reasonably good specificity for ruling it in.[1] Vertebro-basilar insufficiency (VBI) test was performed in a supine position with the patient's head and neck rotated to the end-range in one direction and held for 10 seconds and then brought to neutral and held for 10 seconds. A repeat of rotation in the opposite direction was done and held for 10 seconds and finally placed back into the neutral position of the neck for 10 seconds.

CASE 9

(Please act out the following findings if working with a learning partner in a laboratory environment.)

Step One: Sinister Findings Assessment

Constant pain is the only red flag noted on the initial evaluation.

Active Physiological Findings

Cervical right rotation was limited at 25° secondary to pain and extension was limited at 25° because of a "sharp" pain. All other motions were within normal limits and pain free. Thoracic mobility was painful and restricted with right rotation, and bilateral side bending. Thoracic extension was severely restricted but not painful.

Passive Physiological Findings

Passive motion behaved the same as active. Significant restriction noted in T1–T2.

Passive Accessory Findings

Passive accessory joint play elicited restriction and pain from T2–T4.

Special Tests

Spurling's test was negative. Vertebrobasilar arterial insufficiency test was negative. Cranio-cervical flexion test was performed at 20mmHg for 10 seconds for 10 trials but the patient was only able to hold 5 at 22mmHg for 10 seconds. Neurodynamic testing was positive bilaterally along the distributions of both median and ulnar nerves. Neurological testing was negative in bilateral upper extremities. Included were dermatome, myotome, and reflex testing.

CASE 10

PATIENT'S PAPER

(Please act out the following findings if working with a learning partner in a laboratory environment)

Step One: Sinister Findings Assessment

This patient's past medical history indicates a history of depression and migraines, both of which are controlled with medication. She denies the following red-flag questions at intake: unexplained recent weight loss/gain, night sweats, clumsiness while walking and changes in vision. Upon subjective interview, she also denies recent illness or any other systemic symptoms.

Active Physiological Findings

Cervical range of motion: Flexion is 45° with cervical stiffness at end-range; extension is 45° with cervical stiffness at end-range; bilateral side bending is 25°

L rotation: 70°

R rotation: 60°

Wrist range of motion: Within normal limits and does not reproduce symptoms into wrist.

Passive Physiological Findings

Overpressure during passive cervical flexion reproduces some discomfort across the lower cervical spine.

Passive Accessory Findings

Passive accessory intervertebral movements were performed from C3–T7 with the patient in the prone position. She had tenderness noted over the unilateral transverse processes of T2–T3 on the right and T1–T4 centrally. She also had complaints of stiffness from C5–T1 but reported the manual pressure during the examination "felt good."

Special Tests

Classification of special tests:

1. *Normal*
2. *Clinical Physiologic Result: Provocative but doesn't reproduce chief complaint*
3. *Neurogenic: Provocative and reproduces chief complaint*

Special Test Results:

a. *Positive (Neurogenic) ULNT-1. This reproduces her chief complaints bilaterally and sensitizes with contra-lateral cervical side bending of the cervical spine.*
b. *Negative ULNT-2b, c*
c. *Negative Hoffman's sign*
d. *DTRs for C5/6/7 and L4/S1 were 2+*
e. *Deep neck flexor endurance was > 10 seconds*

After ruling out sinister pathology, the clinician provided education and then a thrust manipulation to the cervicothoracic junction and mid-thoracic spine in a seated position. This was followed by gentle cervical active motions. This resulted in a within-session change of symptoms.

Upon reassessment at the beginning of the second session, the patient reported a significant decrease of symptoms into bilateral wrists. She also demonstrated a significant improvement in cervical motion.

CASE 11

PATIENT'S PAPER

(Please act out the following findings if working with a learning partner in a laboratory environment.)

Step One: Sinister Findings Assessment

Vital Signs: Blood pressure = 140/82, Heart rate = 94, respiration rate = 28 breaths per minute.

Active Physiological Findings

Active flexion, abduction, and extension of the left shoulder do not reproduce his symptoms, and range of motion for all planes is nearly normal. External and internal rotation, both feel "tight" but do not reproduce his concordant pain.

Manual Muscle Testing

Flexion is 4+/5; extension is 4/5 internal rotation and 4–/5 external rotation for the left shoulder.

Passive Physiological Findings

As with active movements, none of the movements reproduce his concordant pain. Internal and external rotation at 90° of abduction is restricted but is not concordant.

Passive Accessory Findings

An anterior-posterior, posterior-anterior, and lateral glide all do not reproduce the patient's symptoms, nor are these concordant.

Special Tests

The patient demonstrates a negative Neer's test and Hawkins-Kennedy test for impingement of the shoulder. He demonstrates only marginal weakness in all plane-based testing positions.

CASE 12

PATIENT'S PAPER

(Please act out the following findings if working with a learning partner in a laboratory environment.)

Step One: Sinister Findings Assessment

Although not suspected, if the clinician performs a neurological testing such as upper extremity reflexes, there would be negative findings throughout. It may be beneficial to be attentive to a possible underlying genetic component related to connective tissue dysfunction, such as Ehler's Danlos Syndrome Type III (hypermobility). One could screen for this by guiding one's subjective history as well as assessing for general hypermobility in other joint locations other than the patient's shoulders.

Active Physiological Findings

Active cervical range of motion screen is within normal limits and there are no signs of concordant pain. Bilateral active movements at the glenohumeral joint show hypermobility with all glenohumeral movements, especially ER, FLEX, and ABD noted bilaterally. Scapular dyskinesia with excessive winging is noted with active flexion and abduction of the glenohumeral joint bilaterally. Bilateral strength of rotator cuff musculature and scapular stabilizers was 3+/5.

Manual Muscle Testing

Glenohumeral flexion, abduction, extension, and internal rotation are 4+/5 in both shoulders, and external rotation is 3+/5 in both shoulders.

Passive Physiological Findings

Passive physiological findings are similar to those found during the active examination with excessive movement and winging of the patient's bilateral scapula.

Passive Accessory Findings

Hypermobility/laxity noted with inferior, posterior, and anterior glides of the glenohumeral joint and reproduces the patient's concordant symptoms. Hypermobility of the scapula is noted bilaterally with all movements.

Special Tests

The patient demonstrates negative Hawkins-Kennedy test, painful arc, infraspinatus test, biceps load II, and Speed's test. She demonstrates positive jerk test, Kim test, load and shift test, anterior and posterior drawer, and sulcus sign as well as apprehension test.

CASE 13

PATIENT'S PAPER

(Please act out the following findings if working with a learning partner in a laboratory environment.)

Step One: Sinister Findings Assessment

Although not suspected, the clinician may want to rule out contributions of the neck. Provide negative findings to subjective history to rule out possibility of fracture or cardiac involvement.

Active Physiological Findings

Active range of motion of the cervical spine is limited in all directions but there are no reports of pain in the neck or the shoulder by the patient during neck movements. The patient demonstrates concordant pain and limited range of motion with glenohumeral flexion, abduction, and internal and external rotation. Greater limitation with flexion and abduction was observed with examination.

Manual Muscle Testing

Shoulder flexion is 3+/5; abduction is 3+/5; external rotation is 3+/5; internal rotation is 4–/5; and extension 4+/5.

Passive Physiological Findings

Passive physiological findings are similar to those found during the active examination. Passive shoulder movements on the right are painful.

Passive Accessory Findings

There are no passive accessory test findings that are concordant to the patient.

Special Tests

The patient demonstrates a positive painful arc test, drop arm test, and infraspinatus muscle test. If tested, there is a negative finding with the Spurling's compression test and distraction of the cervical spine.

CASE 14

PATIENT'S PAPER

(Please act out the following findings if working with a learning partner in a laboratory environment.)

Step One: Sinister Findings Assessment

Although not suspected, if the clinician performs a neurological test (such as cranial nerve testing) it will show negative findings throughout. Provide negative findings for tumor- or fracture-related questions, as x-ray is negative. No subjective or medical history suggest trauma or tumor.

Active Physiological Findings

Active cervical motions are within normal limits. Shoulder movements are painful and decreased in all directions, most limited in external rotation (10°), followed by abduction (78°), internal rotation (56°), and flexion (96°) (capsular pattern). Flexion and abduction both cause the patient to move her scapula excessively in order to compensate for glenohumeral stiffness. This compensation compromises scapulohumeral rhythm.

Manual Muscle Testing

Shoulder flexion is 4–/5; abduction is 3+/5; external rotation is 4–/5; internal rotation is 4+/5; and extension is 4+/5. All strength measures are noted within available range of motion.

Passive Physiological Findings

Passive physiological findings were similar to those found during the active examination. Passive movements of the cervical spine were within age-related limits and did not provoke symptoms. Passive range of the right shoulder was limited in all directions, most severely in external rotation followed by abduction, internal rotation, and flexion. Scapular movements were decreased in all planes. The end-feel of all passive shoulder movements is a hard capsular feel.

Passive Accessory Findings

Right glenohumeral joint mobility was decreased in all directions. Anterior and inferior capsule showed greatest restriction. Cervical and thoracic posterior-anterior testing were within normal limits for her age but stiffness was noted through the mid-thoracic spine.

Special Tests

The patient demonstrated negative Spurling's test, and painful Hawkins-Kennedy, Yergason's, and Speed's tests.

CASE 15

(Please act out the following findings if working with a learning partner in a laboratory environment.)

Step One: Sinister Findings Assessment

Although not suspected, if the clinician performs a neurological test, it will display negative findings throughout.

Active Physiological Findings

Active glenohumeral joint range of motion was globally restricted secondary to pain. Patient reports feeling of "instability" with glenohumeral extension, horizontal abduction, and external rotation. Concordant pain produced with abduction, horizontal adduction, and internal rotation. The patient used his scapula more during the earlier ranges of motion in order to take some of the movement away from the glenohumeral joint to protect it. This created observable alterations in scapulohumeral rhythm.

Manual Muscle Testing

Shoulder flexion is 3+/5; abduction is 3+/5; external rotation is 3/5; internal rotation is 4−/5; and extension is 4−/5. All testing performed closer to neutral position to avoid the apprehension position.

Passive Physiological Findings

Passive physiological findings are similar to those found during the active examination.

Passive Accessory Findings

Posterior to anterior force produces concordant pain and is hypermobile.

Special Tests

The patient demonstrates a positive apprehension test and relocation test. Infraspinatus muscle test, painful arc, and drop arm sign are all negative.

CASE 16

(Please act out the following findings if working with a learning partner in a laboratory environment.)

Step One: Sinister Findings Assessment

Imaging has ruled out fracture and moderate to severe ligamentous disruption. Initially, one cannot rule out insidious onset of liver, gallbladder, duodenum, or cardiac disease referring to the right shoulder. However, the patient has no history of cardiac disease, no complaints of gastrointestinal pain or disruption, and demonstrates unilateral, localized signs and symptoms provoked by mechanical movement.

Active Physiological Findings

Cervical active physiological movements were within normal limits with no effect on concordant pain. The patient was able to perform full active physiologic movement in all directions with demonstration of decreased scapular upward rotation during flexion and abduction. Concordant pain was present in 150° to 180° of right shoulder flexion and 140° to 170° of abduction. Over-head movement of the right upper extremity increases his concordant pain initially and increases pain with repeated overhead movement. Pain lessens with relative rest.

Passive Physiological Findings

Passive right glenohumeral flexion and abduction reproduced concordant pain at end-range. Passive extension, internal, and external rotation do not produce an increase in concordant pain through normal range of motion. When over-pressure is provided in passive glenohumeral external rotation, concordant pain is present.

Passive Accessory Findings

Passive accessory joint play of the right glenohumeral joint was not limited and did not produce concordant pain. Inferior glide of the glenohumeral joint in a position of end-range flexion and abduction reduced concordant symptoms. Scapulothoracic movement was hypomobile in all directions.

Special Tests

Neer's sign:[1] Positive

Hawkins-Kennedy test[1]: Positive

Painful arc[1]: Positive

Shrug sign[1]: Negative

Distraction test[1]: Negative

CASE 17

PATIENT'S PAPER

(Please act out the following findings if working with a learning partner in a laboratory environment.)

Step One: Sinister Findings Assessment

Imaging has not been performed to rule out fracture or severe ligamentous disruption. One cannot rule out insidious onset of liver, gallbladder, duodenum, or cardiac disease, especially with patient's past medical history of diabetes and no mechanism of injury. However, the patient has no complaints of gastrointestinal pain or disruption or history of cardiac disease. He does demonstrate localized signs and symptoms provoked by movement.

Active Physiological Findings

All movement in the right shoulder is limited, and repeated over-head movement of Right Upper Extremity increases his concordant pain and it decreases with rest. The patient demonstrates weakness (4/5) with right shoulder flexion, internal rotation, and external rotation.

Passive Physiological Findings

Passive physiological movements of shoulder flexion, internal rotation, and external rotation increase concordant pain.

Passive Accessory Findings

Passive accessory motion of right shoulder demonstrates hypermobility anteriorly and hypomobility posteriorly with an increase in concordant pain.

Special Tests

Active compression:[1] Positive

Yergason's test:[2] Positive

Compression-rotation:[2] Positive

Relocation test:[2] Negative

Hawkins-Kennedy:[3] Negative

Neer:[4] Negative

Biceps Load test:[5] Positive

CASE 18

(Please act out the following findings if working with a learning partner in a laboratory environment.)

Step One: Sinister Findings Assessment

Postoperative incision must be watched closely to monitor for infection. Numbness, tingling, or muscle weakness should be evaluated and could represent nerve damage secondary to surgical intervention. Vitals should also be monitored during postoperative physical therapy interventions because of the patient's comorbidities.

Active Physiological Findings

All active physiological movements at the hand, wrist, and elbow are within normal limits without increasing pain. However, active shoulder physiological movements should not be performed.

Passive Physiological Findings

Passive left glenohumeral flexion (35°), extension (25°), abduction (25°), internal (35°), and external rotation (10°) produce an increase in concordant pain through limited range of motion. Over-pressure should not be performed.

Passive Accessory Findings

Passive accessory joint play of the left glenohumeral joint should not be performed this early postoperative TSA.

Special Tests

None performed.

CASE 19

PATIENT'S PAPER

(Please act out the following findings if working with a learning partner in a laboratory environment.)

Step One: Sinister Findings Assessment

Since the patient presents with left shoulder pain, other possible systemic pathologies cannot be ruled out. However, she is a young athlete in overall excellent health and her symptoms act mechanically. The MRI showed a T2 hypersignal to the supraspinatus tendon and it is likely musculoskeletal in origin.

Active Physiological Findings

All active physiological movements of the right shoulder are within normal limits. Active flexion in the left shoulder reproduces concordant sign. Abnormal scapular movements are also noted during arm elevation.

Manual Muscle Testing

Flexion is weak and painful 4/5, extension is strong and painless 5/5, external rotation is weak and painful 4−/5, internal rotation is strong and mildly painful 5/5, and abduction is weak and painful 4−/5.

Passive Physiological Findings

Passive movement of left glenohumeral flexion, extension, internal, and external rotation are within normal limits but are slightly painful.

Passive Accessory Findings

Passive accessory joint play of the left glenohumeral joint and scapula is within normal limits.

Special Tests

Hawkins-Kennedy: Positive

Neer impingement: Positive

Scapular assistance test: Positive

Sulcus sign: Negative

Anterior apprehension: Negative

Jerk test: Negative

CASE 20

PATIENT'S PAPER

(Please act out the following findings if working with a learning partner in a laboratory environment.)

Step One: Sinister Findings Assessment

The patient's symptoms are activity-related and position-specific. She is not complaining of neurological symptoms, and a neurological evaluation is not indicated. If the clinician performs a neurovascular or neurological evaluation, it is likely negative findings will be exhibited throughout. Cervical, thoracic, and elbow screens yield normal results. The noninvolved has normal findings throughout.

Active Physiological Findings

Active shoulder flexion is 150° and abduction 150°, demonstrating excessive scapulothoracic mobility during both. Both motions have concordant pain at end-range. Active shoulder external rotation ROM is 60° with complaint of mid-range and end-range pain, and internal rotation is 50°.

Manual Muscle Testing

Strength for the noninvolved shoulder is grossly 4+/5 throughout, and 5/5 for the elbow and forearm. Right upper extremity strength is as follows:

Shoulder flexion 4−/5; abduction is 4−/5; external rotation is 3−/5 with pain; internal rotation is 3+/5; elbow flexion is 4+/5; elbow extension is 4+/4; lower trapezius is 3−/5, middle trapezius is 3/5; rhomboid 4/5; and forearm and wrist are 5/5 throughout.

Passive Physiological Findings

Passive physiological motion testing of the shoulder produces pain at end-range of flexion (165°) and horizontal adduction (105°).[1] The onset of pain and resistance are at the same point in range. Passive internal rotation is pain-free (55°). External rotation (70°) and horizontal abduction (−5°) examination are limited by muscle guarding. Pectoralis major and minor muscle length is limited on involved side.[1]

Passive Accessory Findings

Passive accessory testing of the glenohumeral joint with the shoulder at the patient's side reveals excessive mobility for anterior to posterior and posterior to anterior glide. Pain and resistance coincide with AP examination, and posterior-anterior examination is limited by pain before resistance. Inferior glide is slightly excessive with pain and resistance at the same point in range. Scapulothoracic joint mobility is excessive in all directions and is pain-free. Acromioclavicular and sternoclavicular joint mobility is normal and pain-free.

Special Tests
Empty can test (−) [2-4]
Full can test (−) [2,3]
Apprehension test for anterior instability (+)[2,5]
Relocation test (+)[5]
Surprise test/Release test (+)[2,5]

CASE 21

PATIENT'S PAPER

(Please act out the following findings if working with a learning partner in a laboratory environment.)

Step One: Sinister Findings Assessment
Negative ulnar stress test was found. Using a stethoscope and tuning fork to assess for wrist fracture, the right wrist did not demonstrate a decrease or absence of sound when compared to the left wrist.[1] Sensation is intact and normal throughout right upper extremity and vascular testing is negative.

Active Physiological Findings
Active wrist ulnar deviation (10°), supination (55°), and pronation (30°) are limited in ROM secondary to swelling and all produce concordant sign. All other motions cause mild pain but are within normal limits. Gripping is weak and causes an increase in pain.

Passive Physiological Findings
Similar to active physiological findings: pain with right wrist ulnar deviation, supination, and pronation. All other motions cause mild wrist pain.

Passive Accessory Findings
There is tenderness to palpation along the triquetrum and distal ulnar joint line. Passive accessory movements of the carpal bones increase pain with anterior-posterior and posterior-anterior.

Special Tests
Triangular fibrocartilage complex injury (TFCC) load test is positive for concordant sign but there is no clicking. The TFCC lift test, Ballottement test, and ulnar grind test were all positive for concordant sign. Piano key test was negative. There was no excessive laxity found.

CASE 22

PATIENT'S PAPER

(Please act out the following findings if working with a learning partner in a laboratory environment.)

Step One: Sinister Findings Assessment
Sinister findings are not likely in this case due to the obvious and straightforward nature of the injury. The clinician should perform neurological and sensory testing to bilateral upper extremities to determine any nerve or vascular involvement from the fracture site but they are all negative.

Active Physiological Findings

The patient has reduced ROM and strength for right wrist flexion (25°) and extension (30°), and is unable to actively perform radial and ulnar deviation. Forearm pronation (60°) and supination (70°) are grossly impaired. All motions elicit concordant pain. She has decreased grip strength on right compared to left (35 lbs versus 85 lbs).

Passive Physiological Findings

The patient has great restriction in all ranges of motion of the wrist, including pronation and supination. She reports experiencing P1 prior to R1 in all ranges of motions. She remains guarded and pulls right extremity away from therapist frequently during assessment.

Passive Accessory Findings

Passive accessory testing was limited due to the patient's tolerance. The clinician is able to perform grade-one mobilizations for right wrist flexion, extension, ulnar, and radial deviation with some reduction of pain.

Special Tests

The patient demonstrates no numbness and tingling with Tinel's Test, Phalen's or Reverse Phalen's; however, she does have increased pain with the last two tests due to moving toward end-ranges of motion.

CASE 23

PATIENT'S PAPER

(Please act out the following findings if working with a learning partner in a laboratory environment.)

Step One: Sinister Findings Assessment

Although not suspected, the clinician should rule out possibility of a fracture since the patient reports a blow to his arm. An undiagnosed fracture could possibly be a source of pain. Provide negative exam findings during a fracture screen. Clinicians should also screen out the possibility of spinal cord involvement through a quick screen of the cervical and thoracic spines, Hoffman's test, and/or the test item cluster for myelopathic conditions[1] (gait deviation, + Hoffmann's, inverted supinator sign, + Babinski, age > 45). All five are negative in this case.

Active Physiological Findings

Normal range of motion throughout cervical spine observed with no concordant pain elicited. Weakness and pain detected in right elbow flexion (4/5), elbow extension (4/5), wrist flexion (4/5), wrist extension (4+/5), pronation and supination (both 4/5). The patient has a loss of ulnar deviation of the wrist with a loss of finger abduction and adduction of the digit. Decreased grip strength was observed using a hand-held dynamometer with right grip strength being significantly decreased compared to left (65 lbs versus 145 lbs). Repetitive elbow AROM increases pain and paresthesia.

Passive Physiological Findings

Passive physiological findings are similar to those found during the active examination. Right wrist PROM is limited by pain.

Special Tests

The patient demonstrates a negative Yergason's and Roos test as well as a negative varus and valgus stress test. He has a positive upper limb tension test of the right ulnar nerve, positive elbow flexion test, and a positive Tinel sign on the right cubital fossa, which elicited his paresthesia in the ulnar nerve distribution. Results showed negative Phalen's and negative Reverse Phalen's.

CASE 24

PATIENT'S PAPER

(Please act out the following findings if working with a learning partner in a laboratory environment.)

Step One: Sinister Findings Assessment

Since the symptoms behave mechanically, the patient is currently in excellent health, and there is a known mechanism of injury, there are no red flags to any sinister disease. However, he does report having multiple migraines per year. The signs and symptoms will need to be monitored throughout the episode of care.

Active Physiological Findings

All active physiological movements of the wrist increase pain. Range of motion was as follows: flexion 60°, extension 65°, radial deviation 20°, ulnar deviation 23°, supination 65°, and pronation 70°. End-range supination and pronation elicit the concordant sign.

Passive Physiological Findings

Passive left wrist movements increase pain, with end-range supination and pronation eliciting the most pain. Over-pressure should be avoided due to pain provocation with passive movements.

Passive Accessory Findings

Passive accessory joint play of the lunotriquetral joint reveals joint laxity and is painful. Scapholunate joint is normal but elicits pain. All passive accessory findings are within normal limits and painless.

Special Tests

Watson test for carpal instability:[1] Negative

Press test: Negative[2]

Reagan test: Positive[1]

Piano key test: Positive[1]

Ballottment test: Positive[1]

CASE 25

PATIENT'S PAPER

(Please act out the following findings if working with a learning partner in a laboratory environment.)

Step One: Sinister Findings Assessment

The pain awakens the patient at night, which may cause a concern because of the possibility of cancer; however, she has a mechanism of injury, imaging showing a dislocation, no history of cancer, and no recent weight loss. Due to the nature of the injury, there are no other red flags of sinister disease. Numbness and tingling should be monitored due to the possibility of nerve damage due to the dislocation.

Active Physiological Findings

Flexion and extension increase the patient's concordant pain initially, but repeated flexion and extension do not worsen symptoms. Pronation and supination do not reproduce her concordant pain. Some of these movements may be contraindicated, depending on physician and time in the sling.

Passive Physiological Findings

These movements need to be assessed carefully due the patient's immobilization while wearing the sling. Flexion and extension reproduce the concordant sign. Supination and pronation do not reproduce the concordant sign. Over-pressure should not be performed at this time.

Passive Accessory Findings
All joint play of radiohumeral, ulnohumeral, and proximal radioulnar joint are too painful to test at this time.

Special Tests
Static valgus stress test: Negative
Static varus stress test: Negative
Moving valgus stress test: Negative
Timed up and go: 15 seconds
Berg balance test: 44/56
Six-minute walk test: 934 ft.

CASE 26

PATIENT'S PAPER

(Please act out the following findings if working with a learning partner in a laboratory environment.)

Step One: Sinister Findings Assessment
Most sinister findings can be ruled out secondary to the fact that there is a mechanism of injury and the concordant sign is reproducible through mechanical movement. Imaging was negative for the effects of a regional tumor. Neurological testing of the ulnar nerve distribution is negative.

Active Physiological Findings
All active physiological movements at the elbow are within normal limits without increasing pain or discomfort.

Passive Physiological Findings
All left passive physiological movements with over-pressure at the elbow are within normal limits.

Passive Accessory Findings
Passive accessory joint play of the left elbow joint is within normal limits except for a valgus stress test performed in both 30° and 90° flexion, which shows medial joint opening and joint laxity.

Special Tests
Valgus stress test: Painful
Moving valgus stress test:[1] Painful

CASE 27

PATIENT'S PAPER

(Please act out the following findings if working with a learning partner in a laboratory environment.)

Step One: Sinister Findings Assessment
Initially, one cannot rule out cervical, thoracic, or shoulder pathology presenting as referred pain to the elbow. After examination, it is clear that the patient's pain is localized to the lateral elbow; she presents with negative neurological signs and symptoms. Imaging has ruled out possible fracture, dislocation, or ligamentous disruption. Systemic pathology can also be ruled out due to strictly unilateral complaints, localized symptoms with the absence of edema and redness, and mechanical presentation.

Active Physiological Findings

Active end-range elbow extension/abduction produced an increase in her lateral elbow pain. Cervical spine, shoulder, and all other elbow range of motion were pain-free. Resisted wrist extension and gripping reproduced the patient's concordant pain. Heavy lifting (>10 lbs.) worsens her concordant pain; relative rest reduces her pain.

Passive Physiological Findings

Passive elbow range of motion in all directions was negative for reproduction of concordant pain. Valgus and varus stresses of the right elbow mildly reproduced her pain in the lateral elbow. All movements were within normal limits.

Passive Accessory Findings

Humeroulnar, humeroradial, and radioulnar accessory joint play revealed mild stiffness with no reproduction of pain. Cervical, thoracic, and shoulder accessory joint play were within normal limits.

Special Tests

To rule out a possible elbow fracture, an elbow extension test and flexion test were performed; results were negative.[1] Maudsley's test revealed positive reproduction of pain.[1]

CASE 28

PATIENT'S PAPER

(Please act out the following findings if working with a learning partner in a laboratory environment.)

Step One: Sinister Findings Assessment

Cancer cannot be ruled out due to the patient's persistent pain and no known mechanism of injury. However, he has no history of cancer, has not lost weight recently, and is in excellent overall health. He also has pain with movement and upon palpation, further validating a musculoskeletal issue. There is no obvious swelling.

Active Physiological Findings

All active physiological movements are within normal range. Repeated wrist flexion and pronation reproduce concordant sign. No other movement reproduces the concordant sign.

Manual Muscle Testing

Wrist extension and radial deviation are 5/5. Wrist flexion and ulnar deviation are 4/5 and painful.

Passive Physiological Findings

Extreme wrist and elbow extension reproduces the concordant sign. All other movements are within normal limits and do not reproduce any pain.

Passive Accessory Findings

All anterior and posterior movements of both the elbow and the wrist are within normal limits and do not cause any pain.

Special Tests

Valgus stress test: Negative

Moving valgus stress test:[1] Negative

Golfer's elbow test: Positive

Tinel's sign: Negative

CASE 29

PATIENT'S PAPER

(Please act out the following findings if working with a learning partner in a laboratory environment.)

Step One: Sinister Findings Assessment

The near constant symptoms are concerning; however, the patient's symptoms can be modulated by position and activity, implying a musculoskeletal issue. A neurological examination is recommended for this patient, including tests for upper motor neuron lesions secondary to bilateral symptoms and occasional gait deviations.

Active Physiological Findings

All active physiological movements are within normal range. Repeated wrist extension into end-range or prolonged positioning into end-range increases symptoms. The patient's cervical ROM is limited in all planes of motion but most notably in lower cervical extension and bilateral side bending.

Passive Physiological Findings

Extreme wrist flexion and extension are provocative. Passive cervical movements are also limited with end-range side bending being mildly provocative.

Passive Accessory Findings

All anterior and posterior movements of the wrist are within normal limits and do not cause any significant pain. Posterior-anterior glides both centrally and bilaterally (left greater than right) at C6–C7 are provocative with unilaterals being more provocative and giving lasting tingling in the hands when taken to the end of available motion (R2).

Special Tests

ULNT-2a: Positive bilaterally (left > right)

Spurling's test: Negative

Sensation should be intact

DTRs: Normal 2+

Distraction test: Negative

Grip strength a little weakened

Inverted supinator reflex: Negative

Suprapatellar reflex: Negative

Hoffman's sign: Negative

Clonus: Negative

Phalen's test: Positive

Flick test: Positive

Wrist ratio index .74: Positive

Tinel's sign: Negative

Carpal compression test: Positive

CPR for carpal tunnel syndrome: 4/5: Positive[1]

  Wrist ratio: >.76

  Flick test: Positive

  Age: >45

  SSS: >1.9

  Sensory deficits in median nerve distribution: Negative in this case

CASE 30

PATIENT'S PAPER

(Please act out the following findings if working with a learning partner in a laboratory environment.)

Step One: Sinister Findings Assessment

This patient's dermatomes, myotomes, and reflexes are normal. Thumb and finger extension strength are slightly limited[1] but are also painful; supination strength is normal but painful. The neurodynamic testing of the radial nerve is positive. There is a 30° difference between sides. This test reproduces the patient's comparable sign for forearm burning on the right and worsens with contralateral cervical lateral flexion.

Active Physiological Findings

Active cervical flexion and extension are restricted;[1] although the patient complains of stiffness, the comparable sign is not reproduced. Cervical rotation ROM is symmetrical and pain-free.

His shoulder ROM is normal and pain-free and his elbow ROM is normal but produces slight forearm pain on the right at end-range of extension. The patient's wrist and finger ROM is normal and produces pain at end-range of wrist flexion on the right, which increases with addition of finger flexion. Forearm pronation with the elbow extended increases pain.[1]

Passive Physiological Findings

Passive physiological findings are similar to those found during the active examination. Passive movements into cervical flexion and extension are slightly restricted at C5–C6 [1-3] but create only local tenderness and do not reproduce the comparable sign.

Passive shoulder ROM is normal and pain-free. Passive physiological elbow extension/adduction combination is slightly hypomobile with local tenderness on the involved side. Passive wrist flexion produces pain at end-range.

Passive Accessory Findings

Posterior to anterior examination at C5–C6 is slightly hypomobile with local tenderness but does not produce elbow symptoms.[1,2] Passive accessory motion of the radiohumeral joint is slightly limited on the involved side with local tenderness. Wrist and shoulder findings are normal.

Special Tests

The patient's elbow/forearm pain is produced with palpation of the radial tunnel laterally along the brachioradialis and extensor carpi radialis brevis as well as the supinator muscle.[1,4] Tenderness is also present over the C5–C6 zygapophyseal joint.[2,3]

Palpation over the lateral epicondyle shows no symptoms. Cervical compression and distraction tests are negative, and Spurling's test is negative.

CASE 31

PATIENT'S PAPER

(Please act out the following findings if working with a learning partner in a laboratory environment.)

Step One: Sinister Findings Assessment

Cancer cannot be ruled out because of the patient's pain at night. However, she has no history of cancer and has not lost weight recently. She has a positive fist test and a finding of 4 of 5 on the clinical prediction rule for compression fractures.[1]

Active Physiological Findings

All movements increase the patient's concordant pain initially but repeated flexion (which is also contraindicated) increases her pain over time, whereas repeated extension decreases her pain. Repeated side flexion has a null finding and rotation increases her pain. Repeated movements worsen her condition. Generally, pain is reduced in all planes of motion. Extension is most limited in motion by stiffness, and flexion is limited by pain.

Manual Muscle Testing

Too painful to perform

Passive Physiological Findings

Flexion should not be performed. There is marginal usefulness of a repeated flexion test.

Passive Accessory Findings

Posterior anterior movements of the spine (central and unilateral) are too painful (and concordant) for the patient to perform.

Special Tests

The clinical prediction rule for a compression fracture and the fist test should be considered. A strength test of the paraspinals may be a useful choice as well. The patient has structural kyphosis when examined using the structural versus flexible kyphosis test.

CASE 32

PATIENT'S PAPER

(Please act out the following findings if working with a learning partner in a laboratory environment.)

Step One: Sinister Findings Assessment
All negative.

Active Physiological Findings

Active repeated flexion worsens the left leg pain (baseline pain of 6 goes to a pain of 7) but does not worsen the back pain. Active repeated extension improves the leg pain (baseline pain of 5 drops to a pain of 4) but worsens the low back pain. Active side flexion and rotation to the right do not influence his condition but side flexion to the left does increase his leg symptoms. Left rotation to the left is unremarkable.

Passive Physiological Findings

A side glide correction in standing (a left glide) worsens his leg pain (pain goes to 7/10). A side glide correction in prone does not influence his leg pain.

Passive Accessory Findings

A unilateral posterior-anterior on the left side at L4–L5 worsens the patient's left leg symptoms with static or repeated pressures (pain 8/10). Repeated pressure at L4–L5 on the right reduces leg pain to 4/10. No other findings are unique.

Special Tests

He demonstrates a positive straight leg raise and slump sit test. He has a negative "well leg raise" test and he has no "hard neurological findings" of sensory loss, reflex loss, or strength loss.

CASE 33

PATIENT'S PAPER

(Please act out the following findings if working with a learning partner in a laboratory environment.)

Step One: Sinister Findings Assessment

Although not suspected, clinicians do a quick neurological screen to rule out cauda equina syndrome (it is negative). Clinicians should also rule out possible fracture by inquiring about pinpoint pain to the spinous process.

Active Physiological Findings

Active thoracic and lumbar movements are painful; however, they do not produce concordant pain. Flexion and rotation to the right appear most painful. All planes of motion are slightly limited due to pain. Active hip movements are negative for concordant symptoms.

Passive Physiological Findings

Passive physiological findings are similar to those found during the active examination. These do not reproduce concordant symptoms.

Passive Accessory Findings

Passive accessory test findings of the thoracic and lumbar spine do not produce concordant symptoms.

Special Tests

The patient demonstrates positive Gaenslen's test, positive sacroiliac shear test, positive sacral thrust, and positive thigh thrust. The straight leg raise test is negative for neurological involvement but painful. Well-leg raise test is negative. The active straight leg raise test is positive. The prone segmental instability test is inappropriate because posterior-anterior glides of the lumbar spine are negative. Hip scour and quadrant are uncomfortable but negative for concordant symptoms.

CASE 34

PATIENT'S PAPER

(Please act out the following findings if working with a learning partner in a laboratory environment.)

Step One: Sinister Findings Assessment

Although not suspected, if the clinician performs sensory or motor testing, negative findings will be exhibited throughout.

Active Physiological Findings

Active lumbar flexion and extension are restricted and concordant for tightness. Active movements are aberrant in all directions. Repetitive active lumbar flexion causes a decrease in pain and stiffness.

Passive Physiological Findings

There were no concordant passive physiological findings.

Passive Accessory Findings

There are no passive accessory test findings that are concordant to the patient, but increased lumbar vertebral mobility (grade 4) was found at L4–L5. Sacrotuberous ligament stress test and sacral apex thrust tests are negative

Special Tests

The patient demonstrates a positive prone instability test, specific spine torsion test, and passive prone extension test. She demonstrates a negative straight leg raise and well-leg raise.

CASE 35

PATIENT'S PAPER

(Please act out the following findings if working with a learning partner in a laboratory environment.)

Step One: Sinister Findings Assessment

Although not suspected, if the clinician performs a neurological test to rule out any spinal cord compression, it is negative.

Active Physiological Findings

Active cervical range of motion is limited but does not produce pain. Thoracic active range of motion (AROM) painful and limited in all directions; greatest degree of limitation is in flexion. Lumbar movements slightly decreased; however, they did not produce concordant symptoms. Lower extremity AROM is unremarkable.

Passive Physiological Findings

Passive physiological findings are similar to those found during the active examination. Passive thoracic movements are also limited by pain.

Passive Accessory Findings

Posterior-anterior joint mobility testing of the cervical spine is mildly painful and hypomobile in the lower cervical segments. Posterior-anterior joint mobility testing of the thoracic spine produces concordant pain at the T9 level. Hypomobility noted throughout the thoracic spine. Posterior-anterior joint mobility testing of the lumbar spine does not produce concordant symptoms.

Special Tests

Thoracic slump test produced back pain along with the Valsalva maneuver; the straight leg raise and the Hoover test was negative.

CASE 36

PATIENT'S PAPER

(Please act out the following findings if working with a learning partner in a laboratory environment.)

Step One: Sinister Findings Assessment

Sensory testing is negative for changes in bilateral lower extremities. All reflexes were normal except bilateral Achilles reflexes were diminished. Diminished Achilles reflexes is not an uncommon finding in spinal stenosis.

Active Physiological Findings

Active lumbar extension is limited and concordant for pain. Lumbar flexion is within normal limits and relieves patient's concordant pain. Hip range of motion in all planes is also within normal limits. Strength testing was normal throughout bilateral lower extremities, and core strength of the abdominals and lumbar extensors were 3/5.

Passive Physiological Findings

Passive physiological findings are similar to those found during the active examination. The patient reports that passive movement into lumbar flexion "feels good."

Passive Accessory Findings

Lumbar central pressures were painful and produced concordant pain in low back. No tenderness with palpation of the lumbar spine.

Special Tests

The patient demonstrates negative straight leg raise and prone segmental instability test. Repetitive active movements into lumbar extension were positive for concordant symptoms and repetitive lumbar flexion was positive for concordant pain relief. Central posterior-anterior's glides at lumbar spine were positive. Thomas test for hip flexor tightness was positive bilaterally. The patient also completed a 2-stage treadmill test and was positive for symptoms with level walking with prolonged recovery but was able to increase her total walking time while on an incline.

CASE 37

PATIENT'S PAPER

(Please act out the following findings if working with a learning partner in a laboratory environment.)

Step One: Sinister Findings Assessment

Although not suspected, if the clinician performs a neurological test (such as dermatome, myotome, and reflex testing) it will exhibit negative findings throughout. The clinician should also consider that muscular pain could be an adverse side effect from the statin medication used to control hyperlipidemia.

Active Physiological Findings

Active lumbar movements both single and repeated were unremarkable. Active hip abduction and external rotation were concordant for pain. When performing loaded hip flexion through a functional squat, the patient demonstrated excessive hip internal rotation and adduction.

Passive Physiological Findings

Passive physiological findings were unremarkable in the lumbar spine and sacroiliac joint (SIJ). Passive hip movements into flexion, adduction, and internal rotation are restricted and concordant for reproduction of symptoms.

Passive Accessory Findings

There are no passive accessory test findings that are concordant to the patient.

Special Tests

The patient demonstrates a negative well-leg raise for lumbar radiculopathy. All tests using Laslett's cluster for the SIJ compression, SIJ distraction, sacral thrust, and sacrotuberous ligament stress test) were negative for reproduction of symptoms. The patient reported tenderness to palpation of the piriformis muscle posterior to the greater trochanter and a sausage-shaped mass was palpable. He also demonstrated a positive piriformis test for pain and tightness.

CASE 38

(Please act out the following findings if working with a learning partner in a laboratory environment.)

Step One: Sinister Findings Assessment
Appendicitis pain is typically located in the right lower quadrant. If tested for appendicitis (Blumberg's sign at McBurney's point), the tests would be negative. Although not suspected, if the examiner performs a neurological screen such as reflexes and sensation, the findings would be negative throughout.

Active Physiological Findings
Range of motion and strength were found to be within normal limits in all extremities. Resisted glenohumeral extension, internal rotation, and adduction elicited and increased the patient's pain. Glenohumeral flexion, external rotation, and abduction yielded no findings of pain. Trunk flexion, extension, side flexion right, and both rotations are within normal limits but side flexion left pulls on the painful area. Muscle length testing of the latissimus on the right side is uncomfortable, especially when performed with knees straight versus in a hook-lying position.

Passive Physiological Findings
Passive physiological findings did not indicate concordant pain.

Passive Accessory Findings
Passive accessory testing is not applicable to this case.

Special Tests
McBurney's point test: Negative
Psoas test: Negative
Rebound tenderness (Blumberg's sign): Pain increased with pressure but rebound was negative
Palpation at Murphy's point: Negative
Liver palpation: Negative

CASE 39

(Please act out the following findings if working with a learning partner in a laboratory environment.)

Step One: Sinister Findings Assessment
There are no sinister findings.

Active Physiological Findings
Increased pain with weight bearing and all active movements noted during the examination. There is not a pattern consistent with mechanical pain.

Passive Physiological Findings
Passive physiological findings were not found during examination.

Passive Accessory Findings

There are no passive accessory test findings that are concordant to the patient.

Special Tests

The patient demonstrates a positive FABER test, Sacroiliac Joint (SIJ) distraction test, SIJ compression test, sacral thrust test, and Gaenslen's test. She also demonstrates a negative Diastasis recti test.

CASE 40

PATIENT'S PAPER

(Please act out the following findings if working with a learning partner in a laboratory environment.)

Step One: Sinister Findings Assessment

All assessments for sinister findings will be negative.

Active Physiological Findings

Lumbar range of motion (ROM) in all directions is not concordant for the patient's pain. Right hip flexion and adduction against gravity are both concordant for her groin pain and generally a grade weak (4/5). End-range right hip abduction causes adductor muscle spasm. The patient demonstrates guarding with end-range hip motion in all directions.

Passive Physiological Findings

End-range right hip abduction was concordant. The patient demonstrated difficulty with relaxing the right lower extremity for passive exam secondary to guarding behaviors.

Passive Accessory Findings

Posterior to anterior at all lumbar segments are "tender" but not concordant. Hip joint passive accessory motion testing in all planes is negative for reproduction of pain.

Special Tests

The following special tests are negative: sacroiliac joint (SIJ) distraction test, Gaenslen's test, thigh thrust, scour test, Patrick's test. Straight leg raise and slump tests are also negative.

The following special test is positive: Resisted hip adduction.

There is also tenderness to palpation over the patient's right inguinal region as well as the pubic symphysis.

CASE 41

PATIENT'S PAPER

(Please act out the following findings if working with a learning partner in a laboratory environment.)

Step One: Sinister Findings Assessment

Although not suspected, if the clinician performs a neurological test (such as dermatome, myotome, reflex testing), exhibit negative findings throughout.

Active Physiological Findings

Active lumbar physiological findings were unremarkable in all directions. Active hip flexion and extension were concordant for pain.

Passive Physiological Findings

Passive physiological findings are similar to those found during the active examination. Passive lumbar movements were unremarkable and hip flexion and extension movements were both concordant for pain. Passive counter-nutation was also concordant for pain and stiffness.

Passive Accessory Findings

Lumbar passive accessory test findings were unremarkable. Posterior-to-anterior mobilization of S1 was concordant to the patient, causing sharp pinpoint pain.

Special Tests

The patient demonstrates a negative femoral nerve tension test. Her symptoms are reproduced with compression test, sacral thrust, and thigh thrust. She displays a positive pubic percussion test on the right and leg length discrepancy of approximately 1 inch on the right.

CASE 42

PATIENT'S PAPER

(Please act out the following findings if working with a learning partner in a laboratory environment.)

Step One: Sinister Findings Assessment

Although chest pain appears to be a reaggravation of her previous musculoskeletal injury and it is right-sided, the patient's vital signs should be examined. The patient is a female with no history of cardiac or pulmonary problems, no family history of such, and is relatively young. She demonstrates no signs of acute distress; she denies nausea and denies shortness of breath.

The patient does not complain of symptoms of neural dysfunction; however, it has been suggested that costochondritis may have a neurogenic component, so a neurological evaluation may be indicated.[1]

Active Physiological Findings

Active thoracic extension is concordant for both anterior pain and posterior stiffness. Active thoracic rotation and lateral flexion ranges of motion (ROM) are full; left rotation is concordant for both anterior pain and posterior stiffness. Cervical active ROM is full in all planes and reproduces anterior chest pain at end-range extension. Shoulder active ROM is normal bilaterally with pain at end-ranges of shoulder elevation and horizontal adduction on the right.

Passive Physiological Findings

Passive physiological examination reveals segmental hypomobility and local tenderness at T1–T2 and T2–T3 with thoracic extension and left rotation passive physiological intervertebral motion (PPIVM). Elevation of right rib 2 is slightly limited upon inspiration compared to left.

Passive Accessory Findings

Posterior-to-anterior (PA) examination of T1–T2 and T2–T3 reveals hypomobility, local tenderness, and produces concordant anterior pain. Posterior stiffness is produced with unilateral PA T1–T2, T2–T3, and T3–T4 on the right. Anterior-to-posterior accessory testing of the chondrosternal and costochondral joints are painful at the level of rib 2 on the right.

Posterior-to-anterior at the costovertebral/costotransverse joints at right rib 2 produces concordant anterior pain. Posterior-to-anterior examination of the cervical spine is pain-free.

Special Tests

Vital Signs: Heart rate, respiration rate, and blood pressure are within normal ranges.

Neurological Screen: This patient has normal findings upon examination of dermatomes, myotomes, reflexes, and neurodynamic testing.

Strength: Concordant anterior pain is reproduced with resisted shoulder flexion, external rotation, and horizontal adduction on the right. Strength is slightly limited, right compared to left. Serratus anterior, middle trapezius, and lower trapezius muscle strength are limited, right compared to left.

Muscle Length: Limited muscle length is present, right compared to left in the pectoralis major and pectoralis minor muscles.

Palpation: Palpation over the costochondral joint of right rib 2 reproduces concordant pain; no noticeable swelling is present.

CASE 43

PATIENT'S PAPER

(Please act out the following findings if working with a learning partner in a laboratory environment.)

Step One: Sinister Findings Assessment

Through neurological examination, the following abnormal findings are noted:

Dermatomal testing: impaired left lateral lower leg and foot, including the fifth digit

Myotomes: impaired left great toe extension, ankle plantarflexion, ankle eversion

Reflexes: left Achilles tendon hyporeflexia

Babinski reflex: negative

Straight leg raise: positive on left for low back pain (LBP) at 25°.[1]

Active Physiological Findings

Active lumbar range of motion is very slow and guarded. Flexion is limited to 25% of full range and concordant for LBP and leg pain. Extension is limited to neutral. Attempts at rotation produce complaint of "spasm" in the lower lumbar paraspinal muscles.

Passive Physiological Findings

The patient is unable to tolerate a side-lying position for passive physiological examination due to difficulty attaining this position and complaints of LBP intensity once there. Muscle spasm is present with attempts at passive movement.

Passive Accessory Findings

Unable to examine due to muscle spasm with attempts at segmental examination.

Special Tests

Palpation of the lumbar region reveals spasm in the left quadratus lumborum muscle and in the lower lumbar paraspinal muscular bilaterally.

CASE 44

(Please act out the following findings if working with a learning partner in a laboratory environment.)

Step One: Sinister Findings Assessment

A neurological exam should be completed on this patient. Strength in the tibialis anterior muscle was 3+/5 bilaterally and the extensor hallicus longus was 4/5 bilaterally. Remaining lower extremity myotomes were normal. Dermatomal testing was slightly impaired on dorsum of great toe and medial lower leg bilaterally, with the patient demonstrating 4 out of 6 correct responses to light touch testing. Deep tendon reflexes were normal with the exception of patellar tendon, which was 1+/2+ bilaterally.

Babinski test: Normal

Slump test: Negative

Straight leg raise: Negative for back symptoms, and limited to 65° bilaterally

   For gait assessment, the patient walks in slight excessive forward flexion of the trunk, moderately limited trunk rotation, and limited hip extension bilaterally. In assessing his gait over 100 feet, the patient's plantar forefoot drags on the surface 4 times.

Active Physiological Findings

Active lumbar flexion is restricted and concordant for stiffness. Active extension is asymptomatic; however, limited intersegmental mobility is observed. Upon active hip range of motion (ROM), the patient demonstrates compensation with hip hiking/lumbar lateral flexion. Hip ROM is limited to 100° of flexion and 5° of internal rotation. Passive ankle dorsiflexion ROM is 2° bilaterally.

Passive Physiological Findings

Passive physiological findings are similar to those found during the active examination. Passive movements into lumbar flexion are restricted but "feel good" to the patient. Rotation at L4–L5 and L5–S1 are painful into rotation bilaterally. The talo-crural joint mobility is limited into dorsiflexion and is not painful.

Passive Accessory Findings

Posterior-anterior mobility testing centrally at L4 and L5 as well as unilaterally on both sides at L4–L5 and L5–S1 are concordant to the patient.
   Anterior-posterior glide of the talo-crural joint is hypomobile and not painful.

Special Tests

Repeated motion testing for lumbar flexion produces a decrease in LBP intensity that remains better. The patient reports no change in symptoms with repeated extension ROM; however, he demonstrates very limited lumbar segmental mobility during this test.

CASE 45

(Please act out the following findings if working with a learning partner in a laboratory environment.)

Step One: Sinister Findings Assessment

No imaging was performed prior to the examination. The patient demonstrated only 1 red flag finding and that was interrupted sleep 2 times/night due to his symptoms. It has been estimated that 80% of individuals with acute LBP will demonstrate at least 1 red flag finding on examination.[1] The patient is a young, healthy, and active individual with an unremarkable past medical history. The neurological tests conducted included deep tendon reflexes as well as myotome and dermatome testing. They were negative for any neurological signs that would indicate the presence of a radiculopathy.

Neurodynamic Testing
A slump test was performed on the patient that resulted in a positive test. Reproduction of the patient's concordant sign occurred after lower cervical flexion and lumbar flexion. It was sensitized by then moving the patient's head back to neutral from the flexed position. The patient demonstrated a full slump position on the opposite extremity.

Active Physiological Findings
Trunk flexion and either rotation or side-bending right reproduced the comparable sign and worsened the pain intensity on the right side of the low back. Standing extension was painful and stiff but did not worsen symptoms on the right side. When performed repeatedly, symptoms centralized and reduced overall pain level.

Passive Physiological Findings
Similar to active physiological movements.

Passive Accessory Findings
Central posterior-anterior (PA) glide produced a stiff and painful response on L4–L5 but right unilateral PA was most provocative at that level.

Special Tests
Shift correction was trialed in an unloaded, right side-lying position so that the lumbar spine was extended, side-bent right, and rotated left. This resulted in an abolishment of the patient's pain.

CASE 46

PATIENT'S PAPER

(Please act out the following findings if working with a learning partner in a laboratory environment.)

Step One: Sinister Findings Assessment
Vital signs should be examined in this patient. Although the problem appears to be musculoskeletal in nature based on her history, the patient does report pain with deep inspiration and this should be examined.

Active Physiological Findings
Cervical range of motion (ROM): full without symptoms.

Shoulder ROM: flexion limited to about 60% range right versus left and reproduces back pain; external rotation is limited about 20% right versus left and reproduces back pain

Thoracic ROM: pain with extension, right rotation, and left lateral flexion

Bucket-handle elevation of the right 7th rib is limited with deep inspiration.

Passive Physiological Findings
Passive physiological findings are similar to those found during the active examination. Passive intervertebral movements of thoracic extension, right rotation, and left lateral flexion are restricted and painful at T6–T7 and T7–T8. The costovertebral joint at the patient's right rib 7 is painful and restricted with inspiration and right thoracic rotation. Bucket-handle elevation of the right 7th rib is limited, with passive shoulder abduction, and it produces mild pain.

Passive Accessory Findings

The posterior-to-anterior (PA) mobility of T6–T7 and T7–T8 is limited and painful. The PA to right rib 7 is also hypomobile and reproduces the patient's comparable sign both when applied at the costotransverse joint and at the rib angle. Ribs are pain-free with anterior-to-posterior mobility testing. The patient's scapulothoracic joint mobility is limited for protraction and upward rotation, but these motions are pain-free.

Special Tests

Palpatory findings reveal pain and prominence of the right 7th rib posteriorly at the rib angle; when palpated anteriorly, the right 7th rib feels slightly deep compared to the left but is pain-free. The patient experiences tenderness in the iliocostalis muscle in the region of ribs 6–8. Intercostal muscles were not painful to palpation. Resistance testing produces comparable sign with right shoulder horizontal abduction, external rotation, flexion, and extension.

CASE 47

PATIENT'S PAPER

(Please act out the following findings if working with a learning partner in a laboratory environment.)

Step One: Sinister Findings Assessment

This patient has a current episode of non-Hodgkins lymphoma that is being treated medically. The MRI indicates a potential neoplasia and current symptoms may or may not be related to this. This stated, the clinician has been cleared by the physician to treat this patient, and due to uncertainty on the MRI, the physician requested that no large amplitude, manual techniques are performed.

Active Physiological Findings

The patient experiences discomfort when actively flexing forward, with her knees extended. This diminishes when she flexes forward with her knees bent as well as active extension, past neutral. Side bending to her right also provokes symptoms in the low back but does not reproduce her chief complaint.

Passive Physiological Findings

The patient experiences provocation of pain down her right lower extremity with the passive straight leg raise test on the right. Onset of symptoms occurs at 25° and those symptoms are sensitized with dorsiflexion and slight hip adduction.

Passive Accessory Findings

The patient has tenderness with mobilizations over the right side of her low lumbar vertebrae. This tenderness improves with PA mobilizations with her propped onto her elbows, taking her into slight extension. She reports that this "feels really good."

Special Tests

The patient experiences onset of symptoms around 25° of the passive SLR test.

The patient has a positive slump test on the right, which reproduces her chief complaint.

Distraction of the right lower extremity does not improve nor worsen symptoms.

Deep tendon reflexes are absent at the knee on the right and 1+ on the left.

Negative Hoffmann's sign.

CASE 48

PATIENT'S PAPER

(Please act out the following findings if working with a learning partner in a laboratory environment.)

Step One: Sinister Findings Assessment

Because of recent surgery and relative immobility the patient is at risk for deep vein thrombosis (DVT). She is also at risk for posterior dislocation, and therefore needs to follow proper positioning and mobility guidelines of hip flexion no greater than 90°, no hip adduction past midline, and no hip internal rotation past neutral.

Lower Quarter Screen

The patient has a very limited active range of motion: Flexion is 25°; abduction is 11°; adduction to neutral, external rotation is 28°; and internal rotation to neutral and extension to neutral. Her strength is also limited function below 3/5 for all hip planes of motion. There are no sensory deficits.

Bed Mobility

The patient requires minimal assistance of 1 person with lines and tubes along with verbal cueing for technique and safety (particularly to maintain total hip precautions). Minimal assist of 1 is necessary to go from supine to sitting.

Transfers

The patient requires minimum to moderate assistance of 1 person in order to go from sitting at edge of bed to chair via stand pivot transfer.

Balance

The patient is unable to stand unsupported and requires a close contact guard and standard walker to maintain standing upright. She is able to close eyes for 2 seconds with minor swaying while holding onto a walker.

Ambulation

When performing the TUG test, the patient requires a standard walker and close contact guarding as well as verbal cueing to complete the test.

CASE 49

PATIENT'S PAPER

(Please act out the following findings if working with a learning partner in a laboratory environment.)

Step One: Sinister Findings Assessment

The patient demonstrates a negative pubic percussion test for fracture of the hip and a negative finding for the sign of the buttock (if tested). She is unable to stand in side-to-side or tandem stance for Romberg testing. She cannot get her feet into the position.

Active Physiological Findings

All hip movements are limited by strength. The patient cannot bring her hip into flexion or abduction against gravity. All other movements are limited to 60 to 70% of total range. The movements are concordant for her pain, which she indicates is minor.

Passive Physiological Findings

Her movement ranges while supine are within normal limits for her age. She has slight tightness with flexion and internal rotation, which is also concordant.

Passive Accessory Findings

The passive accessory movements of traction and glides (multiple directions) are all negative for pain.

Special Tests

The flexion-internal rotation, adduction test is concordant and painful. Her strength is 3/5 to 3+/5 throughout for the right hip. All other tests are negative.

CASE 50

PATIENT'S PAPER

(Please act out the following findings if working with a learning partner in a laboratory environment.)

Step One: Sinister Findings Assessment
All sinister findings negative.

Active Physiological Findings

Active hip flexion and internal rotation on the left were not limited but produced the patient's concordant groin and buttock pain. Hip external rotation felt "tight" but not painful. Active lumbar ROM is within functional limits. Manual muscle testing (MMT) of the bilateral lower extremities yielded grossly 4+ to 5/5 with all motions. There were no sensory deficits noted.

Passive Physiological Findings

Hip flexion and internal rotation produced the patient's concordant pain. There was decreased hamstring flexibility noted bilaterally.

Passive Accessory Findings

Posterior-anterior glides at all lumbar spinal levels do not reproduce her concordant pain. Posterior-anterior as well as anterior-posterior glides in the left hip reproduce concordant pain.

Special Tests

The patient demonstrates negative findings with the following: Ober's test, log roll test, sacroiliac joint (SIJ) compression, sacral thrust, SIJ distraction, and thigh thrust. She demonstrates positive findings with the hip scour test and hip quadrant test (femoral acetabular impingement test).

CASE 51

PATIENT'S PAPER

(Please act out the following findings if working with a learning partner in a laboratory environment.)

Step One: Sinister Findings Assessment
All findings negative throughout.

Active Physiological Findings

All lumbar spine, hip, and knee active range of motion (ROM) are not concordant for patient's pain. Strength testing measurements are as follows: 4–/5 for bilateral hip extension, 4+/5 for bilateral knee flexion, and 5/5 for remaining lower extremity musculature. Sensory testing is within normal limits for all dermatome patterns in both lower extremities.

Passive Physiological Findings

All SIJ, lumbar spine, hip, and knee passive ROM are not concordant for patient's pain.

Passive Accessory Findings

All SIJ, lumbar spine, hip, and knee passive accessory motion testing are not concordant for patient's pain.

Special Tests

The patient demonstrates negative findings with the following: prone instability test, passive straight leg raise, hip scour test, and Patrick test. The only significant finding is decreased hamstring length bilaterally (testing position supine with hip flexed to 90°).

CASE 52

PATIENT'S PAPER

(Please act out the following findings if working with a learning partner in a laboratory environment.)

Step One: Sinister Findings Assessment

Although suspected, if Homan's sign test is performed, the patient should have a negative finding. He does not have an infection and all other findings would be attributed to the surgery alone.

Active Physiological Findings

Active right hip movement is decreased and painful. Flexion is 34°, abduction is 16°, adduction and internal rotation to neutral only, and extension is 7°. Hip strength is functioning <3/5 all planes and painful. Knee flexion is 100° and extension is full with strength of at least 4/5 (hip pain alters maximum effort). Active right dorsiflexion is restricted (5°) and the patient complains of tightness during dorsiflexion. Strength at the ankle is 4/5.

Passive Physiological Findings

Passive physiological findings they are similar to "active movements" at the hip, knee, and ankle.

Passive Accessory Findings

Passive accessory testing is not necessary for this case.

Special Tests

Homan's sign test is negative. According to the Well's clinical prediction rule, there are 2 major criteria and 2 minor criteria noted, indicating a negative likelihood of a DVT being present.[1]

Functional Assessment

Bed mobility requires minimum assistance to roll and moderate assistance for supine to sit. The patient requires moderate assistance to stand with a standard walker and to take a few steps to a bedside chair.

CASE 53

PATIENT'S PAPER

(Please act out the following findings if working with a learning partner in a laboratory environment.)

Step One: Sinister Findings Assessment and Further Patient History
Are you experiencing any numbness or tingling? No
Perform sensation testing and LE reflex testing: Negative findings
Do you have pain that wakes you up at night? No
Have you had unexpected change in weight over the last two weeks? No

Active Physiological Findings
The patient has no limitations or concordant pain with active knee flexion and extension with over-pressures. She demonstrates decreased range of motion (ROM) and strength grossly 3/5 for hip flexion, internal rotation, and abduction with concordant pain in groin and anterior knee.

Passive Physiological Findings
There are no restrictions or concordant findings with passive knee ROM. End-range assessment of the patient's left hip elicited pain in the anterior/medial hip, with anterior knee revealing flexion to 90°, internal rotation to 5°, and external rotation to 45°.

Passive Accessory Findings
Anterior-posterior (AP) and posterior-anterior (PA) glides of knee are normal with no concordant findings.

Special Tests
Patient demonstrates positive Trendelenburg test on left.

CASE 54

PATIENT'S PAPER

(Please act out the following findings if working with a learning partner in a laboratory environment.)

Step One: Sinister Findings Assessment
Although unlikely, clinicians should rule out a possible hip fracture. Clinicians should also rule out spinal cord compression, which can be quickly screened with a neurological exam. With known hyperlipidemia, performance of vital signs is a very good idea, and in this case was found to be at acceptable levels to complete the physical examination.

Active Physiological Findings
Active right hip range of motion (ROM) limited in flexion, extension, abduction, and internal and external rotation as compared to left lower extremity. Pain was noted with internal rotation. Weakness was also noted in all planes of motion functioning at 4/5 level. No restriction or concordant pain in lumbar spine was noted with McKenzie exam. Active knee range of motion is slightly limited bilaterally.

Passive Physiological Findings

Passive physiological findings are similar to those found during the active examination. Internal rotation is more restricted than external rotation

Passive Accessory Findings

No concordant pain or restriction in mobility was noted with posterior-anterior glides (PA) of the lumbar spine. Reduction of pain was noted with right hip distraction. The patient did note pain with a PA glide to the right hip.

Special Tests

No concordant pain was noted with sacroiliac compression, distraction, thigh thrust, or sacral thrust. The patient also demonstrates a negative straight leg raise and a positive FABER and Scour test with concordant pain reported. Muscle length testing demonstrates a positive Ober's test and Thomas test.

CASE 55

PATIENT'S PAPER

(Please act out the following findings if working with a learning partner in a laboratory environment.)

Step One: Sinister Findings Assessment

Although not suspected, the patient is negative for Wells criteria for a deep vein thrombosis (DVT); she also has no palpable warmth, erythema, or tenderness to her right posterior calf. Cardiorespiratory assessment reveals that her blood pressure is 138/87 with a pulse rate of 74 and respiratory rate of 18. Pulse oximetry is 95%.

Active Physiological Findings

Active physiological findings were concordant for the patient's symptoms with AAROM of all hip movements. The patient demonstrated increased pain with adduction and flexion. End-range was not attainable secondary to pain. All movements have greater than 50% limitation in range of motion. Muscle strength testing revealed significant limitations and a general unwillingness to provide much effort. It would appear that strength is less than 4/5 in all planes of motion.

Passive Physiological Findings

The patient reports pain with all right passive hip movements. Again, pain was greatest with adduction and flexion. Firm end feel was noted in all directions.

Passive Accessory Findings

Passive accessory motions are not appropriate during initial evaluation.

Special Tests

Special tests are not appropriate in this patient situation

Functional Assessment

Moderate assistance is required for all bed mobility, to stand and transfer to a geri-chair, and for <10 feet of gait with a standard walker.

CASE 56

PATIENT'S PAPER

(Please act out the following findings if working with a learning partner in a laboratory environment.)

Step One: Sinister Findings Assessment

Hip complex problems can be difficult to differentiate.[1,2] Even though radiographs may have been negative for a stress fracture, the patient's difficulty with weight bearing, very low BMI, and activity history combine as a risk factor for fractures;[3] therefore, a clinical test is warranted. Low back pain history with potential referral into the leg also warrants a neurological examination. The neurological exam and pubic percussion test will be negative.

Active Physiological Findings

Trunk flexion in standing is within normal limits. Extension in standing is limited at end-range and painful locally but not in the lower extremity. Repeated flexion in standing is painful in her back and her left buttock but not in the patient's lateral thigh or knee. Her hip ROM is full but end-range adduction produces her characteristic pain. Trunk strength is 4+/5 but she has limited endurance as measured by plank (28 seconds) and Biering-Sorensen test (53 seconds). Her hip strength is generally 4/5.

Passive Physiological Findings

Passive end range adduction in extension and internal rotation is very provocative. FADIRS test is not provocative.

Passive Accessory Findings

Left unilateral PA glides in the lumbar spine produce back and buttock pain. Hip and SIJ accessories are not provocative.

Special Tests

Slump test: Positive for buttock symptoms

Thigh thrust for SIJ: Negative

Distraction test: Negative

Compression test: Negative

Sacral thrust test: Positive

Ober's test: Negative

Little's sign (deep palpation in extension, adduction and IR): Negative

Palpation of hip flexor tendons: Positive for groin pain

Pubic percussion test: Negative

Fulcrum test: Negative

One-legged stance on left for 30 seconds: Painful in lateral hip

Manual muscle testing of external rotators in 90° of flexion: Painful and weak

FABER to extension and IR: Creates snapping of hip

Thomas test: Positive for mild tightness in left iliopsoas

CASE 57

PATIENT'S PAPER

(Please act out the following findings if working with a learning partner in a laboratory environment.)

Step One: Sinister Findings Assessment

The purely mechanical behavior of the symptoms make it highly unlikely that sinister pathology plays a role in this case, but with the pain pattern in the posterior thigh, a neurological examination would be an acceptable clinical strategy. Straight leg raise (SLR) testing is positive (see below) but any testing for hard neurological signs is negative.

Active Physiological Findings

Lumbar ROM and repeated movements are full and negative. Active right hip flexion with a bent knee is WNL. If the knee is straightened, it is limited to 65° and provocative.

Passive Physiological Findings

While passively performing an SLR exam, dorsiflexion of the ankle or flexing the neck increases symptoms. The opposite leg is within normal limits and non-provocative. These findings on the SLR indicate a positive neurodynamic test.[1]

Passive Accessory Findings

Not needed in the lumbar spine. Hip accessory movements are WNL and equal bilaterally. Translational movement of the hamstring muscle belly yields discomfort.

Special Tests

Straight leg raise: Positive and painful at 65°

Slump test: Positive

Repeated movements for lumbar spine: Negative

Sensory testing and DTRs: Negative

Manual muscle testing (MMT) is weak for the hamstring and gluteal muscle groups on the involved side. Weakness ranges from 4–/5 for the hamstrings to 4/5 for adductors and abductors and 4+ for gluteus maximus.

CASE 58

PATIENT'S PAPER

(Please act out the following findings if working with a learning partner in a laboratory environment.)

Step One: Sinister Findings Assessment

Lateral hip pain can be caused by many different pathologies; reaching a diagnosis of trochanteric bursitis can be difficult.[1] Radiographs have been performed in this case that should rule out avascular necrosis (AVN) and stress fractures; however, any form of neurological testing to be certain that it is not neurogenic and referred from the spine would be acceptable because of the tingling sensation. Chronic low back pain and trochanteric bursitis symptoms have been identified, and appropriate treatment of the bursitis has been associated with improved outcomes.[2]

Sensation: Intact

Myotomes: Intact but hip abduction is weak (4/5)

Deep tendon reflexes (DTRs): 2+ in both lower extremities

Active Physiological Findings

Trunk range of motion (ROM) is within normal limits and equal in all directions. Repeated ROM is normal and non provocative. Hip ROM is full but end-range adduction produces the patient's characteristic pain.

Passive Physiological Findings

Passive ROM is WNL and equal bilaterally for hips. Passive end-range adduction in extension and internal rotation is very provocative. Flexion, adduction, and internal rotations (FADIRs) test is not provocative.

Passive Accessory Findings

No lumbar or hip joint accessory movement reproduces her pain.

Special Tests

Ober's test: Positive
Little's sign (deep palpation in extension, adduction, and internal rotations): Positive
Hip scour: Negative
Flexion, abduction, and external rotation (FABER) test: Negative

CASE 59

PATIENT'S PAPER

(Please act out the following findings if working with a learning partner in a laboratory environment.)

Step One: Sinister Findings Assessment

The patient's integumentary examination, coupled with her past medical history and white blood cell count, may be indicative of a postoperative infection. Vital signs should be screened in every session. The patient's blood pressure was 145/92, heart rate was 68, and respiratory rate was 17. Pulse oximetry was 96%.

Left Knee Range of Motion

–10 degrees of extension to 95 degrees of flexion

Bed Mobility

The patient requires verbal cueing from the therapist for proper technique in order to minimize pain in the left lower extremity (LLE). She requires minimal assistance to move LLE in bed as well as minimum to moderate assistance from 1 person to go from supine to sitting.

Transfers

The patient requires moderate assistance from 1 person to go from sitting at the edge of the bed to the chair via stand pivot transfer.

Balance

The patient is able to stand with a standard walker while maintaining weight bearing as tolerated (WBAT) on right lower extremity. Close contact guarding provided.

Ambulation

The patient requires a standard walker to maintain WBAT during ambulation and close contact guarding with verbal cueing to ambulate distances of 10 feet before requiring a rest break. She is able to do 2–3 sets of this distance.

CASE 60

(Please act out the following findings if working with a learning partner in a laboratory environment.)

Step One: Sinister Findings Assessment
The patient has no blatant considerations that would warrant a red flag assessment. The clinician should check the patient's blood pressure but otherwise it is unlikely there are sinister contributors.

Active Physiological Findings
The patient demonstrates full active range of motion (ROM). He has pain at end-range over-pressure of knee extension and during full flexion while squatting. The pain is lateral on the anterior knee at the joint line.

Passive Physiological Findings
Passive physiological findings are similar to those found during the active examination. Again, the pain is laterally on the joint line of the left knee with both extension and flexion.

Passive Accessory Findings
Concordant pain is reproduced with a lateral shear to the knee and with passive accessory rotations of the knee. The patella does not appear to be a contributor. Hamstrings are tight but bilaterally tight.

Special Tests
The patient demonstrates a positive McMurray's test for a lateral meniscus problem and a positive Thessaly's test. Ege's and all other tests are negative. He has no ligamentous laxity. He has one-third strength loss on his left knee when compared to the right.

CASE 61

(Please act out the following findings if working with a learning partner in a laboratory environment.)

Step One: Sinister Findings Assessment
Tuning fork over painful area does not elicit concordant sign. Vital signs should be monitored in this patient with his medical history. At the time of the examination, his blood pressure was 128/82, heart rate was 66, and respiratory rate was 14.

Active Physiological Findings
Active knee flexion is limited to 120° and causes concordant pain and audible crepitus. Functional testing of squatting and stepping up and down stairs elicited pain; the patient demonstrates slow guarded movement. He leads with left lower extremity going up stairs and right lower extremity going down stairs, and he is unable to ascend and descend when cued to use other lower extremity leading. End-range extension is painful but the patient is able to achieve extension to 0°. He has 10° of hip external rotation with no complaints of pain at the hip. Ankle ROM was unremarkable with no significant findings.

Passive Physiological Findings
Passive knee flexion is limited to 120° and causes concordant pain. End-range knee extension is not painful when the patient performed passively and unloaded of body weight. His hip has external rotation of 10° with no pain. The patient complains of stretching sensation.

Passive Accessory Findings

Tenderness to palpation on the medial joint compartment of right knee was found. His knee internal rotation was painful and hypomobile.

Special Tests

Ligament testings were negative; valgus test, posterior drawer test, and Lachman's test were unremarkable. There was tenderness to palpate at medial compartment of right knee with a positive varus test for concordant pain. His sensation was unimpaired throughout bilateral lower extremities using dermatome sensation testing.

CASE 62

PATIENT'S PAPER

(Please act out the following findings if working with a learning partner in a laboratory environment.)

Step One: Sinister Findings Assessment

Sinister findings are not likely in this case; however, the clinician may choose to complete a neurological and cardiovascular assessment to determine any postsurgical deficits.

Active Physiological Findings

The patient lacks 10° of extension for active ROM with stiff, aberrant movement. At this time she has surgical protocol restrictions to prevent AROM into flexion. She has difficulty with quadriceps contraction and is able to hold a quad set for 2 seconds.

Passive Physiological Findings

The patient is able to achieve full extension with firm PROM, concordant for stiffness and aching joint line pain.

Passive Accessory Findings

No passive accessories were performed to tibiofemoral joint due to acute surgical repair. Patellofemoral joint grades 1 and 2 reveal minimal restrictions and no concordant symptoms.

Special Tests

Completing special tests would not be necessary or appropriate in this patient, as she has a confirmed meniscal lesion, which is now repaired. However, in the case of diagnosing knee pathology, the patient would have positive findings with McMurray's test and paradoxical McMurray's test indicating a meniscal tear. Surface palpation reveals joint line tenderness in the anterior, lateral, and posterior aspects of the knee. It would be desirable to complete circumferential tape measurements of the proximal knee as well as distal calf to monitor effusion.

CASE 63

PATIENT'S PAPER

(Please act out the following findings if working with a learning partner in a laboratory environment.)

Step One: Sinister Findings Assessment

Although not suspected, if the clinician performs an integumentary screen, it will exhibit negative findings for infection.

Active Physiological Findings

Active knee flexion and extension are restricted (−12°–92°) and concordant for pain.

Passive Physiological Findings

Passive physiological findings are similar to those found during the active examination. Passive physiological motion into flexion is 5° greater than with active physiological motion. Muscle guarding is present during all passive physiological movements, along with reports of knee pain.

Passive Accessory Findings

Passive accessory movements are not appropriate at this time.

Special Tests

If tested, a Lachman's test would have increased movement but a firm end-feel and a positive valgus stress test.

CASE 64

PATIENT'S PAPER

(Please act out the following findings if working with a learning partner in a laboratory environment.)

Step One: Sinister Findings Assessment

The patient presents with a right anterior thigh contusion that is somewhat painful to palpation, but no edema is present. There is also no visible increase in muscle bulk or a visible or palpable lump in his quadriceps muscle belly. Although not suspected, if the clinician performs lower extremity sensation and reflex testing for neurological involvement, negative findings would be present throughout. Strength assessment with MMT reveals weakness (3+/5) in his right hamstring and quadriceps muscle groups compared to his left lower extremity.

Active Physiological Findings

The patient's active knee extension is full but painful throughout the range. Discomfort is also present with resisted knee extension with the knee fully flexed. Knee flexion is slightly limited and painful. The patient reports that his knee feels "stiff" in this position.

Passive Physiological Findings

Passive physiological findings are similar to those found during the active examination with passive movements into knee flexion being painful. He has no pain with passive knee extension.

Passive Accessory Findings

There are no passive accessory test findings that are concordant to the patient.

Special Tests

Thomas test and prone hip extension test are positive for hip flexor tightness. Anterior drawer, posterior drawer, and varus and valgus stress tests for MCL and LCL instability were all negative. Vastus medialis coordination test and eccentric step test were positive.

CASE 65

PATIENT'S PAPER

(Please act out the following findings if working with a learning partner in a laboratory environment.)

Step One: Sinister Findings Assessment
It is critical to rule out the possibility of a deep vein thrombosis (DVT) due to the inactivity, recent surgery, and age. A neurological screen is unremarkable with unimpaired sensation.

Active Physiological Findings
She demonstrates active right knee range of motion of 10 to 15° secondary to swelling and pain.

Passive Physiological Findings
Findings are similar to active physiological findings. When the therapist applies over-pressure, the patient complains of pain and a "stretching" sensation in her knee.

Passive Accessory Findings
The knee is tender to palpate across tibia-femoral joint line and patella.

Special Tests
The patient's left knee girth is 5 cm greater than her right knee girth.

CASE 66

PATIENT'S PAPER

(Please act out the following findings if working with a learning partner in a laboratory environment.)

Step One: Sinister Findings Assessment
Wells criteria and Homan's signs should be assessed and reassessed to rule out the presence of deep vein thrombosis (DVT) in the patient. Post operative infection can reasonably be ruled out at this time due to the absence of fever, sweating, rubor, and warmth of the area.

Active Physiological Findings
Her active knee flexion and extension reproduce concordant pain at –25–48°. The pain becomes sharper with knee flexion. She exhibits difficulty with active knee flexion. Quadriceps and hamstrings strength are substantially less on right side compared to left side.

Passive Physiological Findings
More range of motion (ROM) is achieved for both knee flexion and extension but concordant pain is still produced, especially with knee flexion.

Passive Accessory Findings
Passive accessory movements were not tested so soon post-operative.

Special Tests
Special tests were not necessary.

CASE 67

(Please act out the following findings if working with a learning partner in a laboratory environment.)

Step One: Sinister Findings Assessment

Imaging has ruled out possible fracture, dislocation, and ligamentous disruption. Systemic pathology can be ruled out due to the patient's strictly unilateral complaints, localized symptoms with the absence of edema and redness, and mechanical presentation.

Active Physiological Findings

The patient's anterior knee pain is increased by prolonged weight-bearing activities, such as running. Concordant pain is greatly increased by squatting, stair climbing, and prolonged sitting. Walking mildly reproduces symptoms of pain. ROM is within normal limits.

Passive Physiological Findings

Passive knee flexion, extension, internal rotation, and external rotation were negative for reproduction of concordant pain. Valgus and varus stresses of the left knee were also negative for pain reproduction. All movements were within normal limits.

Passive Accessory Findings

Left patella accessory joint play revealed moderate lateral tracking and grade II crepitus. All other patellar, femoral, tibial, and fibular accessory movements were within normal limits.

Special Tests[1]

By arranging tests from sensitive to specific, assessment of this patient was done by using a "diagnosis of exclusion" method. Pain during prolonged squatting, stair climbing, kneeling, and sitting were positive for pain reproduction. Pain during resisted muscle contraction was also positive. Both the patellar compression test and Clark's sign were positive.

CASE 68

(Please act out the following findings if working with a learning partner in a laboratory environment.)

Step One: Sinister Findings Assessment

The patient experienced a trauma to the knee. A neurological evaluation is not indicated. If the clinician performs a neurological evaluation, it will exhibit negative findings throughout. Lumbar, hip, and ankle screens yield negative results with the exception of ankle dorsiflexion range of motion (ROM) on left which is 0°.

Active Physiological Findings

Active left knee flexion is restricted to 110° and concordant for stiffness. Active extension is restricted to −4°.

Passive Physiological Findings

Passive physiological findings for tibiofemoral joint flexion and extension are similar to those found during the active examination with pain and resistance occurring at the same time in the range.

Passive Accessory Findings

Passive accessory tibio-femoral joint mobility for anterior to posterior and posterior to anterior glides are limited by muscle guarding. Patello-femoral joint mobility is slightly limited in inferior and medial directions but this passive accessory test finding is not concordant to the patient. Superior tibio-fibular joint mobility is normal.

Special Tests

Lachman's test is positive with excessive anterior tibial translation. Pivot shift test is positive with gross shift between 10° and 20° of knee flexion.[1,2]

CASE 69

PATIENT'S PAPER

(Please act out the following findings if working with a learning partner in a laboratory environment.)

Step One: Sinister Findings Assessment
The patient has sustained a traumatic injury and subsequent constant pain.

Active Physiological Findings
Active left knee flexion was limited to 110° due to pain and extension was limited to 10° with significant pain lateral/anterior joint line. The patient's hip and ankle AROM were all within normal limits.

Passive Physiological Findings
Findings were similar to those in active physiological findings except passive flexion demonstrated 120° of motion but was still limited by pain.

Passive Accessory Findings
Results from accessory joint play tests revealed concordant pain with an A-P glide of the tibiofemoral joint, external rotation, and lateral glide of the tibia on the femur. All other accessory joint play tests of the tibiofemoral joint were "uncomfortable."
   All accessory tests of the patellofemoral joint were unremarkable, as were all accessory joint play motions of the proximal tibiofibular joint.

Special Tests
Lateral joint line tenderness[1] was positive for the reproduction of the patient's pain. McMurray test,[2] Thessaly test/Disco test,[3] and Ege's test[4] were positive. Dynamic test[5] was negative. Lachman's test and anterior and posterior drawer tests were negative with normal end-feel. The varus and valgus stress tests were negative for instability. Barford's test (tuning fork and stethoscope test) to identify fracture[6] was negative at the lateral tibial condyle.

CASE 70

PATIENT'S PAPER

(Please act out the following findings if working with a learning partner in a laboratory environment.)

Step One: Sinister Findings Assessment
With all suspected PCL injuries, a vascular examination should be performed to rule out potential neurovascular complications that are often associated with these injuries. Distal pulses should be checked and potentially an ankle-brachial index.[1] In this particular circumstance, the type of trauma makes this an unlikely occurrence.

Active Physiological Findings
The patient's sagittal plane knee motion is 0-15-98° and tender.

Passive Physiological Findings
The patient's range improves over active to 0-5-120° and still quite tender.

Passive Accessory Findings
Anterior-posterior displacement is excessive with a very soft end-feel. Posterior-anterior displacement from neutral is normal with a firm end-feel.

Special Tests
The Lachman's test is negative and the reverse Lachman's test is positive. Posterior drawer tested positive for laxity and the posterior drawer with rotation tested negative for rotation adding to laxity.

CASE 71

PATIENT'S PAPER

(Please act out the following findings if working with a learning partner in a laboratory environment.)

Step One: Sinister Findings Assessment
Since there is a mechanism of injury and there is no history that would suggest sinister pathology, most testing here is unnecessary. The patient might have general hypermobility, so an assessment for general mobility (laxity) is in order because it can contribute to the likelihood of patellar dislocation and prognostic for recurrence rates.[1,2]

Active Physiological Findings
Knee ROM is 0–75° on the left and 10-0-145° on the right. End-range movement is painful and a little unsettling but the pain is not too severe. Manual muscle testing is 4/5 for knee extension and 4+/5 for flexion. Pain and sense of patellar movement limits extension.

Passive Physiological Findings
The range of motion of the passive knee is uncomfortable but within normal limits.

Passive Accessory Findings
The patient's patella mobility is hypermobile on the right but very guarded and painful on the left.

Special Tests
Lachman's test reveals increased laxity but was not positive. The varus and valgus stress tests reveal increased laxity, and the Beighton's sign was positive (7/9).

CASE 72

PATIENT'S PAPER

(Please act out the following findings if working with a learning partner in a laboratory environment.)

Step One: Sinister Findings Assessment
With the insidious onset, a therapist should be more concerned with sinister pathology. Due to the fact that the symptoms are consistent with overuse injury and unilateral in nature, a neurogenic or vascular cause is unlikely.

Active Physiological Findings
The sagittal plane ankle motion is 10°–40° and is tender in full dorsiflexion (DF).

Passive Physiological Findings
Range improves over active to 12°–50° and additional pain in end- range DF

Passive Accessory Findings
AP displacement feels normal with firm end-feel. PA displacement from neutral is normal with a firm end-feel.

Special Tests
From the clinical exam, location of subjective complaints and tendon palpation tenderness yield the highest clinical value.[1]
The palpation of pain in the tendon is positive: $\kappa = .74 - .96$, $+ LR = 3.11$, $- LR = .23$. The subjective report of pain is between 2–6cm proximal to tendon insertion, which is positive: $\kappa = .75 - .81$, $+ LR = 3.39$, $- LR = .29$

CASE 73

PATIENT'S PAPER

(Please act out the following findings if working with a learning partner in a laboratory environment.)

Step One: Sinister Findings Assessment
Palpation is painful at the posterior third of the lateral malleolus.

Active Physiological Findings
Active movements are restricted to half the available range (7°–25° sagittal plane 8° eversion and 15° inversion). Dorsiflexion is concordant for pain. Strength is limited to 4/5 DF, 4+/5 PF, 4/5 inversion, and 4−/5 eversion.

Passive Physiological Findings
Passive physiological movements are similar to those found in active movements. Dorsiflexion is substantially restricted.

Passive Accessory Findings
An anterior-posterior movement of the talus is painful and concordant. The right side feels stiffer than the left side.

Special Tests
The medial tilt test (for an inversion sprain) was positive for laxity in the lateral ligaments.

CASE 74

PATIENT'S PAPER

(Please act out the following findings if working with a learning partner in a laboratory environment.)

Step One: Sinister Findings Assessment
The patient complains of tenderness at the base of the fifth metatarsal. Otherwise, there are no lesions or poor healing wounds, despite the diabetes.

Active Physiological Findings

Active movements are restricted to 6° dorsiflexion (DF) and 27° plantarflexion (PF) the available range. Eversion is somewhat uncomfortable and notably stiff at 3°. Manual muscle testing (MMT) is generally weak in the foot and ankle, demonstrating 4–/5 strength throughout the right side and 4/5 on the left.

Passive Physiological Findings

Passive physiological movements are similar to those found in active movements. Stiffness is the chief report during all movements.

Passive Accessory Findings

There is pitting edema throughout the foot during passive accessory movements. No movements are markedly stiff.

Special Tests

The plantar fascia of the foot is very tight during weight-bearing lifting of the first toe. No other soft tissue findings are significant.

CASE 75

PATIENT'S PAPER

(Please act out the following findings if working with a learning partner in a laboratory environment.)

Step One: Sinister Findings Assessment

Because the patient's left calf is larger than his right, edema was initially considered as a potential cause. Since he was held in the hospital for suspected deep vein thrombosis (DVT) of the lower left extremity, it would be imperative to evaluate for the risk of DVT and rule it out at this stage using the Wells criteria.

Active Physiological Findings

Limitations in all ROM include right ankle plantarflexion (PF) = 30°, dorsiflexion (DF) = 8°, inversion = 20°, eversion = 5°. Strength is limited to 4– to 4/5 throughout the ankle and all are painful.

Passive Physiological Findings

Limitations in ROM include ankle DF and eversion with increased pain and "pulling" sensation when moved into DF. There is equal ankle restriction with right knee flexed and extended.

Passive Accessory Findings

All motions are hypomobile with concordant pain during posterior glide of the Talus.

Special Tests

To assess a potential Achilles rupture, one might perform the Thompson's squeeze test. Because this patient has confirmed rupture, this test is not necessary or appropriate. Due to high cholesterol and high blood pressure, a capillary refill test to the affected foot would be imperative to assess for any vascular concerns.

Other

Tape measure recordings of bilateral lower leg circumference measures to compare symmetry.

CASE 76

(Please act out the following findings if working with a learning partner in a laboratory environment.)

Step One: Sinister Findings Assessment
Sinister findings not suspected secondary to negative radiographs.

Active Physiological Findings
All right ankle motions are globally restricted secondary to pain to very little movement in any direction. Concordant sign is confirmed with external rotation and dorsiflexion. Manual muscle testing is inappropriate secondary to his severe pain but would be very limited by the pain if performed.

Passive Physiological Findings
Passive physiological findings are similar to those found during the active examination.

Passive Accessory Findings
Palpation is painful over syndesmosis. Anterior-posterior movement of the talus produces concordant pain.

Special Tests
Positive external rotation test, Cotton test, and syndesmosis squeeze test.

CASE 77

PATIENT'S PAPER

(Please act out the following findings if working with a learning partner in a laboratory environment.)

Step One: Sinister Findings Assessment
Sinister findings are not expected; however, if the clinician palpates for pinpoint pain over the lateral aspect of the ankle, negative findings will be exhibited for a possible fracture. Also, a vibrating tuning fork at the fibular mallelous will exhibit negative findings (no reproduction of pain).

Active Physiological Findings
Active inversion and dorsiflexion are limited by 50% with reports of pain. Eversion is slightly painful and limited to 8° secondary to increased swelling on the lateral aspect of the ankle. Strength is limited in all planes and definitive manual muscle test (MMT) is inappropriate secondary to the pain.

Passive Physiological Findings
Passive physiological findings are consistent with those findings during the active examination.

Passive Accessory Findings
Passive accessory findings demonstrated hypermobility and pain with anterior to posterior mobilization of the tibia on talus. All other passive accessories were unremarkable.

Special Tests
The patient demonstrates a positive anterior drawer test and a positive talar tilt for an inversion sprain.

CASE 78

PATIENT'S PAPER

(Please act out the following findings if working with a learning partner in a laboratory environment)

Step One: Sinister Findings Assessment
Although not suspected, if the clinician performs a neurological, it will display negative findings throughout.

Active Physiological Findings
Active right dorsiflexion is limited to 2 degrees with knee extended and 8 degrees with knee flexed. Strength is limited in dorsiflexion to 4+/5, inversion to 4−/5, eversion is 4+/5, and plantarflexion in 4/5.

Passive Physiological Findings
Passive physiological findings are similar to those found during the active examination. Passive right dorsiflexion and great toe extension is concordant for pain.

Passive Accessory Findings
There are no passive accessory findings that are concordant to the patient.

Special Tests
The patient demonstrates negative Tinel's, sign painful arc, and pinch test. Palpation of the Achilles tendon or the posterior tibialis tendon does not produce concordant sign. Windlass mechanism is positive.

CASE 79

PATIENT'S PAPER

(Please act out the following findings if working with a learning partner in a laboratory environment.)

Step One: Sinister Findings Assessment
Imaging has ruled out possible fracture and dislocation. MRI findings were negative for tendon rupture. Systemic pathology can be ruled out due to strictly unilateral complaints and localized symptoms.

Active Physiological Findings
All weight-bearing activity increases his pain, but the patient's left great toe extension with weight bearing for a sustained period of time or during rapid acceleration greatly reproduces concordant pain. The left great toe flexion only mildly produces discomfort.

Passive Physiological Findings
Passive flexion and extension of the left metatarsal-phalangeal (MTP) reproduces concordant pain with extension producing more severe pain. Valgus and varus stresses of the left MTP produces increased concordant pain.

Passive Accessory Findings
Stiffness and edema limit joint play in all planes of the left MTP.

Special Tests
Tuning fork test and Morton's test for stress fracture should be considered to further rule out fractures that may have been hidden on radiologic testing.[1]

CASE 80

PATIENT'S PAPER

(Please act out the following findings if working with a learning partner in a laboratory environment.)

Step One: Sinister Findings Assessment

Imaging has ruled out a fracture. The patient is in excellent health with no known comorbidities.

Active Physiological Findings

Over-pressure to active left dorsiflexion, inversion, and eversion reproduce concordant pain. Pain is worse with weight bearing and weight-bearing activities, especially those that involve dorsiflexion of the left ankle.

Passive Physiological Findings

Passive dorsiflexion re-creates the patient's concordant pain. Palpation over area of anterior tibiofibular ligament is also provocative.

Passive Accessory Findings

Inversion, eversion, internal rotator, and external rotatory stresses to the left ankle reproduce and increase the patient's concordant pain.

Special Tests

Positive special tests include anterior drawer test, inversion stress test, eversion stress test, external rotation stress test, forced dorsiflexion test, and squeeze test. The left anterior drawer test, in particular, exposed increased laxity compared to the right.

CASE 81

PATIENT'S PAPER

(Please act out the following findings if working with a learning partner in a laboratory environment.)

Step One: Sinister Findings Assessment

A medical screen is performed and is unremarkable for this patient. There is no familial history for sinister diseases related to his current problem.

Active Physiological Findings

Active range of motion of the patient's hip and knee are unremarkable. Ankle dorsiflexion is significantly limited to 5° and plantar flexion to 15°. Eversion is noted to be slightly restricted and inversion produces mild discomfort anterior to the lateral malleolus but range of motion is full.

Passive Physiological Findings

Passive physiological findings indicated an increase in motion for all restricted planes and are limited by pain.

Passive Accessory Findings

Anterior-posterior (AP) glide of the talocrural joint produces the concordant stiffness and was determined by the clinician to be hypomobile compared to the opposite limb. Posterior-anterior (PA) of the talocrural joint produces the same pain found with active inversion (anterior to lateral malleoli). Accessory joint testing of the subtalar joint, mid-foot, and forefoot were negative.

Special Tests

The anterior drawer produced pain anterior to the lateral malleolus but not the concordant stiffness. A trial bout of mobilization with movement of the talocrural joint to improve dorsiflexion could be performed.[1]

CASE 82

PATIENT'S PAPER

(Please act out the following findings if working with a learning partner in a laboratory environment.)

Step One: Sinister Findings Assessment

The medical screen ruled out any systemic cause to the patient's symptoms. The patient denied pain at night or with sleeping, weakness, and changes with bowel or bladder. His prior lab testing as well as past medical history screen were both negative for systemic disease being responsible for his symptoms. Vital signs were tested and stable.

Active Physiological Findings
Unremarkable

Passive Physiological Findings
Unremarkable

Passive Accessory Findings
Unremarkable

Special Tests

Palpation of localized tenderness was noted 9.4 cm above the lateral malleolus. With the Feiss line, grade 1 pes planus with the navicular tuberosity positioned one-third the distance from the line drawn to the floor. Tinel's sign was positive 9.4 cm above the lateral malleolus, causing radiating pain into the foot.

Resisted eversion and dorsiflexion while adding compression to the peroneal tunnel was positive. The ankle brachial index showed a normal value of 1.15, ruling out the presence of peripheral vascular disease (PVD). Initially, the straight leg raise did not elicit symptoms until adding distal ankle inversion and plantar flexion. The patient's knee was then placed into flexion and the symptoms persisted.

Neurological testing showed intact sensory and motor pathways as well as intact deep tendon reflexes in bilateral lower extremities. The patient presented with an unremarkable gait assessment.

CASE 83

PATIENT'S PAPER

(Please act out the following findings if working with a learning partner in a laboratory environment.)

Step One: Sinister Findings Assessment

Because of recent surgery and relative immobility, the patient is at risk for deep vein thrombosis. The nature of this surgery also places the patient at risk for hip dislocation; therefore, the patient needs to follow positioning and mobility guidelines as dictated by the surgeon. In this case, no active straight-leg raising or hip abduction has been ordered. Vital signs were tested and stable.

Range of motion

Lower extremity ROM is limited by pain and the patient's movement is slow. Left hip passive ROM tested in supine was 0° to 30° and limited by pain; extension to neutral, abduction 0° to 5°, and external rotation not tested to prevent dislocation. Muscle strength is functioning 2–/5 with assistance to ensure hip precautions. Upper extremity ROM and strength testing is deferred secondary to fixation and fractures for the right; the left is within normal limits.

Bed Mobility

The patient requires minimal to moderate assistance of 1 person along with verbal cueing for technique and safety (particularly to hip precautions). Minimal to moderate assist of 1 is necessary to go from supine to sitting.

Transfers

The patient requires minimum to moderate assist of 1 to go from sitting at edge of bed to chair via stand pivot transfer.

Balance

Unable to stand unsupported; requires close contact guarding to minimum assist of 1 and standard walker to maintain standing upright and weight-bearing precautions.

Ambulation

The patient requires a standard walker and close contact guarding as well as verbal cueing to ambulate on level surfaces maintaining touch-down weight bearing.

CASE 84

PATIENT'S PAPER

(Please act out the following findings if working with a learning partner in a laboratory environment.)

Step One: Sinister Findings Assessment

The patient's history of diabetes (DM), coronary artery disease (CAD), and hypertension (HTN) puts him at risk for silent cardiac ischemia. Monitoring of vitals is advisable and in this case were found to be stable. Additionally, recent surgery puts this patient at risk for DVT.

Lower Quarter Screen

Right lower extremity range of motion is limited in the hip at 20° flexion, 5° extension, 9° abduction, adduction and internal rotation to neutral and external rotation to 25°. Strength is functioning at 3–/5 in the right hip. The knee is functioning at 4–/5 and the foot and ankle at 4+/5 with good ROM. The left lower extremity is functioning with functional ROM and generally at 4+/5 strength.

Bed Mobility

Requires verbal cueing from therapist for proper technique in order to minimize pain in the right lower extremity. Supervision of 1 is necessary to go from supine to sitting.

Transfers

Requires close contact guarding with occasional minimum assist of 1 to go from sitting at the edge of the bed to a chair via stand pivot transfer.

Balance

The patient is able to stand with a standard walker while maintaining partial weight bearing (PWB) on right lower extremity. Close supervision provided.

Ambulation

The patient requires a standard walker to maintain PWB during ambulation and close contact guarding with verbal cueing to ambulate distances of 25 feet before requiring a rest break. He is able to do 2–3 sets of this distance.

CASE 85

PATIENT'S PAPER

(Please act out the following findings if working with a learning partner in a laboratory environment.)

Step One: Sinister Findings Assessment
Because of the injuries, recent surgery, and relative immobility, the patient is at risk for DVT and pneumonia. Vital signs were tested and stable.

Range of motion
The patient's lower extremity ROM is limited by pain and his movement is slow. Muscle strength is functioning 2+/5 with pain as a limiting factor. Upper extremity ROM and strength testing is deferred secondary to fixation and fractures for the right and left are within functional limits.

Bed Mobility
Requires assistance of 1 with lines and tubes along with verbal cueing for technique and safety. Assist of 1 is necessary to go from supine to sitting.

Transfers
Requires contact guard to minimum assist of 1 to go from sitting at the edge of the bed to a chair via stand pivot transfer.

Balance
The patient is able to stand unsupported with close contact guard but complains of pain in right hip. He is also able to close his eyes for 3 seconds with minor swaying.

Ambulation
When performing the TUG test, the patient requires a rolling walker and close contact guard as well as verbal cueing to complete the test.

CASE 86

PATIENT'S PAPER

(Please act out the following findings if working with a learning partner in a laboratory environment.)

Step One: Sinister Findings Assessment
Because of recent traumatic incident, multiple surgeries, and prolonged intensive care unit stay, the patient is at risk for orthostatic hypotension and DVT.[1,2] Vital signs were tested and stable.

Range of Motion
Left upper extremity has full shoulder ROM and 4–/5 strength, but elbow ROM is limited to 25°–110° actively and 3+/5 strength in available ROM. Left lower extremity ROM is mildly limited at the hip with 3+/5 strength.

Bed Mobility

Requires assistance of 1 and verbal cueing for technique and safety. Patient is utilizing trapeze in the bed. Assist of 1 is necessary to go from supine to sitting.

Transfers

Requires moderate assist of 1 to go from sitting at the edge of the bed to a chair via a slide board transfer.

Balance

With lower extremity prostheses in place, the patient is able to stand supported with a standard walker and close contact guarding. He complains of dizziness and limits his standing tolerance to a few seconds.

Ambulation

He has attempted to begin gait training with bilateral lower extremity prosthetics and upper extremity prosthetic but complaints of dizziness in upright positions limit this activity.

CASE 87

PATIENT'S PAPER

(Please act out the following findings if working with a learning partner in a laboratory environment.)

Step One: Sinister Findings Assessment

Although not suspected, if the clinician performs lymph node palpation and asks about significant weight loss within the last month, negative findings will result.

Active Physiological Findings

Active physiological findings were unremarkable other than stiffness noted throughout.

Passive Physiological Findings

Passive physiological findings are unremarkable.

Passive Accessory Findings

The patient exhibits "tenderness" with unilateral passive accessories at C1–C2 and L5–S1. Otherwise, passive accessories were unremarkable.

Special Tests

She demonstrates 12/18 tender points: medial aspect of bilateral knees, bilateral elbows, bilateral sub-occipitals, bilateral upper trapezius's, low back, and bilateral sternocleidomastoids. In general, she is tender everywhere, but the standard focal points for tender/trigger points are the worst.

CASE 88

PATIENT'S PAPER

(Please act out the following findings if working with a learning partner in a laboratory environment.)

Step One: Sinister Findings Assessment

Although not suspected, performing an integumentary screen to assess for proper wound healing and looking for any signs or symptoms associated with an infection of his recent transfemoral amputation would be negative. A thorough neurological screen for this patient yields findings that are common among those who sustain a mild TBI, including difficulty with concentrating on a specific task as well as delayed recall when asked to answer a question utilizing his short-term memory.

Active Physiological Findings

Active ROM of right hip yields poor hip extension and abduction. Left lower extremity ROM is within normal limits. The patient's strength is grossly decreased in his right lower extremity but he uses his trunk and upper extremity to compensate for these deficits.

Passive Physiological Finding

Passive physiological findings are similar to those found during the active examination. Passive movements into hip extension are restricted but feel like a "good stretch" to the patient.

Passive Accessory Findings

Passive accessory motions are inappropriate for this patient.

Special Tests

The patient demonstrates positive Thomas test of his right hip. No other special tests for lower extremities were performed at this time.

CASE 89

PATIENT'S PAPER

(Please act out the following findings if working with a learning partner in a laboratory environment.)

Step One: Sinister Findings Assessment

It may be helpful to know additional blood counts such as WBC, ESR, Hgb, and Hct.[1] These values could substantiate or refute active infections that could alter treatment intervention indications and contraindications.[1] Also, platelet count would be helpful to rule out anemia.[1] Finally, UA for blood cells, casts, and proteins may be helpful to rule out SLE.[1] The physical therapist should be vigilant for side effects of the patient's medications. If the physical therapist is unaware of how his or her interventions will affect medication metabolism or how medication will affect his or her interventions, then outside resources should be consulted.

Active Physiological Findings

AROM	R	L
Shoulder flexion	0–172°	0–170°
Shoulder extension	0–55°	0–50°
Elbow flexion	5–150°	5–148°
Forearm pronation	0–72°	0–71°
Forearm supination	0–67°	0–70°
Wrist flexion	0–54°	0–50°
Wrist extension	0–51°	0–49°
IP joints	Bilateral and significant decrease in finger extension actively	
Hip internal rotation	0–47°	0–45°
Hip eternal rotation	0–43°	0–43°
Knee flexion	2–145°	1–142°
Knee extension	2–0°	1–0°
Ankle PF	0–50°	0–50°
Ankle DF	0–12°	0–10°

Pain is not increased with AROM but is present with and without movement.

Bilateral strength testing is within normal limits for both upper and lower extremities except bilateral shoulder IR and ER are 4/5.

Passive Physiological Findings
End-range motion with passive over-pressure increases concordant pain.

Passive Accessory Findings
Stiffness and edema limit joint play in all planes in bilateral carpals, metacarpals, and phalanges.

Special Tests
None.

CASE 90

PATIENT'S PAPER

(Please act out the following findings if working with a learning partner in a laboratory environment.)

Step One: Sinister Findings Assessment
This patient's past medical history is quite intensive and because the signs do not follow a distinct musculoskeletal pattern, one must rule out all red flags before progressing. She does have pain with lying supine at night but when probing further, she states this has been present for years. She denies having a low-grade fever, recent unexplained weight loss or gain, night sweats, and history of cancer or tumor. She also denies bowel or bladder changes. At this point, the primary concerns are the comorbidities of bipolar disorder, depression, and anxiety; these need to be assessed to determine if they are being properly treated. She reports that she is treated medically by a psychiatrist but does not see a "shrink."

Active Physiological Findings
Active movements produce pain within the first 10 degrees of motion in all directions. She does not have a directional preference and displays hesitancy in moving because of pain.

Passive Physiological Findings
These were not performed secondary to the patient's hypersensitivity to light touch by the therapist.

Passive Accessory Findings
The patient had hypersensitivity to light touch across the entire lumbar region. This sensitivity was not discriminate and lumbar mobility cannot be further assessed secondary to this.

Special Tests
Classification of special tests:

1. *Normal*
2. *Clinical physiologic result: Provocative but doesn't reproduce chief complaint*
3. *Neurogenic physiologic: Provocative and reproduces chief complaint*

Special Test Results

a. *Positive clinical physiologic Slump test: Caused pain in the low back (and pulling into her posterior leg to her knee) but patient could not identify if the pain was her chief complaint.*
b. *Positive clinical physiologic SLR test: Caused pain in her low back and she actively pulls away from the tested position.*

CASE 91

(Please act out the following findings if working with a learning partner in a laboratory environment.)

Step One: Sinister Findings Assessment

Despite this patient fitting several criteria for the Wells criteria for a DVT, he has recently had a Doppler image that was negative. He reports a 2-month bout of constipation, off and on, but reports his physicians have attributed this to his medications and therefore takes a stool softener as needed. The patient is currently under psychiatric care for his depression and anxiety but he reports he does not believe he needs to be medicated, and therefore does not take prescribed medication.

Active Physiological Findings

All active movements produce pain immediately. The patient does not have a directional preference.

Passive Physiological Findings

These could not be performed secondary to the patient not allowing the therapist to touch the lower extremity.

Passive Accessory Findings

Did not assess.

Special Tests

The patient completed laterality testing for the feet. Recognize software tests timely awareness of right from left body parts. Movement and awareness is often diminished in individuals with CRPS. He had 20 images and 5 seconds to correctly identify if that image was a left or right foot. He had 40% accuracy on the left and 65% on the right.
    This patient did not tolerate any other special tests on the date of initial evaluation.

CASE 92

PATIENT'S PAPER

(Please act out the following findings if working with a learning partner in a laboratory environment.)

Step One: Sinister Findings Assessment

This patient's past medical history is only significant for bipolar disorder, depression, and anxiety. Prior to this episode, his left arm was fully functional and it appears that the damage is related to the trauma of direct compression. He denies all red-flag questions, and imaging in the emergency room has ruled out other potential mechanisms. At this time, his arm presents like a brachial plexus lesion. The hand and wrist are concerning with redness/swelling and very superficial tenderness, but it presents very similar to CRPS-2.

Active Physiological Findings

The patient demonstrates very little active motion in his left upper extremity. When asked to lift his arm, the pattern of motion is into horizontal adduction. His wrist and fingers appear to flex with this motion as well. He is unable to move in any other plane.

Passive Physiological Findings

These were not performed secondary to the patient's hypersensitivity to light touch by the therapist.

Passive Accessory Findings
Not assessed due to hypersensitivity.

Special Tests
Due to hypersensitivity of the upper extremity and known diagnostic test results, the majority of special tests were deferred. He did perform the NOIGroups "Recognise" test for iPad for the hand. The specific program was Vanilla Hand. He could perform laterality testing and would score 60% for the left-sided images and 75% for the right-sided images with an average speed of 3.8 seconds per image. This likely demonstrates diminished laterality on the left.

CASE 93

PATIENT'S PAPER

(Please act out the following findings if working with a learning partner in a laboratory environment.)

Step One: Sinister Findings Assessment
Because this patient appeared to be deeply depressed a PHQ-2 was administered. It is a quick and valid way to screen for depression. He had a score of 6, which has been shown to have a specificity of 99.4 for a major depressive episode. He denied any other red-flag questions and diagnostic imaging has ruled out anatomical reasoning for his flaccidity. Treatment will continue with this patient, but with a recommendation that he follows up with a psychiatrist, due to his recent loss as well as his high score on the PHQ-2.

Active Physiological Findings
This patient was unable to perform active movements at the time of initial evaluation.

Passive Physiological Findings
This patient appears to have full passive motion throughout his right upper extremity. The clinician can perform this without eliciting pain.

Passive Accessory Findings
The patient demonstrates significant hypermobility throughout his glenohumeral joint. He has a positive sulcus sign during an inferior humeral glide and appears to have significant atrophy of surrounding shoulder musculature.

Special Tests
Due to flaccidity and nature of symptoms, special testing was done only for the upper extremity and cervical spine.
Deep tendon reflexes: C5/6/7 are 3+ on the right and 2+ on the left
Negative Hoffmann's sign
Negative clonus

CASE 94

PATIENT'S PAPER

(Please act out the following findings if working with a learning partner in a laboratory environment.)

Step One: Sinister Findings Assessment
This patient denies the majority of red-flag questions and has been seen in 2 emergency rooms and by a chiropractor. This stated, the severe symptoms she experiences when she flexes her neck (with slight knee

extension) is very concerning. This position likely tensions the dura but this response is extremely sensitive. In combination with the balance deficits, gait ataxia, and night sweats, the therapist should be quite concerned.

Active Physiological Findings

Active cervical flexion produced pain at end range (around 50°) that intensified with the initiation of knee extension. All other cervical motions were nonprovocative.

Passive Physiological Findings

N/A

Passive Accessory Findings

Due to concerns of potential upper motor neuron (UMN) lesion, mobility assessment is inappropriate.

Special Tests

Classification of special tests:

1. *Normal*
2. *Clinical Physiologic Result—Provocative but doesn't reproduce chief complaint*
3. *Neurogenic Physiologic—Provocative and reproduces chief complaint*

Special Test Results:

a. *Positive neurogenic physiologic Slump test*
b. *Positive neurogenic physiologic SLR test, which causes pain in her "entire" spine*
c. *Deep tendon reflexes of C5/6/7 were 2+ but L4 was 4+*
d. *Negative Hoffmann's reflex*
e. *+ Clonus bilaterally. Approximately 3–4 beats.*
f. *Gait assessment indicated clumsiness and ataxia*

CASE 95

PATIENT'S PAPER

(Please act out the following findings if working with a learning partner in a laboratory environment.)

Step One: Sinister Findings Assessment

This patient's past medical history would not suggest significant pathology. However, since groin pain can be caused by multiple serious pathologies, medical screening becomes necessary to ensure that the problem is mechanical in nature. The patient should be queried for conditions that have a known link to the pain pattern described, including urologic and gynecologic conditions. One study found that 94% of a small sample of females with groin pain had more than one source of pain.[1] In addition, other routine signs and symptoms of sinister pathology—including night pain, night sweats, pain at rest, unexpected weight loss, and bowel and bladder dysfunction—should be queried. Her pain is activity based, which suggests a musculoskeletal origin. There are no reports of recent weight loss, night pain, low-grade fever, night sweats, or history of cancer. There are no overt signs and symptoms of neurologic disorder beyond the potential referred pain pattern.

Active Physiological Findings

Since AP is a syndrome with a diagnosis by exclusion,[2] the examination should begin by first ruling out lumbar, sacroiliac joint, and hip pathology. Therefore, active movements of the lumbar spine with over-pressures as appropriate, and repeated movements[3] should be performed first. In this case, all active movements for the lumbar spine are negative, along with active movements for the hip.

Passive Physiological Findings

Findings were negative for ROM deficits or symptom provocation for lumbar and hip movements. The FADIR test was negative, thus ruling out acetabular impingement and labral tears.[4]

Passive Accessory Findings

Posterior-anterior glides throughout the lumbar spine were not provocative nor were accessories for the hip.

Special Tests

Lower extremity strength ratios for hip adduction/abduction should be tested with objective measurement such as hand-held dynamometry; normal results should be at least .80.[5] In this case, the adductors are weak and the ratio was .65. In addition, the Manual Muscle Test (MMT) for adduction was painful for the concordant sign. The adductor squeeze test[6] and the bilateral adductor test[6] were positive, substantially increasing the likelihood that athletic pubalgia is present.

Lumbar tests such as the straight leg raise test (SLR) and the slump test were negative, along with prone segmental instability test. Provocation tests for the sacroiliac joint (SIJ), including thigh thrust, compression, distraction, and sacral apex stress test: 2/4 should be positive to rule in SIJ in the absence of lumbar pathology.[7] In this case, they are all negative. The active SLR test is mildly painful on the right side.[8]

CASE 96

PATIENT'S PAPER

(Please act out the following findings if working with a learning partner in a laboratory environment.)

Step One: Sinister Findings Assessment

Recent surgery puts this patient at risk for deep vein thrombosis (DVT), and history of osteoporosis puts this patient at risk for fracture.

Bed Mobility

The patient requires verbal cueing from the therapist for proper technique and body mechanics in order to minimize the pain in the thorax. Supervision of 1 is necessary to go from supine to sitting.

Transfers

The patient requires close supervision with occasional contact guard (mostly because of hospital equipment) of 1 to go from sitting at the edge of the bed to a chair via stand pivot transfer.

Balance

The patient is able to stand without an assistive device. Close supervision provided, as this is the first time out of bed.

Ambulation

The patient requires close contact guarding to ambulate distances of 35 feet before requiring a rest break. She is able to do 2–3 sets of this distance.

CASE 97

PATIENT'S PAPER

(Please act out the following findings if working with a learning partner in a laboratory environment.)

Step One: Sinister Findings Assessment

This patient's past medical history would suggest the possibility of significant pathology. A full neurological examination is in order to examine the extent of the small fiber polyneuropathy and to determine if another neurological disorder is possible. The examination should explore lower- and upper-motor neuron lesions.

Active Physiological Findings

The patient was able to demonstrate any functional movement of the trunk, including stooping and bending without additional discomfort. When isolating active movements at the thoracic spine, left-side bending and right rotation were provocative but only mildly limited in range by perceived stiffness. Extension was provocative with overpressure.

The patient's shoulder ROM was within normal limits and equal bilaterally, but there were qualitative abnormalities with the left side, including winging of the scapula with elevation and return at the mid-range position. In addition, strength of all planes of glenohumeral (GH) movement was limited with ER being weakest at 3+/5. All other planes were 4−/5. Serratus anterior was 3+/5.

Passive Physiological Findings

Passive trunk movements were all provocative for the same planes of movement as active movements. GH movements were not painful and not limited.

Passive Accessory Findings

Posterior-anterior glides in the cervical spine were point tender but not provocative for C3–C4 and C5–C6. The thoracic spine examination revealed provocative segments for T3 through T7 but they all were variable in intensity with the most provocative segment being T4. Left unilateral PA glides on T4 were worse than central, and the posterior aspect of the rib was most provocative. This glide actually increased chest pain as well. Unilateral anterior-posterior glides on the costochondral borders of the chest were provocative from ribs 1 to 5, with 4 being the most provocative and creating the most lasting pain.

Special Tests

Empty can test: Positive

Infraspinatus muscle test: Positive

Painful arc: Positive

Drop arm test: Positive

Hoffmann's sign: Negative

Clonus test: 2 beat bilaterally

Inverted supinator sign: Negative bilaterally but hyperreflexia

Suprapatellar reflex: Positive for hyperreflexia bilaterally

CASE 98

PATIENT'S PAPER

(Please act out the following findings if working with a learning partner in a laboratory environment.)

Step One: Sinister Findings Assessment

This patient's past medical history would not suggest the possibility of significant pathology. The negative imaging examination would suggest that no sinister pathology was involved, yet it makes sense to thoroughly examine the patient to be certain changes had not occurred since her last examination.

Deep tendon reflexes (DTRs): Normal

Sensation: Intact

Myotomes: Mild deficits in the hands

Active Physiological Findings

Cervical ROM is limited generally by 20% but is not too painful. Mild over-pressure into side bending reproduces some components of the symptoms down the contralateral upper extremity.[1] Shoulder/elbow/ wrist and hand screening for active movement is normal and over-pressures do not increase symptoms.

Passive Physiological Findings

Passive cervical movements reinforce the loss of mobility with provocation of contralateral symptoms. There was tenderness to palpation in the scalene muscles with positive reproduction of those symptoms when tapped near the first rib.

Passive Accessory Findings

Posterior-anterior (PA) and unilateral posterior-anterior (UPA) glides in the cervical spine can elicit cervical discomfort that is comparable to the patient's usual neck pain at C6–C7 and C7–T1. Unilateral posterior-anterior glides in the mid- to upper-cervical spine provide features of her usual occipital headaches. None of these examinations recreate numbness or tingling in the hands.

Special Tests

ULNT 1: Positive bilaterally

ULNT 3: Positive bilterally

Inverted supinator sign: Negative

ROOS test: Positive

Tinel's test: Positive

Adson's test: Negative

Hyperabduction test: Negative

Wright's test: Positive

Myotomes: Weak in hand intrinsics at approximately 4–/5 and triceps 4/5

Sensory testing mild deficits in the C7 and C8 distributions

Hoffmann's test: Negative

CASE 99

PATIENT'S PAPER

(Please act out the following findings if working with a learning partner in a laboratory environment.)

Step One: Sinister Findings Assessment

No sinister findings were present on the initial assessment.

Active Physiological Findings

Mouth opening was painful and the patient was apprehensive to continue the movement past 27mm; the mandibular left lateral deviation was also painful and self-limiting at 5mm. An audible was heard during right lateral deviation but no pain or limitation was noted.

Passive Physiological Findings

Same as active physiological findings.

Passive Accessory Findings

Passive accessory joint play was determined within normal limits bilaterally. Mild discomfort was elicited during the test of the right temporomandibular joint (TMJ), but no concordant sign was present.

Special Tests

Opening amplitude test was positive with a mandatory cut-off point for females being <30mm.[1] The patient demonstrated opening amplitude of 27mm.

Palpation of the right masseter, temporalis, and medial/lateral pterygoid muscles all elicited pain. Palpation findings are considered necessary in the diagnoses of temporomandibular dysfunction.[1]
Resisted muscle testing reproduced the concordant sign with resisted mouth opening, closing, and mandibular lateral deviation to the right.[2]

CASE 100

PATIENT'S PAPER

(Please act out the following findings if working with a learning partner in a laboratory environment.)

Step One: Sinister Findings Assessment

There is no reason to believe that sinister pathology is involved in this case, but a quick neurological screen to rule out any form of radiating symptoms to the thumb would prove negative. Since the patient does have a history of cholesterol and heart arrhythmia, taking vitals is indicated and they would be found to be within normal limits.

Active Physiological Findings

Thumb range of motion is found to be excessive with discomfort in end-range extension and abduction. The metacarpal phalangeal joint is also hypermobile and mildly uncomfortable in extension.

Passive Physiological Findings

Passive physiological movements are hypermobile in the thumb and also reproduce concordant pain in end range.

Passive Accessory Findings

Posterior-anterior glides of the CMC are hypermobile and painful. General laxity is noted throughout the thumbs bilaterally with mild reproduction of symptoms in the right thumb.

Special Tests

Beighton's sign: Positive (6/9)
Strength testing found good strength for grip and pinch testing, but the left side was 20% stronger than the involved right side.

Endnotes

Case 8:

1. Tong HC, Haig AJ, Yamakawa K. The Spurling test and cervical radiculopathy. *Spine*. 2002;27:156–9.

Case 16:

1. Hegedus E, Goode A, Cook C, Michener L, Myer C, Myer D, Wright A. Which physical examination tests provide clinicians with the most value when examining the shoulder? Update of a systematic review with meta-analysis of individual tests. Br J Sports Med. 2012 Nov;46(14):964–78.

Case 17:

1. Stetson WB, Templin K. The crank test, the O'Brien test, and routine magnetic resonance liaging scans in the diagnosis of labral tears. Am J Sports Med. 2002;30(6):806–9.

2. Hegedus EJ, Goode AP, Cook CE, Michener L, Myer CA, Myer DM, et al. Which physical examination tests provide clinicians with the most value when examining the shoulder? update of a systematic review with meta-analysis of individual tests. Br J Sports Med. 2012;46(14):964–78.

3. MacDonald PB, Clark P, Sutherland K. An analysis of the diagnostic accuracy of the Hawkins and Neer subacromial lipingement signs. J Shoulder Elbow Surg. 2000;9:299–301.

4. Post M, Cohen J. Impingement syndrome: a review of late stage II and early stage III lesions. Clin Orthop. 1986;207:127–32.

5. Kim SH, Ha KI, Ahn JH, Kim SH, Choi HJ. Biceps load test II: a clinical test for SLAP lesions of the shoulder. Arthroscopy 2001;17(2):160–4.

Case 20:

1. Reeser J, Joy E, Porucznik C, Berg R, Colliver E, Willick S. Risk factors for volleyball-related shoulder pain and dysfunction. PM&R. 2010;2:27–36.

2. Cook C, Hegedus E. Orthopedic Clinical Tests: An Evidence-Based Approach. 2nd edition. Upper Saddle River, NJ; Prentice Hall, 2013.

3. Itoi E, Kido T, Sano A, Urayama M, Sato K. Which is more useful, the "full can test" or the "empty can test," in detecting the torn supraspinatus tendon? Am J Sports Med. 1999;27:65–8.

4. Park H, Yokota A, Gill HS, El Rassi G, McFarland E. Diagnostic accuracy of clinical tests for the different degrees of subacromial impingement syndrome. J Bone Joint Surg. AM. 2005;87:1446–55.

Case 21:

1. Moore MB. The use of a tuning fork and stethoscope to identify fractures. J Athl Train. 2009;44(3):272–4.

Case 23:

1. Cook C, Brown C, Isaacs R, Roman M, Davis S, Richardson W. Clustered clinical findings for diagnosis of cervical spine myelopathy. J Man Manip Ther. 2010;18:175–80.

Case 24:

1. Lestayo P, Howell J. Clinical provocative tests used in evaluating wrist pain: a descriptive study. J Hand Ther. 1995;8:10–7.

2. Lester B, Hallbrecht J, Levy IM, Gaudinez R. "Press test" for office diagnosis of triangular fibrocartilage complex tears of the wrist. Ann Plast Surg. 1995;35:41–5.

Case 26:

1. O'Driscoll SW, Lawton RL, Smith AM. The "Moving Valgus Stress Test" for medial collateral ligament tears of the elbow. Am J Sports Med. 2005;33(2): 231–39.

Case 27:

1. Cook C, Hegedus E. Orthopedic Physical Examination Tests: An Evidence-Based Approach. 2nd ed. Upper Saddle River, NJ; Pearson Education, 2013.

Case 28:

1. O'Driscoll S. Richard L. The "moving valgus stress test" for medial collateral ligament tears of the elbow. Am J Sports Med. 2005;33(2):231–40.

Case 29:

1. Wainner RS, Fritz JM, Irrgang JJ, Delitto A, Allison S, Boninger ML. Development of a clinical prediction rule for the diagnosis of carpal tunnel syndrome. Arch Phys Med Rehabil. 2005;86:609–18.

Case 30

1. Ekstrom R, Holden K. Examination of and Intervention for a patient with signs of nerve entrapment. Phys Ther. 2002;82:1077–86.

Case 21 (right column top):

5. Lo I, Nonweiler B, Woolfrey M, Litchfield R, Kirkley A. An evaluation of the apprehension, relocation, and surprise tests for anterior shoulder instability. Am J Sports Med. 2004;33(2):301–7.

2. Berglund KM, Persson BH, Denison E. Prevalence of pain and dysfunction in the cervical and thoracic spine in persons with and without lateral elbow pain. Man Ther. 2008;13:295–9.

3. Fernández-de-las-Peñas C, Ortega-Santiago R, Ambite-Quesada S, Jiménez-García R, Arroyo-Morales M, Cleland J. Specific mechanical pain hypersensitivity over peripheral nerve trunks in women with either unilateral epicondylalgia or carpal tunnel syndrome. J Orthop Sports Phys Ther. 2010;40(11):751–60.

4. Lutz FR. Radial tunnel syndrome: an etiology of chronic lateral elbow pain. J Orthop Sports Phys Ther. 1991;14(1):14–7.

Case 31:

1. Roman M, Brown C, Richardson W, Isaacs R, Howes C, Cook C. The development of a clinical decision making algorithm for detection of osteoporotic vertebral compression fracture or wedge deformity. J Man Manip Ther. 2010;18:44–9.

Case 42:

1. Rabey MI. Costochondritis: Are the symptoms and signs due to neurogenic inflammation? Two cases that responded to manual therapy directed towards posterior spinal structures. Manual Ther. 2007;13:82–6.

Case 43:

1. Deville W, van der Windt D, Dzaferagic A, et al. The test of Lasègue. Systematic review of the accuracy in diagnosing herniated discs. Spine. 2000;25:1140–7.

Case 45:

1. Henschke N, Maher CG, Refshauge KM, Herbert RD, Cumming RG, Bleasel J, et al. Prevalence of and screening for spinal pathology in patients presenting to primary care settings with acute low back pain. Arthritis Rheum. 2009;60:3072–80.

Case 52

1. Wells PS. Advances in the diagnosis of venous thromboembolism. J Thromb Thrombolysis. 2006;21(1):31–40.

Case 56:

1. Ho GW, Howard TM. Greater trochanteric pain syndrome: more than bursitis and iliotibial tract friction. Curr Sports Med Rep. 2012;11:232–8.

2. McSweeney SE, Naraghi A, Salonen D, Theodoropoulos J, White LM. Hip and groin pain in the professional athlete. Can Assoc Radiol J. (Journal l'association canadienne des radiologistes) 2012;63:87–99.

3. Duckham RL, Peirce N, Meyer C, Summers GD, Cameron N, Brooke-Wavell K. Risk factors for stress fracture in female endurance athletes: a cross-sectional study. BMJ open 2012;2.

Case 57:

1. Nee RJ, Butler D. Management of peripheral neuropathic pain: integrating neurobiology, neurodynamics, and clinical evidence. Phys Ther Sport. 2006;7:36–49.

Case 58:

1. Ho GW, Howard TM. Greater trochanteric pain syndrome: more than bursitis and iliotibial tract friction. Curr Sports Med Rep. 2012;11:232–8.

2. Sayegh F, Potoupnis M, Kapetanos G. Greater trochanter bursitis pain syndrome in females with chronic low back pain and sciatica. Acta Orthopaedica. Belgica 2004;70:423–8.

Case 67:

1. Cook C, Mabry L, Reiman M, Hegedus E. Best tests/ clinical findings for screening and diagnosis of patellofemoral pain syndrome: a systematic review. Physiotherapy. 2012;98:93–100.

Case 68:

1. Benjaminse A, Gokeler A, van der Schans CP. Clinical diagnosis of an anterior cruciate ligament rupture: a meta-analysis. J Orthop Sports Phys Ther. 2006;36:267–88.

2. Cooperman JM, Riddle DL, Rothstein JM. Reliability and validity of judgements of the integrity of the anterior cruciate ligament of the knee using the Lachman's test. Phys Ther. 1990;70:225–33.

Case 69:

1. Eren OT. The accuracy of joint line tenderness by physical examination in the diagnosis of meniscal tears. Arthroscopy. 2003;19:850–4.

2. McMurray TP. The semilunar cartilages. Br J Surg. 1942;29:407–14.

3. Harrison BK, Abell BE, Gibson TW. The Thessaly test for detection of meniscal tears: validation of a new physical examination technique for primary care medicine. Clin J Sports Med. 2009;19:9–12.

4. Akseki D, Özcan Ö, Boya H, Pinar H. A new weight-bearing meniscal test and a comparison with McMurray's test and joint line tenderness. Arthroscopy. 20.9 2004;20:951–8.

5. Mariani PP, Adriani E, Maresca G, Mazzola CG. A prospective evaluation of a test for lateral meniscus tears. Knee Surg Sports Traumatol Arthroscopy 1996;4:22–6.

6. Moore MB. The use of a tuning fork and stethoscope to identify fractures. J Athl Train. 2009;44:272–4.

Case 70:

1. Wind WM, Jr., Bergfeld JA, Parker RD. Evaluation and treatment of posterior cruciate ligament injuries: revisited. Am J Sports Med. 2004;32:1765–75.

Case 71:

1. Cash JD, Hughston JC. Treatment of acute patellar dislocation. Am J Sports Med. 1988;16:244–9.

2. Beasley LS, Vidal AF. Traumatic patellar dislocation in children and adolescents: treatment update and literature review. Current opinion in pediatrics. 2004;16:29–36.

Case 72:

1. Hutchinson AM, Evans R, Bodger O, Pallister I, Topliss C, Williams P, et al. What is the best clinical test for Achilles tendinopathy? Foot Ankle Surg. 2013;19:112–7.

Case 79:

1. Cook CE, Hegedus EJ. Physical examination tests for the lower leg, ankle, and foot. In Orthopedic Physical Examination Tests: An Evidence-Based Approach. 2nd ed. 2013;503–31.

Case 81:

1. Mulligan, B. Manual therapy: Nags, snags, mwms, etc. 6th ed. Minneapolis: MN Orthopedic Physical Therapy Products;2010:95.

Case 86:

1. Goff BJ, Bergeron A, Ganz O, Gambel JM. Rehabilitation of a US Army soldier with traumatic triple major limb amputations: a case report. J Prosthetics Orthotics. 2008;20(4):142–9.

2. Wells PS, Anderson DR, Bormanis J, Guy F, Mitchell M, Gray L, et al. Value of assessment of pretest probability of deep-vein thrombosis in clinical management. Lancet. 1997;350:1795–8.

Case 89:

1. Goodman CC, Kelly Snyder TE. Screening for immunologic disease. In Differential Diagnosis for Physical Therapists: Screening for Referral. 4th ed. (Philadelphia, Saunders, Publishing), 2007:517–57.

Case 95:

1. Meyers WC, Foley DP, Garrett WE, Lohnes JH, Mandlebaum BR. Management of severe lower abdominal or inguinal pain in high-performance athletes. PAIN (Performing Athletes with Abdominal or Inguinal Neuromuscular Pain Study Group). Am J Sports Med. 2000;28:2–8.

2. Hegedus EJ, Stern B, Reiman MP, Tarara D, Wright AA. A suggested model for physical examination and conservative treatment of athletic pubalgia. Phys Ther Sport. 2013;14:3–16.

3. Donelson R, Aprill C, Medcalf R, Grant W. A prospective study of centralization of lumbar and referred pain. A predictor of symptomatic discs and anular competence. Spine. 1997;22:1115–22.

4. Cook CE, Hegedus EJ. Orthopedic Physical Examination Tests: An Evidence-Based Approach. 2nd ed. Upper Saddle River, NJ; Prentice Hall, 2013.

5. Tyler TF, Nicholas SJ, Campbell RJ, Donellan S, McHugh MP. The effectiveness of a preseason exercise program to prevent adductor muscle strains in professional ice hockey players. Am J Sports Med. 2002;30:680–3.

6. Verrall GM, Slavotinek JP, Barnes PG, Fon GT. Description of pain provocation tests used for the diagnosis of sports-related chronic groin pain: relationship of tests to defined clinical (pain and tenderness) and MRI (pubic bone marrow oedema) criteria. Scand J Med Sci Sports. 2005;15:36–42.

7. Laslett M, Aprill CN, McDonald B, Young SB. Diagnosis of sacroiliac joint pain: validity of individual provocation tests and composites of tests. Man Ther. 2005;10:207–18.

8. Mens JM, Vleeming A, Snijders CJ, Koes BW, Stam HJ. Validity of the active straight leg raise test for measuring disease severity in patients with posterior pelvic pain after pregnancy. Spine. 2002;27:196–200.

Case 98:

1. Sanders RJ, Hammond SL, Rao NM. Diagnosis of thoracic outlet syndrome. J Vasc Surg. 2007;46:601–4.

Case 99:

1. Dworkin SF, Huggins KH, et al. Epidemiology of signs and symptoms in temporomandibular disorders: clinical signs in cases and controls. J Am Dent Assoc. 1990;120(3):273–81.

2. Truelove E., Sommers E., et al. Clinical diagnostic criteria for TMD. New classification permits multiple diagnoses. J Am Dent Assoc. 1992;123:47–54.

Index